IV Dosage Calculations

Basic to Complex Critical Care IV Dosage Formulas

Sally Fox Harris, BSN, RN

Cover Design by:
Coalescent Creative
www.coalescentcreative.com

Editing by:
Christopher Hall
christopherhall374@gmail.com

Michelle Lehman
Lehman Editing
LehmanEditing@gmail.com
www.facebook.com/LehmanEditing

Disclaimer:
The practice problems are provided to help you improve your dosage calculation skills. Every effort has been made to provide accurate dosage ranges and drug supply mixes within the practice problems. When working in a clinical setting always use APPROVED medication references.
The author and publishers of this book accept no responsibility for any issues that may arise from the use of this book.

Dedication

To my husband Dan,
Thank you for building an office space just for me; a seized opportunity to decorate—I mean, work on this book.

To my twin sister Sue,
Your witty input helped infuse this task of generating hundreds of mathematical equations a fun endeavor. OK, so the word fun...it's a stretch.

To my brave kids, Holle, Glory, David, Nate and Nick,
Thank you for your honest and helpful application of red ink onto the many pages of manuscript.

To my Father-in-Law Jack,
"The Wordist: One skilled in the imaginative use of words."

To my childhood friend Linda,
Cheers to you. You got me across the finish line. Cheers to us.

In memory of my friend Mindy,
To your teaching spirit.

Table of Contents

Table of Contents

Information you should already know:
- A basic understanding of medical terminology, medications, and IV administration
- How to round numbers up or down
- How to cancel out like units (Used with unit conversion)
- Division and multiplication

Any questions or comments?
Please send to: comments.ivdosage@yahoo.com

Introduction

As scary as it may have sounded, after passing the nursing board NCLEX examination, I was now an RN. Not only that, but I was entrusted to provide care for patients in the CVICU (Cardiovascular Intensive Care Unit) at a level-one trauma hospital. Most of the CVICU patients required multiple IV lines. Often, over the course of a 12 hour shift, those IV lines would become a huge tangled mess; I was sure this had to be the handiwork of gremlins lurking just underneath the bed.

Gremlins, however, were the least of my worries. I had to calculate flow rates that delivered the *right dose* of medication to the patient. My dosage calculation skills, to put it nicely, lacked proficiency. To my rescue and in the name of patient safety, a fellow RN showed me a quick and easy method for calculating complex IV dosage rates. Today, I call that method The Wrinkle Method.

Wrinkle can mean a change from a customary procedure or method. And, The Wrinkle Method, unlike the customary methods of dimensional analysis and ratio-proportion makes complex IV dosage calculations easy—even when titrating.

There are several other tools that are commonly used to determine *right dose* delivery for critical care IV infusion drugs, in addition to the above mathematical methods.

The most utilized tool is the programmable (smart) IV infusion pump. It has an awesome bedside feature in that it can perform dosage calculations for you; however, to ensure accurate calculations, great caution must be taken when inputting requested information.

Another handy tool is the IV drug dosage chart. It requires excellent hand eye coordination and, when working with non-standard drug mixes, may have limited value.

Whatever method you choose—for patient safety—always double check for *right dose* delivery.

Twelve Rights of Medication Administration

When administering any medication, for patient safety, the *Rights of Medication Administration* must be followed.

The *Rights*, depending on the source, may vary in number and order. However, this book addresses only one—*Right Dose.*

That being said, here are the standard set of rights in Medication Administration.

1. Right Patient
2. Right Time
3. Right Medication
4. Right Expiration Date
5. Right Route
6. *Right Dose*
7. Right Reason
8. Right Client Education
9. Right to Refuse Medication
10. Right Assessment & Evaluation
11. Right Response
12. Right Documentation

Chapter 1

IV Push
The Formula Method

The easiest approach to calculating IV push medications is to use the formula method.

Unlike the traditional methods of dimensional analysis and ratio-proportion, the formula method is simple, straight forward, and bedside friendly. Therefore, to keep IV push dosage calculations easy, only instructions for the formula method are covered here.

Some IV push medications may be supplied in a form that is not suitable for direct administration. A powdered medication will require reconstitution while a concentrated liquid medication may require dilution.

Reconstitution and dilution are skills frequently used and must be done PRIOR to any dosage calculation. For a review, see Chapter, 8 page 85.

IV Push

Drug Concentration

Understanding Drug Concentration

Drug concentration: (Strength)
Drug concentration describes how weak or strong a medication mixture is. It identifies how much drug and how much liquid are in the mixture and is expressed as a ratio.

Example:
There are 20 mg of a drug mixed with 10 mL of a liquid. A 20/10 ratio. The ratio is written: 20 mg/10 mL

Final concentration:
A final concentration describes the drug concentration with a simplified ratio.

Example:
Drug concentration: The ratio of 20 mg/10 mL is simplified to a final concentration of 2 mg/1 mL.
(written 2 mg/mL)

When there is just one mL (1 mL) of liquid it is written as (mL). The one (1) is understood.

Measurements used in drug concentrations:
Drugs are measured in:
- mcg (micrograms)
- mg (milligrams)
- g (grams)
- units (units)

Liquids are measured in:
- mL (milliliters)

IV Push
The Formula Method

The Formula: $\dfrac{\text{(O) Order}}{\text{(H) Have}} \times \text{(V) Volume} = \text{mL to be administered}$

Explanation of formula:
(O) Order = Ordered dose to be administered to patient.
(H) Have = The amount of drug (mcg, mg, g, units).
(V) Volume = The amount of liquid (mL).

IV Push

The Formula Method/Example

A dosage calculation using the drug concentration ratio: Zofran 40 mg/20 mL

(O) Order: Zofran **4 mg** to be given IV push (IVP)
(H) Have: Zofran **40 mg**
(V) Volume: **20 mL**
How many mL will you administer to deliver
the *right dose* 4 mg? _____

$$\frac{(O)\ Order}{(H)\ Have} \times (V)\ Volume = mL\ to\ be\ administered$$

$$\frac{(O)\ 4\ mg}{(H)\ 40\ mg} \times (V)\ 20\ mL = 2\ mL$$

Administer 2 mL

A dosage calculation using the final concentration ratio: Zofran 2 mg/mL

(O) Order: Zofran **4 mg** to be given IV push (IVP)
(H) Have: Zofran **2 mg**
(V) Volume: **1 mL**
How many mL will you administer to deliver the *right dose*
of 4 mg?_____

$$\frac{(O)\ Order}{(H)\ Have} \times (V)\ Volume = mL\ to\ be\ administered$$

$$\frac{(O)\ 4\ mg}{(H)\ 2\ mg} \times (V)\ 1\ mL = 2\ mL$$

Administer 2 mL

IV Push

Practice Problems

The Formula: $\boxed{\dfrac{\text{(O) Order}}{\text{(H) Have}} \times \text{(V) Volume} = \text{mL to be administered}}$

1. Order: Demerol 25 mg IVP
   Have: Demerol 100 mg/2 mL
   Administer: _____ mL

2. Order: Lasix 20 mg slow IVP
   Have: Lasix 100 mg/10 mL
   Administer: _____ mL

3. Order: Benadryl 12.5 mg IVP
   Have: Benadryl 50 mg /mL
   Administer: _____ mL

4. Order: Fentanyl 25 mcg IVP
   Have: Fentanyl 200 mcg /2 mL
   Administer: _____ mL

5. Order: Labetalol 0.25 mg/kg slow IVP
   Have: Labetalol 100 mg/20 mL
   Wt: 84.5 kg
   Ordered dose is: _____ mg
   Administer: _____ mL

Solutions to questions 1-5 found on pages 7-8

Chapter 1

IV Push

Practice Problems

6. Ordered: Romazicon 0.2 mg IVP
   Have: Romazicon 0.5 mg/5 mL
   Administer: _____ mL

7. Order: Vasotec 0.625 mg IVP
   Have: Vasotec 1.25 mg/2 mL
   Administer: _____ mL

8. Order: Digoxin 0.125 mg IVP
   Have: Digoxin 0.5 mg/mL
   Administer: _____ mL

9. Ordered: Fentanyl 75 mcg IVP
   Have: Fentanyl 250 mcg/5 mL
   Administer: _____ mL

10. Order: Bumex 1 mg IVP
    Have: 2.5 mg/10 mL
    Administer: _____ mL

Solutions to questions 6-10 found on pages 8-9

IV Push

Practice Solutions

The Formula: $\boxed{\dfrac{\text{(O) Order}}{\text{(H) Have}} \times \text{(V) Volume} = \text{mL to be administered}}$

1. **0.5 mL**
   Order: Demerol 25 mg IVP
   Have: Demerol 100 mg/2 mL

   $$\boxed{\dfrac{25\ \text{mg}}{100\ \text{mg}} \times 2\ \text{mL} = 0.5\ \text{mL}}$$

2. **2 mL**
   Order: Lasix 20 mg slow IVP
   Have: Lasix 100 mg/10 mL

   $$\boxed{\dfrac{20\ \text{mg}}{100\ \text{mg}} \times 10\ \text{mL} = 2\ \text{mL}}$$

3. **0.25 mL**
   Order: Benadryl 12.5 mg IVP
   Have: Benadryl 50 mg/mL

   $$\boxed{\dfrac{12.5\ \text{mg}}{50\ \text{mg}} \times 1\ \text{mL} = 0.25\ \text{mL}}$$

4. **0.25 mL**
   Order: Fentanyl 25 mcg IVP
   Have: Fentanyl 200 mcg/2 mL

   $$\boxed{\dfrac{25\ \text{mcg}}{200\ \text{mcg}} \times 2\ \text{mL} = 0.25\ \text{mL}}$$

IV Push

Practice Solutions

5. **21 mg**
   4.2 mL
   Order: Labetalol 0.25 mg/kg slow IVP
   Have: Labetalol 100 mg/20 mL
   Wt: 84.5 kg
   Calculate Ordered Dose:

   $$0.25 \text{ mg} \times 84.5 \text{ kg} = 21 \text{ mg}$$

   Dosage Calculation:

   $$\frac{21 \text{ mg}}{100 \text{ mg}} \times 20 \text{ mL} = 4.2 \text{ mL}$$

6. **2 mL**
   Order: Romazicon 0.2 mg IVP
   Have: Romazicon 0.5 mg/5 mL

   $$\frac{0.2 \text{ mg}}{0.5 \text{ mg}} \times 5 \text{ mL} = 2 \text{ mL}$$

7. **1 mL**
   Order: Vasotec 0.625 mg IVP
   Have: Vasotec 1.25 mg/2 mL

   $$\frac{0.625 \text{ mg}}{1.25 \text{ mg}} \times 2 \text{ mL} = 1 \text{ mL}$$

IV Push

Practice Solutions

8. **0.25 mL**

   Order: Digoxin 0.125 mg IVP
   Have: Digoxin 0.5 mg/mL

   $$\frac{0.125 \text{ mg}}{0.5 \text{ mg}} \times 1 \text{ mL} = 0.25 \text{ mL}$$

9. **1.5 mL**

   Order: Fentanyl 75 mcg IVP
   Have: Fentanyl 250 mcg/5 mL

   $$\frac{75 \text{ mcg}}{250 \text{ mcg}} \times 5 \text{ mL} = 1.5 \text{ mL}$$

10. **4 mL**

    Order: Bumex 1 mg IVP
    Have: 2.5 mg/10 mL

    $$\frac{1 \text{ mg}}{2.5 \text{ mg}} \times 10 \text{ mL} = 4 \text{ mL}$$

Chapter 2

Basic IV Dosage Formulas

Gravity and IV Pump Systems

There are two delivery systems used to administer IV infusion medications.

The Gravity System
When using the gravity system calculate a drip rate (gtt/min).

The IV Pump System
When using the IV pump system calculate a flow rate (mL/hr).

Chapter 2

The Gravity System

Drops Per Minute (DPM) Formula

The Gravity System uses a drip rate (gtt/min) to regulate how fast or slow the IV fluid infuses. To calculate a drip rate (gtt/min), use the **Drops Per Minute (DPM) Formula.**

Drops Per Minute (DPM) Formula

$$\frac{\text{total volume to be infused (mL)} \times \text{drop factor (gtt/mL)}}{\text{total infusion time in minutes}} = \text{drip rate (gtt/min)}$$

Drops Per Minute (DPM) terms:

- The **drip rate (gtt/min)** is how fast or slow the medication is infusing.
- The **drop factor,** also called drip factor, is the number of drops of fluid per mL (gtt/mL). When selecting IV tubing, look for the drop factor (gtt/mL) on the IV tubing package.

Common Drop Factors (gtt/mL) for IV tubing:

A. **Mini or Micro drip set:**
   Used for infants, children, and sensitive medications.
   60 gtt/mL

B. **Macro drip set:**
   Used to deliver large volumes or to infuse quickly.
   10 gtt/mL
   15 gtt/mL
   20 gtt/mL

The Gravity System

Drops Per Minute (DPM)/Example

Using the (DPM) Formula to calculate the drip rate (gtt/min)

$$\frac{\text{total volume to be infused (mL)} \times \text{drop factor (gtt/mL)}}{\text{total infusion time in minutes}} = \text{drip rate (gtt/min)}$$

Example:

Order: Zantac 50 mg/100 mL to infuse over 20 minutes
IV tubing: 10 gtt/mL (drop factor)
What is the drip rate (gtt/min)? _______

$$\frac{100 \text{ mL} \times 10 \text{ gtt/mL}}{20 \text{ minutes}} = 50 \text{ gtt/min}$$

The drip rate is 50 gtt/min.

Mechanical devices are used to control drip rates (gtt/min)

- The most common device is the roller clamp. It's part of the IV tubing.
- The flow regulator, added onto the IV tubing, uses a dial to set the drip rate.

* In some clinical settings when an exact drip rate may not be critical, like an ER, the speed is approximated instead of calculated.

Slow speed: TKO or To Keep Open
Medium speed
Fast speed: WO or Wide Open

If the drip rate has been calculated, the drops should be counted for one minute to ensure accuracy.

Chapter 2

Gravity System

Pump Rate to Gravity Drip Rate

To change a flow rate (mL/hr) to a gravity drip rate (gtt/min), use the formula below.

Pump Rate (mL/hr) to Gravity Drip Rate (gtt/min)

$$\frac{\text{infusion rate (mL/hr)} \times \text{drop factor (gtt/mL)}}{60 \text{ minutes}} = \text{drip rate (gtt/min)}$$

Example:

The pump is infusing at 50 mL/hr, using a 10 gtt/mL tubing, what will the drip rate (gtt/mL) be?

$$\frac{50 \text{ mL/hr} \times 10 \text{ gtt/mL}}{60 \text{ min}} = 8 \text{ gtt/min}$$

The drip rate is 8 gtt/min.

Practice Problem:

Order: Infuse LR at 125 mL/hr
IV tubing: 10 gtt/mL
Drip rate (gtt/min): _____

Practice Solution:

21 gtt/min

Order: LR at 125 mL/hr

IV tubing: 10 gtt/mL

$$\frac{\text{infusion rate (mL/hr)} \times \text{drop factor (gtt/mL)}}{60 \text{ minutes}} = \text{drip rate (gtt/min)}$$

$$\frac{125 \text{ (mL/hr)} \times 10 \text{ (gtt/mL)}}{60 \text{ minutes}} = 21 \text{ (gtt/min)}$$

14

The Gravity System

Calculate the following drip rates (gtt/min)
using the Drops Per Minute (DPM) Formula:

$$\frac{\text{total volume to be infused (mL)} \times \text{drop factor (gtt/mL)}}{\text{total infusion time in minutes}} = \text{drip rate (gtt/min)}$$

1. Order: Infuse 50 mL IVPB (IV piggy back) over 30 minutes
   IV tubing: 10 gtt/mL (drip factor)
   Drip rate (gtt/min): _____

2. Order: Infuse 1 liter Normal Saline over 8 hours
   IV tubing: 15 gtt/mL
   Drip rate (gtt/min): _____

3. Order: Infuse 1 liter Normal Saline over one hour
   IV tubing: 10 gtt/mL
   Drip rate (gtt/min): _____

Solutions on page 16

Chapter 2

Gravity System

Practice Solutions

Solutions ... **Drip Rate (gtt/min)**

$$\frac{\text{total volume to be infused (mL)} \times \text{drop factor (gtt/mL)}}{\text{total infusion time in minutes}} = \text{drip rate (gtt/min)}$$

1. **17 gtt/min**

   Order: 50 mL over 30 minutes

   IV tubing: 10 gtt/mL

   $$\frac{50 \text{ mL} \times 10 \text{ gtt/mL}}{30 \text{ minutes}} = 17 \text{ (gtt/min)}$$

2. **31 gtt/min**

   Order: 1 liter over 8 hours

   IV tubing: 15 gtt/mL

   $$\frac{1,000 \text{ mL} \times 15 \text{ gtt/mL}}{8 \text{ hr} \times 60 \text{ minutes (480 minutes)}} = 31 \text{ (gtt/min)}$$

3. **167 gtt/min**

   Order: 1 liter over one hour

   IV tubing: 10 gtt/mL

   $$\frac{1,000 \text{ mL} \times 10 \text{ gtt/mL}}{60 \text{ minutes}} = 167 \text{ (gtt/min)}$$

IV Pump System

Basic IV Infusion Formulas

The IV infusion pump system uses a programmable IV pump. The flow rate (mL/hr) is controlled electronically—based on the users input.

Three Basic IV Pump System Formulas

1. **Flow Rate (mL/hr)**

$$\frac{\text{total volume to infuse (mL)}}{\text{time in hours (hr)}} = \text{mL/hr}$$

2. **Infusion Time**

$$\frac{\text{total volume to infuse (mL)}}{\text{mL/hr}} = \text{infusion time}$$

3. **Infusion Volumes**

$$\text{infusion rate (mL/hr)} \times \text{infusion time (hr)} = \text{infusion volumes}$$

Chapter 2

IV Pump System

Basic IV Infusion Formulas/ Examples

Applying the three Basic IV Pump System Formulas

1. **Calculate Flow Rate (mL/hr)**
   Order: 1 Liter to infuse over 12 hours
   Convert: 1 Liter = 1,000 mL

   $$\frac{\text{total volume to infuse (mL)}}{\text{time in hours (hr)}} = \text{mL/hr}$$

   $$\frac{1,000 \ (\text{mL})}{12 \ (\text{hr})} = 83 \ \text{mL/hr}$$

2. **Calculate Infusion Time**
   Order: 1 Liter Normal Saline at 125 mL/hr
   Convert: 1 Liter = 1,000 mL

   $$\frac{\text{total volume to infuse (mL)}}{\text{mL/hr}} = \text{infusion time}$$

   $$\frac{1,000 \ (\text{mL})}{125 \ \text{mL/hr}} = 8 \ \text{hours}$$

3. **Calculate Infusion Volumes**
   Order: Normal Saline 150 mL/hr for 3 hours

   $$\text{infusion rate (mL/hr)} \times \text{infusion time (hr)} = \text{infusion volumes}$$

   $$150 \ (\text{mL/hr}) \times 3 \ (\text{hr}) = 450 \ \text{mL}$$

IV Pump System

Calculate Flow Rate (mL/hr)

$$\frac{\text{total volume to infuse (mL)}}{\text{time in hours (hr)}} = \text{mL/hr}$$

1. Order: Normal Saline 500 mL over 3 hours
   mL/hr: _____

2. Order: Ampicillin 500 mg/100 mL over 30 min
   mL/hr: ____

3. Order: Antibiotic 2 g/100 mL infuse over 45 minutes
   mL/hr: _____

4. Order: LR 1,000 mL over 6 hours
   mL/hr: _____

Solutions on page 22

Chapter 2

IV Pump System

Practice Problems

Calculate Infusion Time

$$\frac{\text{total volume to infuse (mL)}}{\text{mL/hr}} = \text{infusion time}$$

1. Order: 1 Liter Banana Bag at 125 mL/hr
   Infusion Time: _____

2. Order: 40 mEq KcL in 100 mL IV at 75 mL/hr
   Infusion Time: _____

3. Order: Normal Saline 500 mL at 50 mL/hr
   Infusion Time: _____

4. Order: Lasix 100 mg/100 mL at 10 mL/hr
   Infusion Time: _____

Solutions on page 23

IV Pump System

Calculate Infusion Volumes

infusion rate (mL/hr) × infusion time (hr) = infusion volumes

1. Order: LR at 75 mL/hr over 8 hours
   Total Volume Infused: _____

2. Order: Normal Saline at 200 mL/hr over 4 hours
   Total Volume Infusion: _____

3. Order: Lasix at 8 mL/hr times 10 hours
   Total Volume Infused: _____

4. Order: Banana Bag at 125 mL/hr over 8 hours
   Total Volume Infused: _____

Solutions on page 24

IV Pump System

Practice Solutions

Solutions ... **Flow Rate (mL/hr)**

$$\frac{\text{total volume to infuse (mL)}}{\text{time in hours (hr)}} = \text{mL/hr}$$

1. **167 mL/hr**
   Order: Normal Saline 500 mL over 3 hours

   $$\frac{500 \text{ (mL)}}{3 \text{ (hr)}} = 167 \text{ mL/hr}$$

2. **200 mL/hr**
   Order: Ampicillin 500 mg/100 mL over 30 min
   Convert: 30 minutes into hours.

   $$X \text{ (hr)} = \frac{30 \text{ min}}{1} \times \frac{1 \text{ hr}}{60 \text{ min}} = 0.5 \text{ hr}$$

   $$\frac{100 \text{ (mL)}}{0.5 \text{ (hr)}} = 200 \text{ mL/hr}$$

3. **133 mL/hr**
   Order: Antibiotic 2 g/100 mL to infuse over 45 minutes
   Convert: 45 minutes into hours.

   $$X \text{ (hr)} = \frac{45 \text{ min}}{1} \times \frac{1 \text{ hr}}{60 \text{ min}} = 0.75 \text{ hr}$$

   $$\frac{100 \text{ (mL)}}{0.75 \text{ (hr)}} = 133 \text{ mL/hr}$$

4. **167 mL/hr**
   Order: LR 1,000 mL over 6 hours

   $$\frac{1,000 \text{ (mL)}}{6 \text{ (hr)}} = 167 \text{ mL/hr}$$

IV Pump System

Solutions ... **Infusion Time**

$$\frac{\text{total volume to infuse (mL)}}{\text{mL/hr}} = \text{infusion time}$$

1. **8 hours**

   Order: 1 Liter Banana Bag at 125 mL/hr
   1 Liter = 1,000 mL

   $$\frac{1,000 \text{ (mL)}}{125 \text{ mL/hr}} = 8 \text{ hours}$$

2. **1 hour 33 min**

   Order: 40 mEq KcL in 100 mL IV at 75 mL/hr

   $$\frac{100 \text{ (mL)}}{75 \text{ mL/hr}} = 1 \text{ hours } 33 \text{ min}$$

3. **10 hours**

   Order: Normal Saline 500 mL at 50 mL/hr

   $$\frac{500 \text{ (mL)}}{50 \text{ mL/hr}} = 10 \text{ hours}$$

4. **10 hours**

   Order: Lasix 100 mg/100 mL at 10 mL/hr

   $$\frac{100 \text{ (mL)}}{10 \text{ mL/hr}} = 10 \text{ hours}$$

Chapter 2

IV Pump System

Practice Solutions

Solutions ... **Infusion Volumes**

infusion rate (mL/hr) × infusion time (hr) = infusion volumes

1. **600 mL**
   Order: LR infuse at 75 mL/hr over 8 hours
   $75\ (mL/hr) \times 8\ (hr) = 600\ mL$

2. **800 mL**
   Order: Normal Saline at 200 mL/hr over 4 hours
   $200\ (mL/hr) \times 4\ (hr) = 800\ mL$

3. **80 mL**
   Order: Lasix at 8 mL/hr times 10 hours
   $8\ (mL/hr) \times 10\ (hr) = 80\ mL$

4. **1,000 mL**
   Order: Banana Bag at 125 mL/hr over 8 hours
   $125\ (mL/hr) \times 8\ (hr) = 1{,}000\ mL$

Chapter 3

A Comparison Study
Dimensional Analysis, Ratio-Proportion, Non-traditional

Traditionally, complex critical care IV dosage calculations are solved using dimensional analysis and/or ratio-proportion methods. There is, however, an easier method; The Wrinkle Method.

The Wrinkle Method is a name given to a group of formulas that are easy to remember and simple to use.

To demonstrate how much easier The Wrinkle Method is, a comparison study is used.

This comparison study shows how dimensional analysis, ratio-proportion and The Wrinkle Method are used to calculate a flow rate (mL/hr). Each method will use the same critical care IV dosage calculation problem.

Since the focus of this chapter is to compare the three methods above, The Wrinkle Method is not introduced in detail. Chapter 4 will explain, step-by-step, how The Wrinkle Method works.

Chapter 3

The Comparison Study

Comparison Problem

The Comparison Problem

Order: **Dopamine** to infuse at **10 mcg/kg/min**
Have: **Dopamine 400 mg in 250 mL**
Wt: **65 kg**

Solve for the flow rate (mL/hr) using:
- Dimensional Analysis
- Ratio-Proportion
- Wrinkle Method

The Comparison Study
Dimensional Analysis Method

Dimensional analysis is a mathematical system using conversion factors to move from one unit of measurement to a different unit of measurement.

Dimensional Analysis Formula: $X = \dfrac{a}{b} \times \dfrac{b}{c} \times \dfrac{c}{d} \times \dfrac{d}{e} \times \dfrac{e}{f}$

Comparison problem:
Order: Dopamine 10 mcg/kg/min
Have: Dopamine 400 mg in 250 mL
Wt: 65 kg
Solve for the flow rate (mL/hr): _____

1. **Draw a line with desired units at the end.**

   $$\rule{4cm}{0.4pt}\ \text{mL/hr}$$

2. **Place known values and conversion factors on the line.**
   Position them either on the top or bottom to facilitate the cancellation of undesired units.
   Order: 10 mcg/kg/min
   Drug concentration: 400 mg/250 mL
   Wt: 65 kg
   Conversion Factors: 1 mg = 1,000 mcg
   60 minutes = 1 hr

   $$\frac{10\ \text{mcg}}{\text{kg} \times \text{minutes}} \times \frac{250\ \text{mL}}{400\ \text{mg}} \times \frac{65\ \text{kg}}{1} \times \frac{60\ \text{minutes}}{1\ \text{hr}} \times \frac{1\ \text{mg}}{1{,}000\ \text{mcg}} = \text{mL/hr}$$

3. **Cancel out like units.**
   Leave only desired units.

   $$\frac{10\ \cancel{\text{mcg}}}{\cancel{\text{kg}} \times \cancel{\text{minutes}}} \times \frac{250\ \text{mL}}{400\ \cancel{\text{mg}}} \times \frac{65\ \cancel{\text{kg}}}{1} \times \frac{60\ \cancel{\text{minutes}}}{1\ \text{hr}} \times \frac{1\ \cancel{\text{mg}}}{1{,}000\ \cancel{\text{mcg}}} = \text{mL/hr}$$

4. **Multiply / Divide**

   $$\frac{10}{1} \times \frac{250\ \text{mL}}{400} \times \frac{65}{1} \times \frac{60}{1\ \text{hr}} \times \frac{1}{1{,}000} = 24.4\ \text{mL/hr}$$

The flow rate is 24 mL/hr

The Comparison Study

Ratio-Proportion Method

Ratio is used to make a comparison between two things.

A ratio can be written several ways: $\dfrac{a}{b}$ or $\dfrac{b}{a}$ | a / b or b/a

Proportion is when two ratios are equal.

A proportion is written: $\dfrac{a}{b} = \dfrac{c}{d}$

Ratio-Proportion Formula: $\dfrac{\text{known value}}{\text{known value}} = \dfrac{\text{known value}}{\text{desired value}}$

Comparison problem:
Order: Dopamine 10 mcg/kg/min
Have: Dopamine 400 mg in 250 mL
Wt: 65 kg
Solve for the flow rate (mL/hr): _____

1. **Convert** mg to mcg (1 mg = 1,000 mcg)
   Have: Dopamine 400 mg/250 mL

   $400 \text{ mg} \times 1{,}000 = 400{,}000 \text{ mcg}$

   Now Have: Dopamine 400,000 mcg in 250 mL

2. **Multiply to determine ordered dose**

   $10 \text{ mcg} \times 65 \text{ kg/min} = 650 \text{ mcg/min}$

   Total dose to be infused is 650 mcg/min.
   Will need to know how many mL's contain 650 mcg/min.

Continued on page 29

The Comparison Study

Ratio-Proportion Method ... *continued*

3. **Set up a Ratio-Proportion formula**

   a.

   $$\frac{400{,}000 \text{ mcg}}{250 \text{ mL}} = \frac{650 \text{ mcg}}{(x) \text{ mL}}$$

   b. **Cross Multiply**

   $$400{,}000 \text{ mcg} \times (x) \text{ mL} = 250 \text{ mL} \times 650 \text{ mcg}$$

   c. **Divide both sides by 400,000 mcg**

   $$\frac{\cancel{400{,}000} \text{ } \cancel{\text{mcg}}}{\cancel{400{,}000} \text{ } \cancel{\text{mcg}}} \times (x) \text{ mL} = \frac{250 \text{ mL} \times 650 \text{ } \cancel{\text{mcg}}}{400{,}000 \text{ } \cancel{\text{mcg}}}$$

   $$(x)\text{mL} = \frac{250 \text{ mL} \times 650}{400{,}000}$$

   $$\text{mL} = 0.40 \text{ mL}$$

   The Order is 650 mcg/min.
   There are 650 mcg/min in 0.40 mL.
   What is the flow rate(mL/hr)?

4. **Set up a Dimensional Analysis formula.**

   $$\overline{} | \text{mL/hr}$$

   $$\frac{0.40 \text{ mL}}{1 \text{ } \cancel{\text{minutes}}} \times \frac{60 \text{ } \cancel{\text{minutes}}}{1 \text{ hr}} = \text{mL/hr}$$

   $$0.40 \text{ mL} \times \frac{60}{1 \text{ hr}} = 24 \text{ mL/hr}$$

The flow rate is 24 mL/hr

29

The Comparison Study

Non-traditional Wrinkle Method

The Wrinkle Method consists of seven formulas. Each formula corresponds to a dosage rate.

mcg/kg/min: $\boxed{\text{mcg} \div \text{mL} \div 60 \text{ minutes} \div \text{kg} = \text{BedsideValue (BV)}}$

Comparison problem:
Order: Dopamine 10 mcg/kg/min
Have: Dopamine 400 mg in 250 mL
Wt: 65 kg
Solve for the flow rate (mL/hr): _____

The Wrinkle Method has three easy steps:

1. **Convert** mg to mcg (1 mg = 1,000 mcg)
   Have: Dopamine 400 mg/250 mL
   $\boxed{400 \text{ mg} \times 1,000 = 400,000 \text{ mcg}}$

   Now Have: Dopamine 400,000 mcg/250 mL

2. **Calculate the BedsideValue (BV)**
   $\boxed{400,000 \text{ mcg} \div 250 \text{ mL} \div 60 \text{ minutes} \div 65 \text{ kg} = 0.41 \text{(BV)}}$
   BedsideValue (BV) = 0.41

3. **Calculate the flow rate (mL/hr)**
   Use the BedsideValue (BV) 0.41 to calculate the flow rate (mL/hr).

   Flow Rate (mL/hr) = $\boxed{\dfrac{\text{Order}}{\text{(BV)}} = \text{mL/hr}}$ $\boxed{\dfrac{10}{0.41} = 24 \text{ mL/hr}}$

The flow rate is 24 mL/hr

The Comparison Study
How to Check Flow Rate (mL/hr) Accuracy

To ensure the *right dose* **of medication** is delivered to the patient, all flow rates (mL/hr) must be checked for accuracy.

If the flow rate was calculated using the dimensional analysis or ratio-proportion methods, the dosage calculations must be repeated to check for flow rate accuracy. This approach is time consuming and the same mistake(s) could be repeated.

If The Wrinkle Method was used to calculate a flow rate, a simple multiplication problem is all that is required to check flow rate accuracy. This is a significant advantage over the traditional methods.

Example:
Using the dosage rate formula below, check for flow rate (mL/hr) accuracy.

Dosage Rate Formula: $\boxed{(\text{mL/hr}) \times (\text{BV}) = \text{dosage rate}}$

Order: **Dopamine 10 mcg/kg/min**
Flow Rate: **24 mL/hr**
Bedside Value: **(BV) 0.41**

$\boxed{(\text{mL/hr}) \times (\text{BV}) = \text{dosage rate}}$ $\boxed{24 \text{ mL/hr} \times (\text{BV}) \, 0.41 = 9.8 \text{ mcg/kg/min}}$

A flow rate of 24 mL/hr has a calculated dosage rate of 10 mcg/kg/min.

Chapter 4

The Wrinkle Method
Critical Care IV Dosage Formulas

INTRODUCING: A refreshing alternative from the customary methods of dimensional analysis and ratio-proportion. Once again, it's The Wrinkle Method.

The Wrinkle Method, unlike the traditional methods that can be confusing to use, makes solving and titrating complex critical care IV dosage calculations easy.

Chapter 4

The Wrinkle Method

Overview

The Wrinkle Method is a collection of seven formulas.
- Two basic formulas
- Five formulas that have slight variations from the basic formulas

Each formula corresponds to a specific dosage rate.
They are located on pages 36 and 37.

The goal of each formula is to calculate a value.
- That value is called BedsideValue (BV)
- The BedsideValue (BV) represents:
    The drug concentration you have on hand
    (i.e., 50 mg/250 mL) and, if required,
    the patient's weight in kilograms (kg).

The BedsideValue (BV) is used to calculate both:
- Flow Rate (mL/hr)
- Dosage Rate

The Wrinkle Method has three easy steps:

Step One: **Convert**, if required
    Example:
    Convert mg to mcg

Step Two: **Calculate the BedsideValue (BV)**
    To calculate the BedsideValue (BV),
    use one of The Wrinkle Method formulas.

Step Three: **Calculate both:** (Use the BV)
    Flow Rate (mL/hr)
    Dosage Rate

* To check for *right dose* delivery, always calculate both the
flow rate (mL/hr) and the dosage rate.

The Wrinkle Method

Critical Care IV Dosage Rates

Dosage Rates for critical care continuous IV infusion medications are written:

- mg/min
- mcg/min
- mcg/kg/min
- units/min

- mg/hr
- units/hr
- units/kg/hr

They are divided into two groups:
1. The first group ends with "**min**", the abbreviation for minute.
2. The second group ends with "**hr**", the abbreviation for hour.

Each dosage rate requires a flow rate (mL/hr).

To calculate a flow rate (mL/hr) use The Wrinkle Method formula that corresponds to the dosage rate.

* Some IV pumps require the use of whole numbers for flow rate (mL/hr) input. Since flow rates affect dosage rates, always use sound clinical judgment when rounding up or down.

Chapter 4

The Wrinkle Method

Dosage Rate Formulas/"min"

Dosage Rate Formulas ending with **"min"**

Divide by 60 minutes.

- mg/min
- mcg/min
- mcg/kg/min
- units/min

The basic formula: **mg/min**

mg/min

> mg ÷ mL ÷ 60 minutes = BedsideValue (BV)

mcg/min

> mcg ÷ mL ÷ 60 minutes = BedsideValue (BV)

mcg/kg/min

> mcg ÷ mL ÷ 60 minutes ÷ kg = BedsideValue (BV)

units/min

> units ÷ mL ÷ 60 minutes = BedsideValue (BV)

The Wrinkle Method

Dosage Rate Formulas/"hr"

Dosage Rate Formulas ending with **"hr"**

Do NOT divide by 60 minutes.

- mg/hr
- units/hr
- units/kg/hr

The basic formula: **mg/hr**

mg/hr

mg ÷ mL = BedsideValue (BV)

units/hr

units ÷ mL = BedsideValue (BV)

units/kg/hr

units ÷ mL ÷ kg = BedsideValue (BV)

* **Caution,** a common error is to divide these formulas by 60 minutes.

Chapter 4

The Wrinkle Method

Using the Bedside Value (BV)

The goal of each Wrinkle Method formula is to generate a BedsideValue (BV).

The BV is calculated to the hundredths place. Do not round. Example: With a calculation of 0.166 the (BV) will be 0.16.

* For patient safety, recalculate the (BV) for accuracy.

The (BV) is used to calculate both the flow rate (mL/hr) and the dosage rate.

Flow Rate = $\dfrac{\text{Order}}{\text{(BV)}} = \text{mL/hr}$

Dosage Rate = $(\text{mL/hr}) \times (\text{BV}) = \text{dosage rate}$

Hint:

For a quick reference at the bedside, write the information given in the example below on a piece of white tape. Stick it onto the IV pump control panel infusing that medication.

Example:

Dopamine: 400 mg/250 mL

Wt: 50 kg

(BV): 0.53

The Wrinkle Method

Example (mg/min)

mg/min

mg ÷ mL ÷ 60 minutes = BedsideValue (BV)

How to use:
1. **This is the basic formula for dosage rates ending in min**
2. **Divided by 60 minutes**

Example:
Order: Cordarone 0.5 mg/min
Have: Cordarone 900 mg/500 mL
Solve for mL/hr: _____ (round to whole number)

Step One: Convert, No conversion required.
Order is in mg, drug concentration is in mg.
(900 mg/500 mL)

Step Two: Calculate the (BV)

mg ÷ mL ÷ 60 minutes = BV

900 mg ÷ 500 mL ÷ 60 minutes = 0.03 BV

Step Three: Calculate both

$$\text{Flow Rate} = \frac{\text{Order}}{\text{(BV)}} = \text{mL/hr} \quad \frac{0.5}{0.03} = 17 \text{ mL/hr}$$

$$\text{Dosage Rate} = (\text{mL/hr}) \times (\text{BV}) = \text{dosage rate} \quad 17 \times 0.03 = 0.5 \text{ mg}$$

Chapter 4

The Wrinkle Method

Example (mcg/min)

mcg/min

| mcg ÷ mL ÷ 60 minutes = BedsideValue (BV) |

How to use:
1. **Use the basic formula**: mg ÷ mL ÷ 60 minutes = (BV)
2. **Convert** mg to mcg
3. **Divided by 60 minutes**

Example:
Order: Nitroglycerin 10 mcg/min
Have: Nitroglycerin 50 mg/250 mL
Solve for mL/hr: _____ (round to whole number**)**

Step One: **Convert,** mg to mcg, (1 mg = 1,000 mcg)
Order is in mcg, drug concentration is in mg.
(50 mg/250 mL)

| 50 mg × 1,000 = 50,000 mcg |

Now Have: 50,000 mcg/250 mL

Step Two: **Calculate the (BV)**

| mcg ÷ mL ÷ 60 minutes = BV |
| 50,000 mcg ÷ 250 mL ÷ 60 minutes = 3.33 BV |

Step Three: **Calculate both**

Flow Rate = $\dfrac{\text{Order}}{\text{(BV)}}$ = mL/hr $\dfrac{10}{3.33}$ = 3 mL/hr

Dosage Rate = (mL/ hr) × (BV) = dosage rate   3 × 3.33 = 10 mcg

The Wrinkle Method

Example (mcg/kg/min)

mcg/kg/min

mcg ÷ mL ÷ 60 minutes ÷ kg = BedsideValue (BV)

How to use:
1. **Use the basic formula**: mg ÷ mL ÷ 60 minutes = (BV)
2. **Convert** mg to mcg
3. **Divide by 60 minutes**
4. **Insert kg**

Example:
Order: Dopamine 10 mcg/kg/min
Have: Dopamine 400 mg/250 mL
Wt: 84.5 kg
Solve for mL/hr: _____ (round to whole number)

Step One: Convert, mg to mcg (1 mg = 1,000 mcg)
Order is in mcg, drug concentration is in mg.
(400 mg/250 mL)

400 mg × 1,000 = 400,000 mcg

Now Have: 400,000 mcg/250 mL

Step Two: Calculate the (BV)

mcg ÷ mL ÷ 60 minutes ÷ kg = BV

400,000 mcg ÷ 250 mL ÷ 60 minutes ÷ 84.5 kg = 0.31BV

Step Three: Calculate both

Flow Rate = $\dfrac{\text{Order}}{\text{(BV)}}$ = mL/hr $\dfrac{10}{0.31}$ = 32 mL/hr

Dosage Rate = (mL/ hr) × (BV) = dosage rate 32 × 0.31 = 10 mcg

The Wrinkle Method

Example (units/min)

units/min

units ÷ mL ÷ 60 minutes = BedsideValue (BV)

How to use:
1. **Use the basic formula**: mg ÷ mL ÷ 60 minutes = (BV)
2. **Change** mg to units
3. **Divide by 60 minutes**

Example:
Order: Vasopressin 0.04 units/min
Have: Vasopressin 100 units/100 mL
Solve for mL/hr: _____ (round to whole number)

Step One: **Convert**, No conversion required.
Order is in units, drug concentration is in units.
(100 units/100 mL)

Step Two: Calculate the (BV)

units ÷ mL ÷ 60 minutes = BV
100 units ÷ 100 mL ÷ 60 minutes = 0.01 (BV)

Step Three: Calculate both

Flow Rate = $\dfrac{\text{Order}}{\text{(BV)}}$ = mL/hr $\qquad$ $\dfrac{0.04}{0.01}$ = 4 mL/hr

Dosage Rate = (mL/ hr) × (BV) = dosage rate $\qquad$ 4 × 0.01 = 0.04 units

The Wrinkle Method

mg/hr

> mg ÷ mL = BedsideValue (BV)

How to use:
1. This is the basic formula for dosage rates ending in hr
2. Do NOT divide by 60 minutes

Example:
Order: Morphine 2 mg/hr
Have: Morphine 50 mg/50 mL
Solve for mL/hr: _____ (round to whole number)

Step One: Convert, No conversion required.
Order is in mg, drug concentration is in mg.
(50 mg/50 mL)

Step Two: Calculate the (BV)

> mg ÷ mL = BV
>
> 50 mg ÷ 50 mL = 1 BV

Step Three: Calculate both

Flow Rate = $\dfrac{\text{Order}}{\text{(BV)}}$ = mL/hr $\dfrac{2}{1}$ = 2 mL/hr

Dosage Rate = (mL/hr) × (BV) = dosage rate   2 × 1 = 2 mg

43

The Wrinkle Method

units/hr

$$\boxed{\text{units} \div \text{mL} = \text{BedsideValue (BV)}}$$

How to use:

1. **Use the basic formula**: $\text{mg} \div \text{mL} = (\text{BV})$
2. **Change** mg to units
3. **Do NOT divide by 60 minutes**

Example:
Order: Heparin 1,300 units/hr
Have: Heparin 20,000 units/500 mL
Solve for mL/hr: _____ (round to whole number)

Step One: Convert, No conversion required.
Order is in units, drug concentration is in units.
(20,000 units/500 mL)

Step Two: Calculate the (BV)

$$\boxed{\begin{array}{l} \text{units} \div \text{mL} = \text{BV} \\ 20{,}000 \text{ units} \div 500 \text{ mL} = 40 \text{ BV} \end{array}}$$

Step Three: Calculate both

$$\textbf{Flow Rate} = \boxed{\dfrac{\text{Order}}{(\text{BV})} = \text{mL/hr}} \quad \boxed{\dfrac{1{,}300}{40} = 33 \, \text{mL/hr}}$$

$$\textbf{Dosage Rate} = \boxed{(\text{mL/ hr}) \times (\text{BV}) = \text{dosage rate}} \quad \boxed{33 \times 40 = 1{,}320 \, \text{units}}$$

The Wrinkle Method

Example (units/kg/hr)

units/kg/hr

$$\boxed{\text{units} \div \text{mL} \div \text{kg} = \text{BedsideValue (BV)}}$$

How to use:
1. **Use the basic formula**: $\text{mg} \div \text{mL} = (\text{BV})$
2. **Change** mg to units
3. **Insert kg**
4. **Do NOT divide by 60 minutes**

Example:
Order: Heparin 18 units/kg/hr
Have: Heparin 25,000 units/250 mL
Wt: 55 kg
Solve for mL/hr: _____ (round to whole number)

Step One: Convert, No conversion required.
Order is in units, drug concentration is in units.
(25,000 units/250 mL)

Step Two: Calculate the (BV)

$$\text{units} \div \text{mL} \div \text{kg} = \text{BV}$$
$$25{,}000 \text{ units} \div 250 \text{ mL} \div 55 \text{ kg} = 1.81 \text{ BV}$$

Step Three: Calculate both

$$\textbf{Flow Rate} = \boxed{\dfrac{\text{Order}}{(\text{BV})} = \text{mL/hr}} \quad \boxed{\dfrac{18}{1.81} = 10 \text{ mL/hr}}$$

$$\textbf{Dosage Rate} = \boxed{(\text{mL/hr}) \times (\text{BV}) = \text{dosage rate}} \quad \boxed{10 \times 1.81 = 18 \text{ units}}$$

Chapter 5

Building Confidence: Practice Problems
The Wrinkle Method Approach

It's easy to solve complex critical care IV dosage calculations when using The Wrinkle Method formulas. They're easy to remember, simple to work with, and powerful at the bedside.

* Some IV pumps require the use of whole numbers for
  flow rate (mL/hr) input. Since flow rates affect dosage rates, always use sound clinical judgment when rounding up or down.

  For simplicity, the following practice problems will use whole numbers when calculating mL/hr and dosage rates.

  And always—for patient safety—double check flow rate accuracy.

Building Confidence: Practice Problems

Dosage Rate Formulas ending with "**min** "
Divide by 60 minutes.
- mg/min
- mcg/min
- mcg/kg/min
- units/min

The basic formula: **mg/min**

mg/min

mg ÷ mL ÷ 60 minutes = BedsideValue (BV)

mcg/min

mcg ÷ mL ÷ 60 minutes = BedsideValue (BV)

mcg/kg/min

mcg ÷ mL ÷ 60 minutes ÷ kg = BedsideValue (BV)

units/min

units ÷ mL ÷ 60 minutes = BedsideValue (BV)

Building Confidence: Practice Problems

Dosage Rate Formulas/Review

Dosage Rate Formulas ending with "hr"

Do NOT divide by 60 minutes.

- mg/hr
- units/hr
- units/kg/hr

The basic formula: **mg/hr**

mg/hr

mg ÷ mL = BedsideValue (BV)

units/hr

units ÷ mL = BedsideValue (BV)

units/kg/hr

units ÷ mL ÷ kg = BedsideValue (BV)

Using the Bedside Value (BV)

The BedsideValue (BV) is used to calculate both the flow rate (mL/hr) and the dosage rate.

Calculate the BV to the hundredths place. Do not round. Example: With a calculation of 0.166 the (BV) will be 0.16.

Flow Rate = $\frac{\text{Order}}{\text{(BV)}} = \text{mL/hr}$

Dosage Rate = (mL/ hr) × (BV) = dosage rate

Building Confidence: Practice Problems
The Wrinkle Method Approach

Solve for:

- BedsideValue (BV)—Calculate to the hundredths place.
  Do not round.
  Example: 0.01
- Flow Rate (mL/hr)—Use whole numbers.
- Dosage Rate—Use whole numbers.

1. Order: Amiodarone 0.5 mg/min
   Have: Amiodarone 450 mg/250 mL
   BV: _____
   mL/hr: _____

2. Order: Labetalol 1 mg/min
   Have: Labetalol 500 mg/250 mL
   BV: _____
   mL/hr: _____

3. Order: Procainamide 2 mg/min
   Have: Procainamide 4 g/500 mL
   BV: _____
   mL/hr: _____

4. Order: Lidocaine 2 mg/min
   Have: Lidocaine 2 g/250 mL
   BV: _____
   mL/hr: _____

Solutions to questions 1-4 found on pages 56-58

Building Confidence: Practice Problems

The Wrinkle Method Approach

5. Order: Diltiazem 8 mg/hr
   Have: Diltiazem 100 mg/100 mL
   BV: _____
   mL/hr: _____

6. Order: Furosemide 2 mg/hr
   Have: Furosemide 100 mg/100 mL
   BV: _____
   mL/hr: _____

7. Order: Levophed 8 mcg/min
   Have: Levophed 4 mg/250 mL
   BV: _____
   mL/hr: _____

8. Order: Isuprel 5 mcg/min
   Have: Isuprel 2 mg/250 mL
   BV: _____
   mL/hr: _____
   If the infusion rate is 46 mL/hr, what is the
   dosage rate?_____

9. Order: Norepinephrine 2 mcg/min
   Have: Norepinephrine 8 mg/250 mL
   BV: _____
   mL/hr: _____

10. Order: Epinephrine 2 mcg/min
    Have: Epinephrine 2 mg/250 mL
    BV: _____
    mL/hr: _____

Solutions to questions 5-10 found on pages 58-62

Building Confidence: Practice Problems
The Wrinkle Method Approach

11. Order: Dopamine 15 mcg/kg/min
    Titrate: Decrease by 1 mcg/kg/min every 30
        minutes.
    Have: Dopamine 400 mg/250 mL
    Wt: 50 kg
    BV: _____
    mL/hr: _____
    Titrate: 1 mcg/kg/min = _____ mL/hr

12. Order: Primacor 0.5 mcg/kg/min
    Have: Primacor 40 mg/200 mL
    Wt: 81 kg
    BV: _____
    mL/hr: _____

13. Order: Diprivan 25 mcg/kg/min
    Titrate: Increase 2 mcg/kg/min every 5 minutes to
        desired sedation.
    Have: Diprivan 1,000 mg/100 mL
    Wt: 78 kg
    BV: _____
    mL/hr: _____(Rounding affects dosage rate.)
    Titrate: 2 mcg/kg/min = _____ mL/hr

14. Order: Insulin 10 units/hr
    Have: Insulin 100 units/100 mL
    BV: _____
    mL/hr: _____

Solutions to questions 11-14 found on pages 63-66

Building Confidence: Practice Problems

15. Order: Heparin 800 units/hr
    Have: Heparin 25,000 units/250 mL
    BV: _____
    mL/hr: _____

16. Order: Heparin 18 units/kg/hr
    Have: Heparin 25,000 units/250 mL
    Wt. 88 kg
    BV: _____
    mL/hr: _____

17. Order: Nitroglycerine 16 mcg/min
    Have: Nitroglycerine 50 mg/250 mL
    BV: _____
    mL/hr: _____(Rounding affects dosage rate.)

18. Order: Vecuronium 0.8 mcg/kg/min
    Have: Vecuronium 100 mg in 250 mL
    Wt: 81 kg
    BV: _____
    mL/hr: _____
    If the infusion rate is 15 mL/hr, what is the
    dosage rate? _____

19. Order: Vasopressin 0.3 units/min
    Have: Vasopressin 200 units in 250 mL
    BV: _____
    mL/hr: _____
    If the infusion rate is 19 mL/hr, what is the
    dosage rate? _____

Solutions to questions 15-19 found on pages 66-69

Building Confidence: Practice Problems
The Wrinkle Method Approach

20. Order: Norepinephrine 5 mcg/min
    Have: Norepinephrine 4 mg/250 mL
    BV: _____
    mL/hr: _____
    If the infusion rate is 50 mL/hr, what is the
    dosage rate?_____

21. Order: Neosynephrine 100 mcg/min
    Have: Neosynephrine 50 mg/250 mL
    BV: _____
    If the infusion rate is 75 mL/hr, what is the
    dosage rate? _____

22. Order: Midazolam 1 mg/hr
    Have: Midazolam 100 mg/100 mL
    BV: _____
    mL/hr: _____

23. Order: Vasopressin 0.04 units/min
    Have: Vasopressin 20 units/100 mL
    BV: _____(Calculate to thousandths place. Example: 0.001)
    mL/hr: _____

24. Order: Dobutamine 10 mcg/kg/min
    Have: Dobutamine 500 mg/250 mL
    Wt: 77 kg
    BV: _____
    mL/hr: _____

Solutions to questions 20-24 found on pages 70-74

Building Confidence: Solutions
Solutions for Chapter 5

Each practice problem from Chapter 5 is solved using one of The Wrinkle Method formulas.

Chapter 6

Building Confidence: Solutions

Practice Solutions

1. **BV: 0.03**
   mL/hr: 17
   Order: Amiodarone 0.5 mg/min
   Have: Amiodarone 450 mg/250 mL

   Step One: Convert, No conversion required.
   Step Two: Calculate the (BV)

   450 mg ÷ 250 mL ÷ 60 min = 0.03 BV

   Step Three: Calculate both

   $$\text{Flow Rate (mL/hr)} = \frac{\text{Order}}{\text{BV}} \qquad \frac{0.5}{0.03} = 17 \text{ mL/hr}$$

   Dosage Rate = mL/hr × BV   17 × 0.03 = 0.5 mg

2. **BV: 0.03**
   mL/hr: 33
   Order: Labetalol 1 mg/min
   Have: Labetalol 500 mg/250 mL

   Step One: Convert, No conversion required.
   Step Two: Calculate the (BV)

   500 mg ÷ 250 mL ÷ 60 min = 0.03 BV

   Step Three: Calculate both

   $$\text{Flow Rate (mL/hr)} = \frac{\text{Order}}{\text{BV}} \qquad \frac{1}{0.03} = 33 \text{ mL/hr}$$

   Dosage Rate = mL/hr × BV   33 × 0.03 = 1 mg

Building Confidence: Solutions

3. **BV: 0.13**
   mL/hr: 15
   Order: Procainamide 2 mg/min
   Have: Procainamide 4 g/500 mL

   Step One: Convert g to mg
   (1 g = 1,000 mg)

   $$mg = \frac{4\cancel{g}}{1} \times \frac{1,000 \text{ mg}}{1\cancel{g}} = 4,000 \text{ mg}$$

   Step Two: Calculate the (BV)

   $$4,000 \text{ mg} \div 500 \text{ mL} \div 60 \text{ min} = 0.13 \text{ BV}$$

   Step Three: Calculate both

   $$\text{Flow Rate (mL/hr)} = \frac{\text{Order}}{\text{BV}} \quad \boxed{\frac{2}{0.13} = 15 \text{ mL/hr}}$$

   $$\text{Dosage Rate} = \text{mL/hr} \times \text{BV} \quad \boxed{15 \times 0.13 = 2 \text{ mg}}$$

Building Confidence: Solutions

Practice Solutions

4. **BV: 0.13**
   mL/hr: 15
   Order: Lidocaine 2 mg/min
   Have: Lidocaine 2 g/250 mL

   Step One: Convert g to mg
   (1 g = 1,000 mg)

   $$mg = \frac{2\cancel{g}}{1} \times \frac{1{,}000\ mg}{1\cancel{g}} = 2{,}000\ mg$$

   Step Two: Calculate the (BV)

   $$2{,}000\ mg \div 250\ mL \div 60\ min = 0.13\ BV$$

   Step Three: Calculate both

   $$\text{Flow Rate (mL/hr)} = \frac{\text{Order}}{\text{BV}} \qquad \frac{2}{0.13} = 15\ mL/hr$$

   $$\text{Dosage Rate} = mL/hr \times BV \qquad 15 \times 0.13 = 2\ mg$$

5. **BV: 1**
   mL/hr: 8
   Order: Diltiazem 8 mg/hr
   Have: Diltiazem 100 mg/100 mL

   Step One: Convert, No conversion required.
   Step Two: Calculate the (BV)
   This order/formula ends in hr,
   do not divide by 60 minutes.

   $$100\ mg \div 100\ mL = 1\ BV$$

   Step Three: Calculate both

   $$\text{Flow Rate (mL/hr)} = \frac{\text{Order}}{\text{BV}} \qquad \frac{8}{1} = 8\ mL/hr$$

   $$\text{Dosage Rate} = mL/hr \times BV \qquad 8 \times 1 = 8\ mg$$

Building Confidence: Solutions

6. **BV: 1**
   mL/hr: 2
   Order: Furosemide 2 mg/hr
   Have: Furosemide 100 mg/100 mL

   Step One: Convert, No conversion required.
   Step Two: Calculate the (BV)
         This order/formula ends in hr,
         do not divide by 60 minutes.

   $$100 \text{ mg} \div 100 \text{ mL} = 1\,\text{BV}$$

   Step Three: Calculate both

   $$\text{Flow Rate (mL/hr)} = \frac{\text{Order}}{\text{BV}} \qquad \frac{2}{1} = 2\,\text{mL/hr}$$

   $$\text{Dosage Rate} = \text{mL/hr} \times \text{BV} \qquad 2 \times 1 = 2\,\text{mg}$$

7. **BV: 0.26**
   mL/hr: 31
   Order: Levophed 8 mcg/min
   Have: Levophed 4 mg/250 mL

   Step One: Convert mg to mcg
         (1 mg = 1,000 mcg)

   $$\text{mcg} = \frac{4\,\cancel{\text{mg}}}{1} \times \frac{1,000 \text{ mcg}}{1\,\cancel{\text{mg}}} = 4,000 \text{ mcg}$$

   Step Two: Calculate the (BV)

   $$4,000 \text{ mcg} \div 250 \text{ mL} \div 60 \text{ min} = 0.26\,\text{BV}$$

   Step Three: Calculate both

   $$\text{Flow Rate (mL/hr)} = \frac{\text{Order}}{\text{BV}} \qquad \frac{8}{0.26} = 31\,\text{mL/hr}$$

   $$\text{Dosage Rate} = \text{mL/hr} \times \text{BV} \qquad 31 \times 0.26 = 8 \text{ mcg}$$

Building Confidence: Solutions

8. **BV: 0.13**
   mL/hr: 38
   At 46 mL/hr, dosage rate is 6 mcg/min
   Order: Isuprel 5 mcg/min
   Have: Isuprel 2 mg/250 mL
   If the infusion rate is 46 mL/hr, what is the dosage rate?

   Step One: Convert mg to mcg
   (1 mg = 1,000 mcg)

   $$mcg = \frac{2\,mg}{1} \times \frac{1{,}000\,mcg}{1\,mg} = 2{,}000\,mcg$$

   Step Two: Calculate the (BV)

   $$2{,}000\,mcg \div 250\,mL \div 60\,min = 0.13\,BV$$

   Step Three: Calculate both

   $$\text{Flow Rate (mL/hr)} = \frac{Order}{BV} \quad \frac{5}{0.13} = 38\,mL/hr$$

   $$\text{Dosage Rate} = mL/hr \times BV \quad 38 \times 0.13 = 5\,mcg$$

   Dosage Rate at 46 mL/hr $\quad 46 \times 0.13 = 6\,mcg$

Building Confidence: Solutions

9. **BV: 0.53**
   mL/hr: 4
   Order: Norepinephrine 2 mcg/min
   Have: Norepinephrine 8 mg/250 mL

   Step One: Convert mg to mcg
   (1 mg = 1,000 mcg)

   $$\text{mcg} = \frac{8\ \text{mg}}{1} \times \frac{1{,}000\ \text{mcg}}{1\ \text{mg}} = 8{,}000\ \text{mcg}$$

   Step Two: Calculate the (BV)

   $$8{,}000\ \text{mcg} \div 250\ \text{mL} \div 60\ \text{min} = 0.53\ \text{BV}$$

   Step Three: Calculate both

   $$\text{Flow Rate (mL/hr)} = \frac{\text{Order}}{\text{BV}} \quad \frac{2}{0.53} = 4\ \text{mL/hr}$$

   $$\text{Dosage Rate} = \text{mL/hr} \times \text{BV} \quad 4 \times 0.53 = 2\ \text{mcg}$$

Building Confidence: Solutions

10. **BV: 0.13**
    mL/hr: 15
    Order: Epinephrine 2 mcg/min
    Have: Epinephrine 2 mg/250 mL

    Step One: Convert mg to mcg
    (1 mg = 1,000 mcg)

    $$mcg = \frac{2\,\cancel{mg}}{1} \times \frac{1{,}000\ mcg}{1\,\cancel{mg}} = 2{,}000\ mcg$$

    Step Two: Calculate the (BV)

    $$2{,}000\ mcg \div 250\,mL \div 60\,min = 0.13\,BV$$

    Step Three: Calculate both

    $$\text{Flow Rate (mL/hr)} = \frac{\text{Order}}{\text{BV}} \qquad \frac{2}{0.13} = 15\,mL/hr$$

    $$\text{Dosage Rate} = mL/hr \times BV \qquad 15 \times 0.13 = 2\ mcg$$

Building Confidence: Solutions

11. **BV: 0.53**
     mL/hr: 28
     Titrate 1 mcg/kg/min = 2 mL/hr
     Order: Dopamine 15 mcg/kg/min
     Titrate: Decrease by 1 mcg/kg/min every 30 minutes
     Have: Dopamine 400 mg/250 mL
     Wt: 50 kg

   Step One: Convert mg to mcg
                (1 mg = 1,000 mcg)

$$mcg = \frac{400 \text{ mg}}{1} \times \frac{1,000 \text{ mcg}}{1 \text{ mg}} = 400,000 \text{ mcg}$$

   Step Two: Calculate the (BV)

   $$400,000 \text{ mcg} \div 250 \text{ mL} \div 60 \text{ min} \div 50 \text{ kg} = 0.53 \text{ BV}$$

   Step Three: Calculate both

$$\text{Flow Rate (mL/hr)} = \frac{\text{Order}}{\text{BV}} \quad \frac{15}{0.53} = 28 \text{ mL/hr}$$

$$\text{Dosage Rate} = \text{mL/hr} \times \text{BV} \quad 28 \times 0.53 = 15 \text{ mcg}$$

   Titrate: 1 mcg/kg/min

$$\text{Flow Rate (mL/hr)} = \frac{\text{Order}}{\text{BV}} \quad \frac{1}{0.53} = 2 \text{ mL/hr}$$

$$\text{Dosage Rate} = \text{mL/hr} \times \text{BV} \quad 2 \times 0.53 = 1 \text{ mcg}$$

Building Confidence: Solutions

Practice Solutions

12. **BV: 0.04**
    mL/hr: 13
    Order: Primacor 0.5 mcg/kg/min
    Have: Primacor 40 mg/200 mL
    Wt: 81 kg

    Step One: Convert mg to mcg
    (1 mg =1,000 mcg)

    $$\text{mcg} = \frac{40\,\cancel{\text{mg}}}{1} \times \frac{1{,}000\ \text{mcg}}{1\,\cancel{\text{mg}}} = 40{,}000\ \text{mcg}$$

    Step Two: Calculate the (BV)

    $$40{,}000\ \text{mcg} \div 200\ \text{mL} \div 60\ \text{min} \div 81\ \text{kg} = 0.04\text{BV}$$

    Step Three: Calculate both

    $$\text{Flow Rate (mL/hr)} = \frac{\text{Order}}{\text{BV}}\qquad \frac{0.5}{0.04} = 13\,\text{mL/hr}$$

    $$\text{Dosage Rate} = \text{mL/hr} \times \text{BV}\qquad 13 \times 0.04 = 0.5\ \text{mcg}$$

Building Confidence: Solutions

13. **BV: 2.13**
 mL/hr: 12
 Titrate: 2 mcg/kg/min = 1 mL/hr
 Order: Diprivan 25 mcg/kg/min
 Titrate: Increase by 2 mcg/kg/min every 5 minutes to
 desired sedation.
 Have: Diprivan 1,000 mg/100 mL
 Wt: 78 kg

 Step One: Convert mg to mcg
 (1 mg = 1,000 mcg)

 $$mcg = \frac{1,000 \cancel{mg}}{1} \times \frac{1,000 \text{ mcg}}{1 \cancel{mg}} = 1,000,000 \text{ mcg}$$

 Step Two: Calculate the (BV)

 1,000,000 mcg ÷ 100 mL ÷ 60 min ÷ 78 kg = 2.13 BV

 Step Three: Calculate both

 Flow Rate (mL/hr) = $\dfrac{\text{Order}}{\text{BV}}$ $\dfrac{25}{2.13} = 12 \text{ mL/hr}$

 Dosage Rate = mL/hr × BV   12 × 2.13 = 26 mcg

 Titrate: 2 mcg/kg/min

 Flow Rate (mL/hr) = $\dfrac{\text{Order}}{\text{BV}}$ $\dfrac{2}{2.13} = 1 \text{ mL/hr}$

 Dosage Rate = mL/hr × BV   1 × 2.13 = 2 mcg

Building Confidence: Solutions

Practice Solutions

14. **BV: 1**
    mL/hr: 10
    Order: Insulin 10 units/hr
    Have: Insulin 100 units/100 mL

    Step One: Convert, No conversion required.
    Step Two: Calculate the (BV)
    > This order/formula ends in hr,
    > do not divide by 60 minutes.
    > | 100 units ÷ 100 mL = 1 BV |

    Step Three: Calculate both

    $$\text{Flow Rate (mL/hr)} = \frac{\text{Order}}{\text{BV}} \qquad \boxed{\frac{10}{1} = 10\,\text{mL/hr}}$$

    $$\text{Dosage Rate} = \text{mL/hr} \times \text{BV} \qquad \boxed{10 \times 1 = 10\,\text{units}}$$

15. **BV: 100**
    mL/hr: 8
    Order: Heparin 800 units/hr
    Have: Heparin 25,000 units/250 mL

    Step One: Convert, No conversion required.
    Step Two: Calculate the (BV)
    > This order/formula ends in hr,
    > do not divide by 60 minutes.
    > | 25,000 units ÷ 250 mL = 100 BV |

    Step Three: Calculate both

    $$\text{Flow Rate (mL/hr)} = \frac{\text{Order}}{\text{BV}} \qquad \boxed{\frac{800}{100} = 8\,\text{mL/hr}}$$

    $$\text{Dosage Rate} = \text{mL/hr} \times \text{BV} \qquad \boxed{8 \times 100 = 800\,\text{units}}$$

Building Confidence: Solutions

16. **BV: 1.13**
     mL/hr: 16
     Order: Heparin 18 units/kg/hr
     Have: Heparin 25,000 units/250 mL
     Wt. 88 kg

     Step One: Convert, No conversion required.
     Step Two: Calculate the (BV)
                  This order/formula ends with hr,
                  do not divide by 60 minutes.

     $$25,000 \text{ units} \div 250\,\text{mL} \div 88\,\text{kg} = 1.13\,\text{BV}$$

     Step Three: Calculate both

     $$\text{Flow Rate (mL/hr)} = \frac{\text{Order}}{\text{BV}} \quad \frac{18}{1.13} = 16\,\text{mL/hr}$$

     $$\text{Dosage Rate} = \text{mL/hr} \times \text{BV} \quad 16 \times 1.13 = 18 \text{ units}$$

17. **BV: 3.33**
     mL/hr: 5
     Order: Nitroglycerine 16 mcg/min
     Have: Nitroglycerine 50 mg/250 mL

     Step One: Convert mg to mcg
                  (1 mg = 1,000 mcg)

     $$\text{mcg} = \frac{50\,\cancel{\text{mg}}}{1} \times \frac{1,000 \text{ mcg}}{1\,\cancel{\text{mg}}} = 50,000 \text{ mcg}$$

     Step Two: Calculate the (BV)

     $$50,000 \text{ mcg} \div 250\,\text{mL} \div 60\,\text{min} = 3.33\,\text{BV}$$

     Step Three: Calculate both

     $$\text{Flow Rate (mL/hr)} = \frac{\text{Order}}{\text{BV}} \quad \frac{16}{3.33} = 5\,\text{mL/hr}$$

     $$\text{Dosage Rate} = \text{mL/hr} \times \text{BV} \quad 5 \times 3.33 = 17 \text{ mcg}$$

Building Confidence: Solutions

18. **BV: 0.08**
     mL/hr: 10
     At 15 mL/hr, dosage rate is 1.2 mcg/kg/min
     Order: Vecuronium 0.8 mcg/kg/min
     Have: Vecuronium 100 mg in 250 mL
     Wt: 81 kg
     If the infusion rate is 15 mL/hr, what is the dosage rate?

     Step One: Convert mg to mcg
     (1 mg = 1,000 mcg)

     $$mcg = \frac{100 \text{ mg}}{1} \times \frac{1,000 \text{ mcg}}{1 \text{ mg}} = 100,000 \text{ mcg}$$

     Step Two: Calculate the (BV)

     100,000 mcg ÷ 250 mL ÷ 60 min ÷ 81 kg = 0.08 BV

     Step Three: Calculate both

     Flow Rate (mL/hr) = $\dfrac{\text{Order}}{\text{BV}}$ $\dfrac{0.8}{0.08}$ = 10 mL/hr

     Dosage Rate = mL/hr × BV   10 × 0.08 = 0.8 mcg

     Dosage rate at 15 mL/hr $15 \times 0.08 = 1.2$ mcg

Building Confidence: Solutions

19. **BV: 0.01**
    mL/hr: 30
    At 19 mL/hr, dosage rate is 0.19 units/min
    Order: Vasopressin 0.3 units/min
    Have: Vasopressin 200 units in 250 mL
    If the infusion rate is 19 mL/hr, what is the dosage rate?

    Step One: Convert, No conversion required.
    Step Two: Calculate the (BV)

    $$\boxed{200 \text{ units} \div 250 \text{ mL} \div 60 \text{ min} = 0.01 \text{ BV}}$$

    Step Three: Calculate both

    $$\text{Flow Rate (mL/hr)} = \frac{\text{Order}}{\text{BV}} \quad \boxed{\frac{0.3}{0.01} = 30 \text{ mL/hr}}$$

    $$\text{Dosage Rate} = \text{mL/hr} \times \text{BV} \quad \boxed{30 \times 0.01 = 0.3 \text{ units}}$$

    Dosage rate at 19 mL/hr $\quad \boxed{19 \times 0.01 = 0.19 \text{ units}}$

Building Confidence: Solutions

20. **BV: 0.26**
    mL/hr: 19
    At 50 mL/hr, dosage rate is 13 mcg/min
    Order: Norepinephrine 5 mcg/min
    Have: Norepinephrine 4 mg/250 mL
    BV: _____
    mL/hr: _____
    If the infusion rate is 50 mL/hr, what is the dosage rate?

    Step One: Convert mg to mcg
    $$(1 \text{ mg} = 1,000 \text{ mcg})$$

    $$\text{mcg} = \frac{4 \text{ mg}}{1} \times \frac{1,000 \text{ mcg}}{1 \text{ mg}} = 4,000 \text{ mcg}$$

    Step Two: Calculate the (BV)

    $$4,000 \text{ mcg} \div 250 \text{ mL} \div 60 \text{ min} = 0.26 \text{ BV}$$

    Step Three: Calculate both

    $$\text{Flow Rate (mL/hr)} = \frac{\text{Order}}{\text{BV}} \quad \frac{5}{0.26} = 19 \text{ mL/hr}$$

    $$\text{Dosage Rate} = \text{mL/hr} \times \text{BV} \quad 19 \times 0.26 = 5 \text{ mcg}$$

    Dosage rate at 50 mL/hr $\quad 50 \times 0.26 = 13 \text{ mcg}$

Building Confidence: Solutions

21. **BV: 2**
    mL/hr: 50
    At 75 mL/hr, dosage rate is 150 mcg/min
    Order: Neosynephrine 100 mcg/min
    Have: Neosynephrine 50 mg/250 mL
    If infusion rate is 75 mL/hr, what is the dosage rate?

    Step One: Convert mg to mcg
    (1 mg = 1,000 mcg)

    $$mcg = \frac{30\ \cancel{mg}}{1} \times \frac{1,000\ mcg}{1\ \cancel{mg}} = 30,000\ mcg$$

    Step Two: Calculate the (BV)

    $$30,00\ mcg \div 250\ mL \div 60\ min = 2\ BV$$

    Step Three: Calculate both

    $$\text{Flow Rate (mL/hr)} = \frac{\text{Order}}{\text{BV}} \qquad \frac{100}{2} = 50\ mL/hr$$

    $$\text{Dosage Rate} = \text{mL/hr} \times \text{BV} \qquad 50 \times 2 = 100\ mcg$$

    Dosage rate at 75 mL/hr $\qquad 75 \times 2 = 150\ mcg$

Building Confidence: Solutions

22. **BV: 1**
    mL/hr: 1
    Order: Midazolam 1 mg/hr
    Have: Midazolam 100 mg/100 mL
    BV: _____
    mL/hr: _____

    Step One: Convert, No conversion required.
    Step Two: Calculate the (BV)
    This order/formula ends in hr,
    do not divide by 60 minutes.
    $$100 \text{ mg} \div 100 \text{ mL} = 1 \text{ BV}$$

    Step Three: Calculate both

    $$\text{Flow Rate (mL/hr)} = \frac{\text{Order}}{\text{BV}} \quad \boxed{\frac{1}{1} = 1 \text{ mL/hr}}$$

    $$\text{Dosage Rate} = \text{mL/hr} \times \text{BV} \quad \boxed{1 \times 1 = 1 \text{ mg}}$$

23.   BV: 0.003
   mL/hr: 13
   Order: Vasopressin 0.04 units/min
   Have: Vasopressin 20 units/100 mL
   BV: _____
   mL/hr: _____

   Step One: Convert, No conversion required.
   Step Two: Calculate the (BV)

   $$20 \text{ units} \div 100 \text{ mL} \div 60 \text{ min} = 0.003 \text{ BV}$$

   Step Three: Calculate both

   $$\text{Flow Rate (mL/hr)} = \frac{\text{Order}}{\text{BV}} \quad \boxed{\frac{0.04}{0.003} = 13 \text{ mL/hr}}$$

   $$\text{Dosage Rate} = \text{mL/hr} \times \text{BV} \quad \boxed{13 \times 0.003 = 0.04 \text{ units}}$$

Building Confidence: Solutions

24. **BV: 0.43**
    mL/hr: 23
    Order: Dobutamine 10 mcg/kg/min
    Have: Dobutamine 500 mg/250 mL
    Wt: 77 kg
    BV: _____
    mL/hr: _____

    Step One: Convert mg to mcg
    (1 mg = 1,000 mcg)

    $$mcg = \frac{500 \cancel{mg}}{1} \times \frac{1,000 \text{ mcg}}{1 \cancel{mg}} = 500,000 \text{ mcg}$$

    Step Two: Calculate the (BV)

    $$500,000 \text{ mcg} \div 250 \text{ mL} \div 60 \text{ min} \div 77 \text{ kg} = 0.43 \text{ BV}$$

    Step Three: Calculate both

    $$\text{Flow Rate (mL/hr)} = \frac{\text{Order}}{\text{BV}} \qquad \boxed{\frac{10}{0.43} = 23 \text{ mL/hr}}$$

    $$\text{Dosage Rate} = \text{mL/hr} \times \text{BV} \qquad \boxed{23 \times 0.43 = 10 \text{ mcg}}$$

Chapter 7

Unit Conversion
Changing Units of Measurement

Unit conversion is often the first step when solving an IV dosage calculation problem.

Example:

      Order: Give 0.05 mcg/kg

      Patient's weight: 185 lbs

The patients weight must first be changed from lbs to kg—unit conversion—before any dosage calculations are performed.

Unit Conversion

Terms

Unit Conversion is changing from one unit of measurement to another unit of measurement with the same value.

Units of Measurement common in the medical field:

Units of Measurement	Value
• Fahrenheit to Celsius	Temperature
• Pounds to Kilograms	Weight
• Inches to Centimeters	Length
• Hours to Minutes	Time
• Gallons to Liters	Volume
• Quarts to Milliliters	Volume

Conversion Factors are mathematical tools used to change the units of measurement without changing its value.

Equivalent means equal in value.
Example:
The equivalent of 2.2 lbs (pounds) is 1 kg (kilogram); its used to build a conversion factor.

The **conversion factor is written**: $\dfrac{2.2 \text{ lbs}}{1 \text{ kg}}$ or $\dfrac{1 \text{ kg}}{2.2 \text{ lbs}}$

Unit Conversion

Formula/Example

Conversion Formula:

$$\text{Desired Unit} = \frac{\text{given unit}}{1} \times \frac{\text{Desired Unit}}{\text{given unit}}$$

The **desired unit** (the unit of measure to which you want to convert) will always be placed **on top** of the conversion factor.

Example:

Convert 175 lbs to kg

175 lbs = _____ kg

Conversion factor: 1 kg = 2.2 lbs

Since the **desired unit** is kg, kg is **placed on top** of the conversion factor.

$$kg = \frac{175 \, \cancel{lbs}}{1} \times \frac{1 \, kg}{2.2 \, \cancel{lbs}}$$

$$kg = (175 \times 1 \, kg) \div 2.2$$

$$kg = 79.5 \, kg$$

To check the answer for accuracy, reverse the conversion process. The **desired unit** is placed **on top** of the conversion factor.

$$lbs = \frac{79.5 \, \cancel{kg}}{1} \times \frac{2.2 \, lbs}{1 \, \cancel{kg}}$$

$$lbs = 79.5 \times 2.2 \, lbs$$

$$lbs = 174.9 \, lbs$$

Chapter 7

Unit Conversion
Common Conversion Factors

Weight

1 milligram (mg) = 1,000 micrograms (mcg)
1 kilogram (kg) = 2.2 pounds (lbs)
1 kilogram (kg) = 1,000 grams (g)
1 gram (g) = 1,000 milligrams (mg)
1 gram (g) = 1,000,000 micrograms (mcg)
750 milligrams (mg) = 10 milliequivalent (mEq)
1 grains (gr) = 60 - 65 milligrams (mg)

Volume

1 (mL) = 15 – 16 (gtt) drops
1 (L) liter = 1,000 (mL) milliliters
1 (tsp) teaspoon = 5 (mL) milliliters
1 (tbsp.) tablespoon = 15 (mL) milliliters
1 (oz) ounce = 30 (mL) milliliters
fluid dram (fl dr) = 1/8 fluid ounce
(fl dr is not commonly used today)

Length

1 inch = 2.54 centimeters (cm)
39.4 inches = 1 meter (m)
1 meter (m) = 1,000 centimeters (cm)

Temperature

Fahrenheit to Celsius $\boxed{(^\circ F - 32) \div 1.8 = {}^\circ C}$

Celsius to Fahrenheit $\boxed{(^\circ C \times 1.8) + 32 = {}^\circ F}$

* There are different methods used to convert temperatures.
The formulas above use 1.8 instead of 9/5 or 5/9.

Unit Conversion

Practice Problems

Conversion Formula: $\text{Desired Unit} = \frac{\text{given unit}}{1} \times \frac{\text{Desired Unit}}{\text{given unit}}$

Remember, the **desired unit** (the unit of measurement to which you want to convert) is placed **on top** of the conversion factor.

1. Convert 250 mg to mcg
2. Convert 400,000 mcg to mg
3. Convert 1,500 mL to L
4. Convert 2 g to mg
5. Convert 60 in to cm
6. Convert 210 lbs to kg
7. Convert 49 kg to lbs
8. Convert 5' 7" to in
9. Convert 500 mg to mEq
10. Convert 98.6 Fahrenheit to Celsius, (Use the formula below)

    $(°F - 32) \div 1.8 = °C$

Solutions on pages 80-83

Chapter 7

Unit Conversions

Solutions

1. **250,000 mcg**

   250 mg = _____ mcg

   Conversion factor: 1 mg = 1,000 mcg

   $$mcg = \frac{250\ mg}{1} \times \frac{1,000\ mcg}{1\ mg}$$

   $$mcg = 250 \times 1,000\ mcg$$

   $$mcg = 250,000\ mcg$$

2. **400 mg**

   400,000 mcg = _____ mg

   Conversion factor: 1 mg = 1,000 mcg

   $$mg = \frac{400,000\ mcg}{1} \times \frac{1\ mg}{1,000\ mcg}$$

   $$mg = 400,000\ mg \div 1,000$$

   $$mg = 400\ mg$$

3. **1.5 L**

   1,500 mL = _____ L

   Conversion factor: 1 L = 1,000 mL

   $$L = \frac{1,500\ mL}{1} \times \frac{1\ L}{1,000\ mL}$$

   $$L = 1,500\ L \div 1,000$$

   $$L = 1.5\ L$$

Unit Conversions

Solutions

4. **2,000 mg**

    2 g = _____ mg

    Conversion factor: 1 g = 1,000 mg

    $$mg = \frac{2\,\cancel{g}}{1} \times \frac{1{,}000\ mg}{1\,\cancel{g}}$$

    $$mg = 2 \times 1{,}000\ mg$$

    $$mg = 2{,}000\ mg$$

5. **152.4 cm**

    60 in = _____ cm

    Conversion factor: 1 in = 2.54 cm

    $$cm = \frac{60\,\cancel{in}}{1} \times \frac{2.54\ cm}{1\,\cancel{in}}$$

    $$cm = 60 \times 2.54\ cm$$

    $$cm = 152.4\ cm$$

6. **113.6 kg**

    210 lbs = _____ kg

    Conversion factor: 1 kg = 2.2 lbs

    $$kg = \frac{250\,\cancel{lbs}}{1} \times \frac{1\ kg}{2.2\,\cancel{lbs}}$$

    $$kg = 250\ kg \div 2.2$$

    $$kg = 113.6\ kg$$

Unit Conversions

Solutions

7. **107.8 lbs**

49 kg = _____ lbs

Conversion factor: 1 kg = 2.2 lbs

$$lbs = \frac{49\ \cancel{kg}}{1} \times \frac{2.2\ lbs}{1\ \cancel{kg}}$$

$$lbs = 49 \times 2.2\ lbs$$

$$lbs = 107.8\ lbs$$

8. **67 in**

5'7" = _____ in

Conversion factor: 1 ft = 12 in

$$in = \frac{5\ \cancel{ft}}{1} \times \frac{12\ in}{1\ \cancel{ft}} + 7\ in$$

$$in = (5 \times 12\ in) + 7\ in$$

$$in = 60 + 7\ in$$

$$in = 67\ in$$

9. **6.66 mEq**

500 mg = _____ mEq

Conversion factor: 750 mg = 10 mEq

$$mEq = \frac{500\ \cancel{mg}}{1} \times \frac{10\ mEq}{750\ \cancel{mg}}$$

$$mEq = (500 \times 10\ mEq) \div 750$$

$$mEq = 5{,}000\ mEq \div 750$$

$$meq = 6.66\ meq$$

Unit Conversions

Solutions

10. **37 degrees Celsius**

98.6 ° Fahrenheit = _____ ° Celsius

This conversion uses a formula instead of a conversion factor.

$$(°F - 32) \div 1.8 = °C$$
$$(°98.6 - 32) \div 1.8 = 37°C$$

37 ° Celsius

Reconstitution, Dilution
Powder and Liquid Medications

To put your mind at ease, when working with medications that require reconstitution or dilution, there are two basic steps to follow.

Step One: **Add a liquid** to the medication.

Step Two: Solve the **Dosage Calculation.**

$$\frac{\text{(O) Order}}{\text{(H) Have}} \times \text{(V) Volume} = \text{mL to be administered}$$

* Dosage calculations are done *after* reconstituting or diluting.

Reconstitution, Dilution

Terms

Reconstitution is adding a liquid to a powder medication prior to administering.

Dilution is adding a liquid to a liquid medication prior to administering.

Solute: (Drug)
A powder or liquid medication that is dissolved or diluted in a liquid.

Solute is measured in:
- mcg (micrograms)
- mg (milligrams)
- g (grams)
- units (units)

Diluent: (liquid)
When diluting medications, the liquid used is called the diluent. When reconstituting medications, the liquid used may be referred to as either the diluent or solvent.

Common Diluents:
- Sterile Water with or without preservative
- Normal Saline (NS), also called 0.9% Sodium Chloride
- Bacteriostatic Sterile Water

Diluents are measured in mL (milliliters).

Solution:
The result of mixing a solute and a diluent (solvent).

Reconstitution, Dilution
Terms

Drug concentration: (Strength)
Drug concentration describes how weak or strong a medication mixture is. It identifies how much drug and how much liquid are in the mixture and is expressed as a ratio.

Example: 10 mg of a drug mixed with 10 mL of a liquid.
Written: 10 mg/10 mL

A final concentration describes the drug concentration with a simplified ratio.

Example:
Drug concentration: The ratio of 10 mg/10 mL is simplified
to a final concentration of 1 mg/1 mL.
(Written as 1 mg/mL)

When there is just one mL (1 mL) of liquid it is written as (mL). The one (1) is understood.

* Drug concentration is defined *after* you have added the liquid to the medication.

87

Reconstitution, Dilution
Guidelines

To reduce the risk of medication errors or other adverse patient outcomes associated with reconstitution or dilution of medications, always follow the current guidelines:
- Drug manufacturer's recommendation (medication label or insert)
- Hospital's guidelines
- Pharmacist's instructions

Medication labels will tell you:
- If reconstitution or dilution is required prior to administration.
- What kind of liquid (diluent) to add
- How many (mL) to add
- The resulting concentration after reconstitution or diluting
  Example: 2 mg/mL

Properly label the syringe with:
- Patient name:
- Drug name:
- Drug concentration: *after* reconstitution or dilution
- Dose ordered:
- Directions for administration:
- Expiration date & time:
- Preparer's Initials:

Reconstitution, Dilution
When to Dilute

Dilution is adding a liquid to a liquid medication prior to administration.

Not all IV Push (IVP) medications require dilution prior to administration.
[1] **Unnecessary diluting practices** can lead to:
- Unlabeled syringes
- Mislabeled syringes
- Potential contamination
- Dosage errors
- Other drug administration errors

Dilute if:
- Drug manufacturer or hospital guidelines recommend.
- Dilution will increase accurate dosage control during administration.
- Dilution will improve patient comfort or reduce risk of injury at injection site.

[1] Dilution guidelines:
- Follow drug manufacture and/or hospital guidelines for *Standard Volume Diluent* with resulting concentrations.
- Properly label the drug concentration *after* diluting.
- Always conduct a double check of drug dose before administering.

1. ISMP, Institute for Safe Medication Practices. Acute Care, ISMP Medication Safety Alert. Some IV Medications Are Diluted Unnecessarily In Patient Care Areas, Creating Undue Risk. 2014, June 19.

Reconstitution, Dilution

Dilution Example

Order: Morphine 2 mg IV push
Have: Morphine 10 mg/1 mL (written 10 mg/mL)

Dilution is recommended because:
- Diluting will increase accurate *right dose* delivery.
  A drug concentration of 10 mg/mL is too
  concentrated for an accurate dose to be administered.
- Diluting will improve patient comfort.
  Morphine may burn during administration.

Goal: Drug concentration 10 mg/10 mL
Final concentration 1 mg/mL

You will need to know:
A. What is the diluent?
B. How many mL of diluent must be added to the medication?
C. What is the final concentration (mg/mL)?
D. How many mL must be administered for a 2 mg dose?

Step One: **Add the liquid** (diluent) to the medication.
Per medication guidelines, use sterile water or normal saline.
Have: 10 mg of medication in **1 mL** of liquid
Goal: 10 mg/10 mL
Add: 9 mL plus 1 mL = 10 mL
Now Have: 10 mg/10 mL or 1 mg/mL

Step Two: **Dosage Calculation** (may use either concentration)

$$\frac{\text{(O) Order}}{\text{(H) Have}} \times \text{(V) Volume} = \text{mL to be administered}$$

$$\frac{\text{(O) 2 mg}}{\text{(H) 10 mg}} \times 10\,\text{mL (V)} = 2\,\text{mL} \quad \text{or} \quad \frac{\text{(O) 2 mg}}{\text{(H) 1 mg}} \times 1\,\text{mL (V)} = 2\,\text{mL}$$

Answers:
A. Diluent is sterile water or normal saline.
B. Add 9 mL
C. Final concentration is 1 mg/mL
D. Administer 2 mL for a 2 mg dose

Reconstitution, Dilution

Order: Ampicillin 500 mg IV
Have: Ampicillin 500 mg sterile powder
Per the medication label, reconstitution is required prior to administration.

You will need to know:
A. What is the diluent?
B. How many mL of diluent must be added to the medication?
C. What is the final concentration (mg/mL)?
D. How many mL must be administered for a 500 mg dose?

Medication label reads:
Add 1.7 mL sterile water
Final concentration: 250 mg/mL

Step One: **Add the liquid** (diluent) to the medication.
Per the medication label add 1.7 mL of sterile water to the medication bottle.

Step Two: **Dosage Calculation**

$$\frac{\text{(O) Order}}{\text{(H) Have}} \times \text{(V) Volume} = \text{mL to be administered}$$

$$\frac{\text{(O) 500 mg}}{\text{(H) 250 mg}} \times 1\,\text{mL} = 2\,\text{mL to be administered}$$

Answers:
A. Diluent is sterile water
B. Add 1.7 mL
C. Final concentration is 250 mg/mL
D. Administer 2 mL for a 500 mg dose

Reconstitution, Dilution

Advanced Reconstitution Example

Order: Penicillin G 1,000,000 units IV
Have: Penicillin G 5,000,000 units sterile powder
Per the medication label, reconstitution is required prior to administration.

You will need to know:
A. What is the diluent?
B. How many mL of diluent must be added to the medication?
C. What is the final concentration (units/mL)?
D. How many mL must be administered for a 1,000,000 units dose?

Step One: **Add the liquid** (diluent) to the medication.
Per the medication label the diluent is normal saline.
Instructions read:

For a **Final Concentration**	**Add** normal saline
250,000 units/mL	20 mL
500,000 units/mL	10 mL
1,000,000 units/mL	5 mL

GoaL: Select the final concentration that best matches the order of 1,000,000 units.
For a final concentration of 1,000,000 units/mL, add 5 mL of normal saline.

Step Two: **Dosage Calculation**
Order: 1,000,000 units
Now Have: 1,000,000 units/mL

$$\frac{(O)\ Order}{(H)\ Have} \times (V)\ Volume = mL\ to\ be\ administered$$

$$\frac{1,000,000\ units}{1,000,000\ units} \times 1\ mL = 1\ mL$$

Answers:
A. Diluent is normal saline
B. Add 5 mL
C. Final concentration is 1,000,000 units/mL.
D. Administer 1 mL for a 1,000,000 units dose.

Reconstitution, Dilution

Practice Problems

1. Order: Cefazolin 500 mg IV
   Have: Cefazolin 1 g powder
   Per medication label: Add 2 mL sterile water or normal saline.
   Final Concentration: 250 mg/mL
   How many mL will you administer for a 500 mg dose? _____

2. Order: Zithromax 400 mg IV
   Have: Zithromax 500 mg powder
   Per medication label: Add 4.8 mL sterile water.
   Final Concentration: 100 mg/mL
   How many mL will you administer for a 400 mg dose? _____

3. Order: Versed 1 mg IV
   Have: Versed 5 mg/mL
   Dilute for accurate dosage administration.
   Per medication guidelines, use normal saline for a diluent.
   A. How many mL will you need to add for a drug concentration of 5 mg/5 mL? _____
   B. How many mL will you administer for a 1 mg dose? _____

4. Order: Morphine 2 mg IV
   Have: Morphine 10 mg/mL
   Dilute for accurate dosage control and increased patient comfort.
   Per medication guidelines, use normal saline for a diluent.
   A. How many mL will you need to add for a final concentration of 1 mg/mL? _____
   B. How many mL will you administer for a 2 mg dose? _____

Solutions to questions 1-4 found on pages 96-98

Reconstitution, Dilution

Practice Problems

5. Order: Ampicillin 750 mg IV
   Have: Ampicillin 1 g powder
   Per medication label: Add 2 mL sterile water.
   Final Concentration: 500 mg/mL
   How many mL will you administer for a 750 mg
   dose? _____

6. Order: Methylprednisolone 75 mg IV
   Have: Methylprednisolone 125 mg vial
   Per medication label: Add 2 mL of bacteriostatic water.
   Final Concentration: 125 mg/2 mL
   How many mL will you administer for a 75 mg
   dose? _____

7. Order: Solu-Medrol 100 mg IV
   Have: Solu-Medrol 500 mg powder
   Per medication label: Add 8 mL bacteriostatic water.
   Final Concentration: 62.5 mg/mL
   How many mL will you administer for a 100 mg
   dose? _____

8. Order: Methicillin 1 g IV
   Have: Methicillin 1,000 mg powder
   Per medication label: Add 5 mL of sterile water.
   Final Concentration: 1,000 mg/5 mL
   How many mL will you administer for a 1 g
   dose? _____

Solutions to questions 5-8 found on pages 99-100

Reconstitution, Dilution
Practice Problems

9. Order: Zithromax 250 mg IV
   Have: Zithromax 1 g powder
   Per medication label: Add 9.8 mL sterile water.
   Final Concentration: 100 mg/mL
   How many mL will you administer for a 250 mg
   dose? _____

10. Order: Penicillin G Sodium 1,000,000 units IV
    Have: Penicillin G Sodium 5,000,000 units sterile powder
    Per the medication label, reconstitution is required prior
    to administration.

    You will need to know:
    A. What is the diluent?
    B. How many mL of diluent will you need to add to the
       medication for a final concentration of 500,000
       units/mL? _____
    C. How many mL will you administer for a 1,000,000
       unit dose?_____

    Instructions read:

For a **Final Concentration**	**Add** normal saline
250,000 units/mL	20 mL
500,000 units/mL	10 mL

Solutions to questions 9-10 found on page 101

Reconstitution, Dilution

Practice Solutions

1. **Administer 2 mL**
   Order: Cefazolin 500 mg IV
   Have: Cefazolin 1 g powder
   Add: 2 mL of diluent
   Final Concentration: 250 mg/mL

   Step One: **Add** 2 mL of sterile water or normal
   saline
   Step Two: **Dosage Calculation**

   $$\frac{O}{H} \times V = \text{mL to administer}$$

   $$\frac{500 \text{ mg}}{250 \text{ mg}} \times 1 \text{ mL} = 2 \text{ mL}$$

2. **Administer 4 mL**
   Order: Zithromax 400 mg IV
   Have: Zithromax 500 mg powder
   Add: 4.8 mL of diluent
   Final Concentration: 100 mg/mL

   Step One: **Add** 4.8 mL of sterile water
   Step Two: **Dosage Calculation**

   $$\frac{O}{H} \times V = \text{mL to administer}$$

   $$\frac{400 \text{ mg}}{100 \text{ mg}} \times 1 \text{ mL} = 4 \text{ mL}$$

Reconstitution, Dilution

3.   A. **Add 4 mL**
     B. **Administer 1 mL**
     Order: Versed 1 mg IV
     Have: Versed 5 mg/mL

Step One: **Add** 4 mL of normal saline
          Goal: 1 mg of Versed for each mL of liquid.
            (5 mg/5 mL)
          Have: 1 mL of liquid in medication bottle
            (5 mg/mL)
          Add: ____**mL** + 1 mL = 5 mL
          Drug Concentration: 5 mg/5 mL
          Final Concentration: 1 mg/mL

Step Two: **Dosage Calculation**

$$\frac{O}{H} \times V = mL \text{ to administer}$$

$$\frac{1 \text{ mg}}{5 \text{ mg}} \times 5 \text{ mL} = 1 \text{ mL} \quad \text{or} \quad \frac{1 \text{ mg}}{1 \text{ mg}} \times 1 \text{ mL} = 1 \text{ mL}$$

Reconstitution, Dilution
Practice Solutions

4. **Add 9 mL**
    Administer 2 mL
    Order: Morphine 2 mg IV
    Have: Morphine 10 mg/mL

    Step One: **Add** 9 mL of normal saline

    GOAL: 1 mg of Morphine for each mL of liquid.
    (10 mg/10 mL)
    Have: 1 mL of liquid in the medication bottle
    (10 mg/mL)
    Add: _____**mL** plus 1 mL = 10 mL
    Drug Concentration: 10 mg/10 mL
    Final Concentration: 1 mg/mL

    Step Two: **Dosage Calculation**

    $$\frac{O}{H} \times V = mL \text{ to administer}$$

    $$\frac{2 \text{ mg}}{10 \text{ mg}} \times 10 \text{ mL} = 2 \text{ mL} \quad \text{or} \quad \frac{2 \text{ mg}}{1 \text{ mg}} \times 1 \text{ mL} = 2 \text{ mL}$$

Reconstitution, Dilution

Practice Solutions

5. **Administer 1.5 mL**
    Order: Ampicillin 750 mg IV
    Have: Ampicillin 1 g powder
    Add: 2 mL sterile water
    Final concentration: 500 mg/mL

    Step One: **Add** 2 mL of sterile water
    Step Two: **Dosage Calculation**

    $$\frac{O}{H} \times V = \text{mL to administer}$$

    $$\frac{750 \text{ mg}}{500 \text{ mg}} \times 1 \text{ mL} = 1.5 \text{ mL}$$

6. **Administer 1.2 mL**
    Order: Methylprednisolone 75 mg IV
    Have: Methylprednisolone 125 mg vial
    Add: 2 mL of bacteriostatic water
    Final Concentration: 125 mg/2 mL

    Step One: **Add** 2 mL of bacteriostatic water
    Step Two: **Dosage Calculation**

    $$\frac{O}{H} \times V = \text{mL to administer}$$

    $$\frac{75 \text{ mg}}{125 \text{ mg}} \times 2 \text{ mL} = 1.2 \text{ mL}$$

Chapter 8

Reconstitution, Dilution

Practice Solutions

7. **Administer 1.6 mL**
   Order: Solu-Medrol 100 mg IV
   Have: Solu-Medrol 500 mg powder
   Add: 8 mL bacteriostatic water
   Final Concentration: 62.5 mg/mL

   Step One: **Add** 8 mL of bacteriostatic water
   Step Two: **Dosage Calculation**

   $$\frac{O}{H} \times V = \text{mL to administer}$$

   $$\frac{100 \text{ mg}}{62.5 \text{ mg}} \times 1 \text{ mL} = 1.6 \text{ mL}$$

8. **Administer 5 mL**
   Order: Methicillin 1 g IV
   Have: Methicillin 1,000 mg powder
   Add: 5 mL of sterile water
   Final Concentration: 1,000 mg/5 mL

   Step One: **Add** 5 mL of sterile water
   Step Two: **Dosage Calculation**

   $$\frac{O}{H} \times V = \text{mL to administer}$$

   $$\frac{1,000 \text{ mg}}{1,000 \text{ mg}} \times 5 \text{ mL} = 5 \text{ mL}$$

Reconstitution, Dilution

Practice Solution

9. **Administer 2.5 mL**
Order: Zithromax 250 mg IV
Have: Zithromax 1 g powder
Add: 9.8 mL sterile water
Final Concentration: 100 mg/mL

Step One: **Add** 9.8 mL of sterile water
Step Two: **Dosage Calculation**

$$\frac{O}{H} \times V = mL \text{ to administer}$$

$$\frac{250 \text{ mg}}{100 \text{ mg}} \times 1 \text{ mL} = 2.5 \text{ mL}$$

10. **A. Diluent is normal saline**
B. Add 10 mL
C. Administer 2 mL
Order: Penicillin G Sodium 1,000,000 units IV
Have: Penicillin G Sodium 5,000,000 units sterile powder

Instructions read:

For a **Final Concentration:**	**Add** normal saline
250,000 units/mL	20 mL
500,000 units/mL	10 mL

Step One: **Add** 10 mL of sterile water
Final Concentration: 500,000 units/mL

Step Two: **Dosage calculation**

$$\frac{O}{H} \times V = mL \text{ to administer}$$

$$\frac{1,000,000 \text{ units}}{500,000 \text{ units}} \times 1 \text{ mL} = 2 \text{ mL}$$

Notes

72014028R00064

Made in the USA
Columbia, SC
10 June 2017

Only in Heaven

william Hazlerigg

Only in Heaven

The Life and Campaigns
of Sir Arthur Hesilrige, 1601-1661

Barry Denton

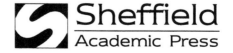

Copyright © 1997 Sheffield Academic Press

Published by Sheffield Academic Press Ltd
Mansion House
19 Kingfield Road
Sheffield S11 9AS
England

Printed on acid-free paper in Great Britain
by Bookcraft Ltd
Midsomer Norton, Bath

British Library Cataloguing in Publication Data

A catalogue record for this book is available
from the British Library

ISBN 1-85075-645-7

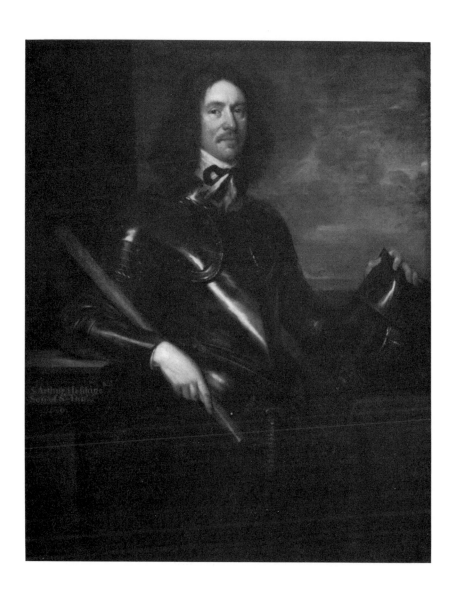

Sir Arthur Hesilrige, the Hazlerigg Collection.

∽ **Contents** ∾

∽ **Prologue** ∾

I had spent many years in researching my friend Sir Arthur's life. With the last words typed, could I leave him without one final goodbye? Of course not. My search for Sir Arthur's story began in the Chapel of St Mary at Noseley, and it is fitting perhaps that it should end there. Entering once more this small family chapel, I remembered the words of that other historian, John Nichols, who like myself lived in a time removed from that of Sir Arthur, yet possibly knew him better than most. From his eighteenth-century study, the pen of John Nichols rested with the words:

> Such are the memorials we have from an immense mass of history been able to collect of our illustrious Republican whose name must defend to posterity as one of the heroes of the age in which he lived, the whole offences to the state were amply expiated by his death; for his remains were permitted to be honourably conveyed to Noseley with great funeral pomp, and interred among his ancestors in the collegiate church belonging to his family.

John Nichols understood the importance of Sir Arthur Hesilrige's stand upon liberty and the people's right to live without fear of oppression. It can only be to the eternal shame of the Restoration that, following Sir Arthur's death, his enemies thought it honest to find him guilty of high treason. If treason can be found in Hesilrige's words to Richard Cromwell's Protectorate, then such treason is a glorious thing. Men who dared not accuse him in life, attacked him in death. Exaggerated stories were circulated of Hesilrige's treatment of Scottish prisoners after Dunbar, and pure fabrications were invented of crimes against the state which history cannot support. Only by the help of George Monck did Sir Arthur's children receive their inheritance.

Moving towards Sir Arthur's resting place, I looked at the figure on the tomb. We had travelled many miles together, and I wondered if my story of liberty would meet with his approval. Unlike Sir Arthur, I live in an age where the 'third estate' of Parliament—the Commons—is free to be elected and sit. It was what Sir Arthur desired, what he had opposed first a King and then a Protector for. The sword had opened the gates of a free Parliament, yet as ever had been the undoing of liberty. Sir Arthur Hesilrige had maintained that no assembly could sit and no nation could flourish without the people; he paid for that belief with a lifetime of work.

The Restoration saw a great boom in trade and adventure into the New World, and was an age of the theatre and art. But within 30 years the Stuarts were Kings of England no more. King Charles II was restored by a popular wave of support, yet had learned little from the fate of his father. Likewise, the last of the Stuart Kings, James II, cared nothing for Parliament. During the last 10 years' reign of these monarchs, Parliament sat for only 20 weeks. It is no surprise therefore that Parliament once more rebelled and ended the Stuart monarchy forever. This was the end Sir Arthur had foretold for all who denied the people's liberty and took the power unto themselves.

I looked up at the inscription above Sir Arthur's tomb. What better way is there to leave him than with these final words. They said:

Here lyes Sir Arthur Haslerig Baronet
Who injoyed his portion of this life
In ye times of greatest civil troubles
Yt ever this nation had
He was a lover of liberty
And faithfull to his country
He delighted in sober company
And departed this life 7th JANUARY
In Englands peaceable Year
Anno Dom 1661

∽ Acknowledgments ∽

In the writing of history, one meets and corresponds with a very large number of people. They are the keys to one's subject, and unlock the doors of research. Often people introduced in study become good friends, and what greater pleasure is there than to thank one's friends:

To the present Lord Hazlerigg and his family for their hospitality during my visits to Noseley. I am extremely grateful to Lord Hazlerigg for his interest in my work on his ancestor, and for his kind permission to quote from his family papers and reproduce letters from the Hazlerigg Collection (Cromwell Letters) at Leicestershire Record Office. Also for the loan of various tracts and reproduction of portraits.

To the late Brigadier Peter Young, for the initial suggestion to write this volume, and his encouragement in its research with open access to his library.

To Dr John Adair—the biographer of Sir William Waller—for advice and encouragement. Also the loan of various notes from Public Record Office SP 28.

To the late Sir Gyles Isham bart, of Lamport Hall, Northamptonshire.

To the staff of Northamptonshire Record Office.

To the staff of Leicestershire Record Office for extensive assistance during the research involving the Hazlerigg Collection.

To the staff of Tyne and Wear Record Office.

To the staff of Durham, West Sussex, Worcester and Herefordshire Record Offices.

To the library staff of York Minster.

To the Department of Palaeography and Diplomatic, University of Durham, for information from the Weardale Chests.

To the staff of Newcastle City Library for help with tracts in their own and the Richardson Collection.

To the late Revd Lawrence Wood (Alderton) for his assistance with the Church Registers.

To Peter B. Boyden and the National Army Museum.

To Dr Williams's Library.

To the Bodleian Library for permission to quote from the Tanner and Clarendon MSS.

To Northampton Central Library.

To Miss Anne West for her kindness in referencing of the Calendar of State Papers, Lords and Commons Journals, in the early stages of research, for smoothing the path through countless bibliographic problems, and in general for being Anne.

To all ranks and fellow members of the Sealed Knot Society, for supplying the taste of black powder, the smell of sweating horseflesh, and for a little light relief from research and writing. And to my North Americans (Col. Walter Lloyd's) for recreating what Sir Arthur and George Fenwick began 350 years ago.

To the Cromwell Association.

To the British Library.

To the Ven. Bazil Marsh, Professor G.E. Aylmer, Lady Antonia Fraser, the Pepysian Library, Cambridge, the Department of the Environment (Hannibal House), Magdalene College, Cambridge.

To the late Tony Partridge for driving me around numerous battle-fields, and Bob Partridge for making photographic records of these days.

And lastly, but certainly not least, to my parents Irene and Raymond Denton, who have had Sir Arthur living with us for many years, in spirit at least. For acting as unpaid secretaries, making notes and generally finding more hours in a day than is usual. Without their help the writing of *Only in Heaven* would have been impossible.

❧ Abbreviations ❧

Cal. Clar. SP	Clarendon State Papers, Bodleian Library, Oxford
CJ	Journals of the House of Commons
CSP Dom	Calendar of State Papers Domestic
CSP Ven	Calendar of State Papers Venetian
DNB	Dictionary of National Biography
E	Thomason Tracts, British Library, London
LJ	Journals of the House of Lords
LRO	Leicestershire Record Office
SP	State Papers, Public Office, London
TTE	Thomason Tracts, British Library, London

⧼ 1 ⧽

A Gentleman of Alderton

O Give thanks unto the Lord; for he is good: for his mercy endeareth for
ever.

(Ps. 136.1)

During the peaceful Elizabethan spring of 1601, a son was born to
Thomas Hesilrige of Noseley in the county of Leicestershire, and
Frances daughter and heir of Sir William Gorges of Alderton.[1] The
boy, born at his mother's home at Alderton in Northamptonshire, was
soon taken to the small village Church of St Margaret, and baptized
Arthur—the church register recording without fuss or detail: 'Arthur
Haselrigge, gent, was baptised the xxiij of July 1601'.

In the seventeenth century it was quite normal to baptize children
within a short period after birth, to safeguard the child's immortal soul
should any of the time's ills carry the infant prematurely to his maker.
Other Hesilrige children were baptized at Alderton: Donald, the eldest
son and heir to Thomas Hesilrige, being baptized 24 January 1600,
and the eldest child Mary on 14 June 1595. When the marriage of
Thomas and Frances took place is unknown, but it is reasonable to
assume it was during the spring of 1594, a year before the birth of
their daughter.

The Hesilriges were at this time living at the Alderton estate of Sir
William Gorges. They were not of established Northamptonshire
stock. Their earliest history shows them to have moved into neigh-
bouring Leicestershire from the far north in the late fourteenth century, with the marriage of another Thomas Hesilrige of Fawdon in
Northumberland, to Isabel, the eldest daughter and heir of Margaret
Hastings of Noseley. Isabel was born to Margaret Hastings from her
marriage to Sir Roger Heron, who had died before 1402.[2] Margaret
was, however, wealthy in her own right, having inherited Noseley

from a very ancient Leicestershire family called Martival, through her grandmother Joyce Sadington, who was either a sister or niece of Roger Martival Bishop of Salisbury.[3] The Hesilrige family strengthened its position in Leicestershire, purchasing land and generally climbing the social ladder over a period of two centuries. By the reign of Henry Tudor, the Hesilriges were established and respected pillars of the community.

Despite these deep roots in Leicestershire, baby Arthur's story began firmly at Alderton, where his branch of the Hesilrige family tree had planted itself.[4] An initial link with Northamptonshire was forged by Arthur's grandfather, yet another Thomas, with his marriage to Ursula, daughter of Sir Thomas Andrew, knight of Charwelton.[5] The Andrew family held a social position in Northamptonshire equal to that enjoyed by the Hesilriges' in Leicestershire, being merchants during the Middle Ages, steadily improving their status to become 'Knights of the Shire'. A marriage between the Hesilrige family and that of the Andrews' was a fine match, Ursula's family was stronger being already knights, but Thomas Hesilrige was possibly wealthier. Arthur never knew his grandfather, the old man dying on 31 May 1600.

The whole social structure of family marrying into family had been the backbone of the Tudor period. Ties of blood were the strength of the social system, where landowner married landowner, peerage married peerage, until power lay in a few hands, and each class of the gentry became a strong unit in its own right. Consequently the marriage between the Hesilrige and Gorges families had bolstered up the ties between Northamptonshire and Leicestershire landowners.

By the time Arthur was born, the family of Thomas and Frances Hesilrige was settled at Alderton, and enjoying the lifestyle of the seventeenth-century middle-class landowner. Arthur was certainly not born into hardship or poverty, indeed his standard of life was very good, food was plentiful and clothing of comfortable quality. With the exception of fevers and plague, which recognized no social barrier, young Arthur could expect to mature to manhood amid the narrow country lanes and fresh green fields around Alderton. The manor house at Alderton was situated at the north-east end of the village. The site was acquired by King Henry VIII, and then demised on lease. In 1567 Edward Cornwell Esq. had a grant for twenty-one years, and appears to have assigned this interest to William Gorges, whose widow Cecilia renewed the lease in 1590.[6] The leasehold then passed to Frances upon her marriage to Thomas Hesilrige. Such a wedding gift might well have been a portion of Frances's dowry, and indeed the estate remained her main home throughout her long life. The house was described as 'a very large mansion house' and 'to have been a noble structure'.[7]

Queen Elizabeth died in 1603, her reign having supplied a few years of social stability. True there had been plots, struggles for power, and a war with Spain, but Elizabeth, through her semi-isolationist approach to commerce and government, had strengthened England within its own shores and, after years of bitter doctrinal dispute, settled the nation to be at peace with itself and its God. Her death brought to the throne the Scottish family of Stuart in the guise of King James VI of Scotland—James I of England.

The infant Arthur Hesilrige would one day be in conflict with a son of this new Scottish monarch. Of course, in 1603 it was impossible to predict that the Stuart temperament would lead to the agony of civil war, although the blood of Scottish monarchy had long stained Queen Elizabeth's reign. In 1603 James was king, and to most godly men this was justification enough for him to sit upon the throne. A quiet and peaceful life was all Englishmen desired, to grow their crops, breed their cattle and horses and trade. Queen Elizabeth had ruled by the power of her will, with justice, but with a single-minded authority which allowed little room for question of her rule, or right to rule. This strength was inbred from her father the daunting Henry VIII, Elizabeth was perhaps the last of those who could rule through personality alone. The Stuarts had strength but they were foreign to the English ideal of constitutional strength within monarchy. The Stuart view of divinity within kings—or 'divine right'—was a theory left behind in history, and unfitting to a world emerging from the Middle Ages. A new framework of religion and commerce was evolving to change the face of England, and it widened the thoughts of those who followed it. The young Hesilrige grew up in this changing culture, and could hardly fail to be influenced by it.

During the 'Royal Progress' of 1605, Queen Anne of Denmark was entertained at Alderton between 16 and 20 August, the King staying at the nearby manor at Grafton. Obviously this shows the importance of the Hesilriges and the quality of their home. The Progress of 1608 found King James himself at Alderton on 4 August, where he knighted Henry Anderson of London 'having just before bestowed the same honour at Grafton, on his host Thomas Hasilrig esq.'[8] It is not difficult to imagine the growing Arthur being presented to his majesty, nor the stark contrasts there must have been between the pomp of James's travelling court and the practical style of the country landowner. The richly trimmed clothes of the King and his entourage would differ sharply to the less pretentious dress of his host. It is a family tradition that Dame Frances Hesilrige dressed her family in fine 'cloth of her own spinning'.[9] What little is known of Dame Frances suggests she was a woman of some ability, certainly a very capable administrator of the house, and with a practicality found in her class. An example of her cloth is represented in a portrait of a young boy, once thought to be Arthur, with his mother. The cloth is plain of a country cut and colour, Dame Frances wearing a small ruff about her neck in the style of early Jacobean England. The boy in dark grey clothes carries himself like a miniature adult, a little proud, perhaps even absurdly bold, but not childlike in the artistic interpretation.

The days at Alderton must have given the growing Arthur Hesilrige a pleasant and happy childhood, and there is no reason to believe any serious social problems disturbed the peace of the Northamptonshire countryside. Even the trauma of the 'Gunpowder Plot' sidestepped the Hesilriges, although its birth and death were conceived and executed in Northamptonshire. No, Arthur's father, now Sir Thomas, was increasing his social importance in the county, and contentment must have surrounded the thriving family.

The education of Arthur Hesilrige is something of a mystery, and the lack of detail for this vital period of his life a great disappointment. It is possible that young Arthur received some private tutoring from one of the many Northamptonshire teachers of Greek and Latin, but his first recognized education was at Westminster School, a good grounding for a future republican and member of the puritan hierarchy. It is difficult to say that the Hesilrige family was at this time of a puritan persuasion, indeed the word itself covers a multitude of religious beliefs, but they certainly accepted the plain Anglican service with ease. At Easter 1617, Arthur matriculated from Magdalene College, Cambridge, along with his brothers Donald and John.[10] Further research into Arthur's time at Magdalene proves fruitless, because no record of academic standards were kept at this time, it being less of an education and more of a social necessity to attend college. Likewise to suggest that Hesilrige underwent a great religious conversion whilst at Cambridge would be stretching the facts to improve the narrative. No, the great conversion in his ideology would come with his association with Lords Brooke, Saye and Sele, and St John, and principally John Pym. How wonderful for a biographer had the young Hesilrige been interested in such delights of college life as drink, gambling or the charms of the 'ladyes' of Cambridge—charges often laid at the college door of his contemporary Oliver Cromwell. Alas none of these simple pleasures of academia can be included to brighten the text.

The next stage in the education of Arthur Hesilrige, however, was training in one of the professions befitting a second son. In Hesilrige's case, he was admitted to Grey's Inn on 29 January 1623—his older brother Donald having been admitted the previous March.[11] His time at the Inns of Court proved invaluable to Arthur, a knowledge of the law being the doctrine of Parliaments past and present, and the very lifeblood of the politician. Grey's Inn taught Arthur Hesilrige the art of debate, the sharp-tongued rhetoric of the political duellist, an invaluable tool in years to come. Throughout his life, Hesilrige would pay due honour to the 'Worthy Gentlemen of the Long Robe'.

It is quite possible that it was during Hesilrige's time at Grey's Inn that he first met George Fenwick, son and heir of George Fenwick of Brinkburn, co. Northumberland.[12] Fenwick was slightly younger than Hesilrige, having matriculated from Queen's College, Cambridge, at Easter 1619. Their friendship lasted throughout their lifetimes, and if Hesilrige had a true friend, it must be Fenwick.

While Arthur Hesilrige grew into manhood, his father had busied himself with developing the family estate in Leicestershire. In the period between the knighting of Sir Thomas Hesilrige and 1613, the branch of the family moved back into Leicestershire. The estate at Noseley was highly profitable with its farmland and tenancies, and more time would now be spent in its development. In accordance with this fact, Sir Thomas Hesilrige executed the office of High Sheriff of Leicestershire in 1613, was chosen Knight of the Shire in 1614 and again in 1623. In 1622 Sir Thomas had been advanced to the title of baronet, successfully fighting the elections of 1615 and 1624, when he duly represented the county.[13]

By 1624 Arthur Hesilrige had become a captain of horse in the Leicestershire Trained Bands.[14] During this time England had no regular army, and each county was responsible for its own defence. Hesilrige, being the son of an MP and notable landowner, equipped himself as a cavalryman with a fine buff coat and the arms befitting his rank. He was a good horseman, and the monthly service with the trained bands was a great opportunity to play soldier while exercising a good hunter. The experience of at least some cavalry training would be valuable in future years, although the battles of civil war England would be somewhat more serious than the gentleman's game in the trained bands.

To Arthur Hesilrige the game of soldiers in Leicestershire must have been pure escapism after a few months at Grey's Inn. But if the trained bands were his joy, he had a more serious campaign on his mind. On 24 May 1624, Arthur Hesilrige married Frances Elmes, a bride of a mere eighteen years of age, having been baptized at Greens Norton in Northamptonshire on 3 June 1606. Frances was the daughter of Thomas Elmes of Greens Norton, a man of some quality and well respected in the county. Arthur received with his bride a portion, or dowry, of £3,000, a considerable sum meant to secure the girl's future. It is unknown if the marriage was a love match, but it is only a short horse ride from Alderton to Green Norton, and it is therefore probable that Hesilrige knew Frances for many of his childhood years. His period at Cambridge and Grey's Inn had given Frances time to mature and blossom into womanhood. In the seventeenth century the arranged marriage was the usual form of courtship for the gentry. Frances belonged to a strong Northamptonshire family which owned not only the small Greens Norton estate but a larger home and land at Lilford in the same county.

Arthur and Frances had two sons and two daughters, but the name of only one son is known, another Thomas. It would seem that Hesilrige's other children with Frances died before him and were unprolific.[15] The young age of Frances, together with her small-framed body, possibly indicates that childbearing was difficult for her and the children were weak.

Political thinking was changing in England. In 1621 and 1627, Sir Thomas Hesilrige and Thomas Elmes both opposed the county loans— Elmes suffering arrest.[16] The ill feeling growing within the 'petty gentry' and men of commerce against the court had reached a point where men like Sir Thomas were questioning the treasury's right. It was against this background that Arthur Hesilrige, encouraged by his father, fought the election of 1625 for the borough seat of Leicester. Despite the enormous influence of his father (Hesilrige's youth was against him), he could not carry Sir Thomas's county support into the borough, consequently failing to gain his first parliamentary seat.

The same year that Arthur failed in his political baptism saw the death of King James, bringing to the throne the ill-fated and equally ill-advised Charles I. In many respects Arthur Hesilrige and Charles Stuart were much alike: both were the same age and small in physical stature, stubborn but true to their beliefs, and furthermore both men were influenced during their early careers by men of strong opinion. In the case of Charles and the royal court, it was the likes of the earls of Buckingham and Strafford, and latterly Archbishop Laud, who framed his policy. Hesilrige and the puritan faction had their own men of ideals in the likes of John Pym and the incorruptible champion against oppressive government, John Hampden. Had Charles in future years been inclined to listen to Pym and the staunchly patriotic Hampden, they might well have built a country for all classes and persuasions. However, during their formative political years, Charles and Hesilrige were merely puppets, and not until after the deaths of their puppetmasters can the real men be seen.

Donald Hesilrige, the elder brother of Arthur, died before 1630, the date and year being unfortunately lost.[17] It is not unlikely that Donald indeed died before 1625, because, from the time of his marriage to Frances Elmes, it was Arthur who took the responsibilities of the heir.

The death of Sir Thomas Hesilrige came, it would seem, without warning in the sixty-sixth year of his life, a good age for the seventeenth century. The death of this important man is recorded on his tomb in the small yet beautiful Chapel of St Mary in the grounds of the Noseley estate:

> Here lyes Sir Thomas Hesilrige Kt & Baron
> who while he lived was trusted with ye places of greatest
> Honour & Power in ye County.
> He was prudent & of impartial Justice, of Great Temperance
> and Sobriety.
> He died ye 11th day of January 1629. Aged 66.[18]

Sir Thomas was now succeeded in title and estate by his eldest surviving son, the second baronet of Noseley—Sir Arthur Hesilrige.

NOTES

1.   Some old references to this small Northamptonshire village refer to Aldrington. For clarity the modern spelling of Alderton has been adopted throughout the text.

2.   *Transactions of the Leicestershire Archaeological Society*, 17 (1855–1917), p. 86.

3.   G.F. Farnham, *Leicestershire Medieval Pedigree*, pp. 56-57.

4.   For an early history of Noseley, see *Transactions of the Leicestershire Archaeological Society*, 12 (1917).

5.   J. Nichols, *History and Antiquities of Leicestershire* (1795–1815), vol. II, pt ii, p. 743.

6.   G. Baker, *History and Antiquities of Northamptonshire* (2 vols.; Northampton, 1822–1841), I, p. 120.

7.   Baker, *History and Antiquities*, I, p.120.

8.   J. Nichols, *Progressive Processions and Magnificent Festivities of King James I* (London, 1828), II, p. 203.

9.   Taken from the tomb of Sir Thomas and Dame Frances, Chapel of St Mary, Noseley.

10. J. Venn and J.A. Venn, *Alumni Cantabrigenses* (4 vols.; Cambridge, 1922–1927), II, pt i, p. 359.

11. Venn and Venn, *Alumni Cantabrigenses*, I, pt i, p. 359.

12. DNB (George Fenwick): this should be used with care.

13. Nichols, *Leicestershire*, II, pt ii, p. 743. According to the Revd. Sergeantson in his 'History of the Church of St Peter', Northampton, Thomas Hesilrige was created a baronet on 21 July 1622. In the 1660s this church became the family church to the Hesilriges, and still stands next to Hazlerigg House in Marefair.

14. SP 16 70/70.

15. The official family pedigree is inconclusive.

16. SP 14 127/82; SP 16 89/5; J. Rushworth, *Historical Collections* (7 vols.; 1680), I, p. 473.

17. Nichols, *Leicestershire*, II, pt ii, p. 743.

18. 1630 by the revised calendar.

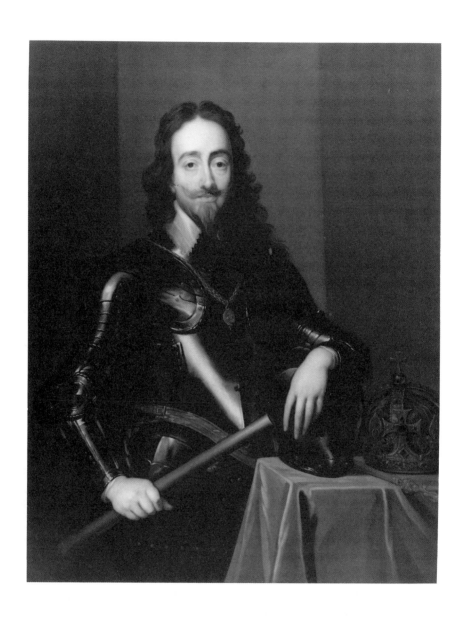

Charles I, by an unknown artist.
By courtesy of the National Portrait Gallery, London.

∞ 2 ∞

New Worlds, New Friends

And I am come down to deliver them out of the land of the Egyptians, and to bring them out of that land and at large, unto a land flowing with milk and honey.

(Exod. 3.8)

The death of Sir Thomas Hesilrige was the beginning of a series of unhappy events within the family. That same year, 1629, Bertin Hesilrige, a second cousin to Sir Arthur, was killed in a duel in London. Duelling was common in the seventeenth century, although strictly illegal, and for Bertin to fight a duel may suggest Sir Arthur was not the only man of quick temper in the family.

There followed in 1632 the death of Thomas Elmes, who departed his earthly body on 8 July, at the rather respectable age of seventy-nine. Old Thomas left a wife, Christian, who lived a further two years, dying 19 April 1635, aged seventy-three. Both Thomas and Christian Elmes were laid to rest at their family's estate at Lilford. If Thomas and his wife had lived to old age, this blessing was not upon their daughter Frances, Sir Arthur's wife, for at her untimely death in 1632, Dame Frances was merely a young woman of twenty-six. The monument inscription to Dame Frances Hesilrige at Noseley describes her as being 'charitable prudent virtuous and a loving wife'. Little more is known of this tragic young woman. Without doubt this marriage had given Hesilrige the foundation upon which to build his political destiny, but Dame Frances's death had great bearing upon the way that destiny would turn.

The thought of a second marriage quite close to the death of a first wife has a certain taboo in later times, but in the seventeenth century marriage had social undertones, leaving love to the poets and romance to the playwright. It was socially necessary for Sir Arthur to marry again, his wife could be of enormous help with the estate, and her role of social administrator in the family was no small one.

If puritan marriages were made in the dour heaven of political intrigue, then Sir Arthur's second marriage was blessed by the angels of the debating chamber, for to the political animal what better match could there possibly be than in Dorothy Greville, the lovely sister to the influencial puritan Lord Robert Brooke. Dorothy was the daughter of Fulke Greville of Thorpe Latimer in Lincolnshire, and a lady of both breeding and social acceptability.[1] Robert Greville, her brother, had been adopted by his elder cousin, the first Lord Brooke, and received an education befitting his future class. In 1627–28 Robert Greville sat in Parliament for the Borough of Warwick, but vacated this Commons seat upon reaching his majority on 30 January 1629 and suceeded to the barony of Brooke of Beauchamp Court, Warwickshire.[2] That same year the young Brooke married Lady Catherine Russell, eldest daughter of Francis Earl of Bedford, and, considering Brooke's own mother was twice descended from the old Earls of Warwick, it must be realized that Sir Arthur Hesilrige had, with his marriage to Dorothy, married into the very heart of English puritanism.

Hesilrige was highly influenced by his new brother-in-law. Under this strength of puritanism, Sir Arthur began to question the laws of the Stuarts. In November 1632, Hesilrige found himself in trouble for a refusal to pay a mustermaster's fee. As a captain in the trained bands of Leicestershire, Hesilrige had to pay a fee any time he 'failed to muster', which went towards arms for the 'Untrayned Militia'. The actual paying of the fee was in reality not in dispute (Hesilrige, like any Englishman, knew it was vital), no, the refusal was simply part of the political standpoint of the puritans against the authority of the King and the old gentry. Hesilrige was simply declaring his colours for all to see. Records of his case say:

> Sir Arthur Haslerig and Sir William Faunt having been sent for on a complaint made by the Earl of Huntingdon Lord Lieutenant of co. Leicestershire, that they refused to pay the levies made for the Muster-Master, on the 23rd inst, made their appearance and at the same time were present Sir Henry Skipwith and Sir John Skeffington, two of the Deputy Lieutenants of that county. When the case had been heard and and order made to refer the examination thereof to a committee, Sir Arthur urged these words to Sir John Skeffington: 'If such gentlemen as you shall be suffered to shark the country of their money, it will be a very

pretty thing.' When Sir John complained to the Lords, Sir Arthur replied softly, 'I do not say to the Lords, but only to you in private.' Sir Arthur was thereupon committed, but returning into the chamber on his knees he humbly craved pardon.[3]

Hesilrige undertook to pay the fee two days later on 30 November. The words 'if such gentlemen as you' can be regarded as characteristic of Hesilrige's tongue. He had no respect for this lackey of Stuart authority, and Sir Arthur could be extremely hard on those he dis-respected. Later in his career, Sir Arthur would find age and political respect a shield against the penalty of a quick temper and fiery tongue, but in 1632 this brash young firebrand held no power and therefore had to pay the price.

If Sir Arthur learned the fire and high puritanism from Lord Brooke, he would gain his political finesse from the arch-enemy of the Court, John Pym. Hesilrige's association with Pym appears to date from their connexion with the Providence and Saybrooke Colonising Companies owned by the puritan traders. The pro-Royalist Edward Hyde, later Earl of Clarendon, calls Hesilrige 'an absurd, bold man, brought up by Mr Pimm'.[4] Of course Hyde refers to a political adop-tion and not in any way a personal interest.[5] There was no better man than John Pym for a political education: few other men during the period could claim the same authority in debate, balanced by good sense and a strictness in his cause. Puritanism to Pym was only a lifestyle, but his religion was the political debate. This attitude was passed on to the inexperienced Hesilrige, implanted into his very heart. To Pym he owed everything that would sustain him through countless speeches, and dark days that would defeat all but those with his kind of inner strength, whether their cause was King, God or Parliament. To the puritan, God and Parliament were so interrelated that the victory of one was a victory to both.

Under the reign of the Stuart kings, it had become more and more difficult to visualize the 'Free Church' held so dear by the puritan brotherhood. With each year that passed, it became more apparent to Pym and his friends that religious freedom could not be found in Stuart England, and that, like Moses and his race before them, the answer was an Exodus to a better, sweeter land.

On 19 March 1632, a grant from Robert Earl of Warwick for a distance of forty leagues from the Narragansett River was made to a group of gentlemen who represented the cream of English puritans.

The most noted of this colonizing group were without doubt William the Viscount Saye and Sele, a man at the forefront of the movement over many years, and Robert Lord Brooke. Others in this illustrious group were Lord Rich, Charles Fiennes, Sir Nathaniel Rich, John Pym, John Hampden and finally the Northamptonshire puritan Richard Knightley. Knightley was a good friend of Sir Arthur and Dame Dorothy Hesilrige, through his associate Lord Brooke. At least two of Hesilrige's children with Dorothy were baptized at Knightley's estate at Fawsley, possibly during great meetings of the party. John Hampden was another rising puritan star, and as he was a relative of Knightley's, it seems likely that Hesilrige knew him well.

In 1633 Brooke, Saye, Hesilrige and others of that Company bought for £2,150 the interest from an association of merchants in Bristol, Shrewsbury and various West Country towns in connexion with their colonization plans.[6] Before any colony could be undertaken, a secondary source of income was needed to sustain the new community in bad years when harvests failed. After all, if the Saybrooke Company was offering new lives to puritans, in return it must offer economic viability to its investors. With this trade route established, it was decided that south Connecticut should be the scene of the new colony, and on 7 July 1633 an agreement was signed with the adventurer John Winthrop junior to lead a pioneer expedition. Winthrop was to build houses and a fortification on the banks of 'the river Connecticutt' for his own men, and then houses fit for gentlemen of quality.[7] This commission was signed on behalf of the patentees by Hesilrige and his close friend George Fenwick, who were appointed to remain in London 'to administer the first stages of the exodus.

From the commission given to John Winthrop, it is clear that some class distinction would prevail between labourers and gentlemen of quality. The puritan colonies should not be confused with the less class-conscious Quaker communes, but be seen to be a transportation of the trading puritans to areas rich in land where, it was hoped, the old-style English Church could not reach.

Hesilrige was in trouble throughout the whole of 1635, appearing before the Court of High Commission on numerous occasions. His case was referred to Sir John Lamb and Doctors Duck and Eden on 30 April with an order to retain or dismiss the charges.[8] Sir Arthur was eventually imprisoned in the Fleet, the warrant for his release being dated 30 December.[9] Imprisonment for what his party deemed political crimes was ideal for Hesilrige; he would certainly enjoy such martyrdom, for it would do nothing but enhance his name.

While Sir Arthur played the political radical, George Fenwick busied himself with the colonization plans. In 1636 he visited Boston in the 'New World' to see the potential of colonial life. He must have found this experience agreeable, for he moved to Connecticut with his wife in 1639 as agent for the patentees and the governor of Saybrooke.[10]

In common with most influential puritans, Hesilrige, during the 1630s, considered leaving old England for the freedom of the colonies. Sir Arthur's new friends like Fenwick had more to gain from a fresh start than they could possibly hope for under the Stuarts. In various stories, Hesilrige planned to leave England with John Pym, Brooke, Hampden and even Oliver Cromwell, but at what time is lost in folk-lore and propaganda. If Sir Arthur had planned to leave for Saybrooke, it must have been before 1636, because the following year a number of land transactions firmly place him back in Leicestershire.

In the years immediately following his father's death, Hesilrige had involved himself in mortgage transactions. Properties and land had been mortgaged in 1630 for £1,800 but were redeemed in 1637.[11] From this it would seem Sir Arthur's thoughts of Saybrooke ended then. Certainly the mortgages were arranged to supply funding of fresh ventures, including colonial ventures, but with the ending of such plans the conservative gentry returned to the security of landowning. By this time Hesilrige was living the life of a seventeenth-century gentleman, moving between his estate of Noseley and the business centre of London, with his brother John administering his mother's estate at Alderton. John Hesilrige is usually called 'John of Alderton', which reflects his greater connexion with that estate.[12] The Hesilriges were becoming major puritan landowners, though as yet not on the scale of the old gentry families, and the whole family knew its destiny was in the puchasing power of land.

National events during the colonization period were involving the puritans in a fight for economic survival. In August 1635 writs for the collection of 'ship money' were issued. This was not a new form of taxation, for the King had introduced a number of such taxes following his dissolution of Parliament in 1629. Taxation without representation was unpopular with all puritans. Many of these unpopular taxes were the brainchild of the King's principle economic adviser, the 'ingenious old lawyer William Noy'.[13] Noy was astute,

and had he lived he may have saved Charles from the terrible consequences his rule was to evoke, for, although he was responsible for
many unpopular measures, he was flexible and did not have the royal
weakness of being beyond question. The unusual, indeed unprecedented, aspect of the Noy writs for ship money was an introduction
of a levy on inland tax payers, whereas this had always been a coastal
tax. In reality it was not totally wrong to expect inland gentry to pay
for ships, because many were now merchant traders of the puritan
group, and enjoyed some protection on the sea. However, this particular tax was chosen by both puritans and monarchists to test each
other's strength. Before the end of 1635 the counties of Essex,
Oxfordshire and Warwickshire had seen civil disorder, and the puritan leaders were busily organizing resistance to payment. Sir Arthur
Hesilrige, although involved in the anti-ship money cases, was not
sufficiently known nationally to lead the legal opposition for the
puritans, and this great task was left principally to John Hampden.
Hampden was certainly a puritan and allied himself with Pym and the
anti-Court group, but he was also known to be honest, patriotic and
indeed all that was good in the English class system. By choosing
John Hampden for the test case against ship money, the puritans were
using a moderate loved by the common people. Had Hesilrige been
used, his temper may have damaged their cause, for although he had
legal training he had not yet learned to control his fiery tongue.

A writ for ship money was issued to the 'Sherriff of Buckingham'
on 4 August 1635,[14] and the sum to be paid by Hampden was no
more than £20, which was hardly ruinous to a gentleman of his
wealth.[15] A mere £20 held to be illegally taxed was enough to bring
forth the most famous civil law case of the decade. The case began
towards the end of 1637 and judgement was finally given on 12 June
1638 in favour of the crown. Although, through this case, ship
money was judged to be legal, it had introduced the idea of opposition to the people of England and done great harm to the King—the
tax was now paid with even more reluctance by the puritans.

During this time of puritan activity, Sir Arthur and Dame Dorothy
had increased their family. Their son, named Arthur after his father,
was baptized on 29 April 1637, and another son, Robert, who was
likely named after Lord Brooke, was baptized on 2 August 1639, both
ceremonies being at Fawsley. A daughter, Catherine, had been born
in 1635.[16]

By the year 1639, events were moving fast, too fast for the good of the nation, it may be concluded. In effect the country was in the grip of a constitutional crisis that the King had little control over, Parliament knowing full well it would be recalled at any time. The monarchy had for some time dabbled in that most dangerous of subjects, an enforced religious doctrine, and now foolishly attempted to impose upon of all peoples the Scots a form of English episcopacy. As the Book of Common Prayer was forcibly sent north, the roar of the Presbyterian Kirks in Scotland could be heard in London. War was clearly only weeks away. If the King had to fight a war of religion, he needed an army; for an army the King needed money—and Parliament held the purse. The King called and broke Parliament's sitting, but Parliament controlled the main money supply. The King held his subjects in his palm, yet his subjects held the purse he so badly needed.

In the Parliament called in April 1640, Hesilrige was chosen for the county of Leicestershire.[17] This Parliament was in an almost rabid frame of mind, and even an offer to suspend the payment of ship money would not sooth the beast. Nothing less than a Parliament with freedom under law to sit would satisfy Pym, and likewise Hesilrige. Also, why should a puritan-controlled Parliament advance money for a King to wage war upon a free Presbyterian people, the Scots? Charles found all this simply too much and dissolved Parliament in early May, ending what history calls the 'Short or Broken Parliament'. This action only embittered the puritans even further, and, when the King found his 'Gentleman Army' could not stop the swarm of Scottish Lowlanders from taking the far north and sweeping ever further southward, the members of yet another hastily assembled Parliament were ready to do or die for their cause.

Once again, in the Parliament that met on 3 November 1640, Sir Arthur Hesilrige sat for Leicestershire. His opponent on this occasion was Sir Richard Halford, a good royalist but an extremely poor loser, for he openly stated of Hesilrige that his countrymen had 'chosen a knight who had more will than wit'. Hearing this the freeholders and inhabitants of the county, who loved Sir Arthur for his assistance in Leicestershire during the whole previous decade, petitioned the Commons, and Halford was judged a delinquent and committed to the Tower for some days.[18]

In contrast to the short-lived assembly of early 1640, the new

Parliament was in no mood to be broken. The King, having totally failed in his holy war, relied upon his new Parliament to seek peace with the Scots, who held Newcastle, Berwick, Carlisle and most of the Bishoprick of Durham. Peace was forthcoming, but only at a terrible price, and this foolhardy monarch would not have his freedom again, because the puritan traders and men of commerce would not willingly pay for kingly wars. Foolhardy Charles knew only too well the mood of Parliament, his Parliament, but listened to his advisers, who perhaps were even more foolhardy than him. This Charles Stuart had inherited a weakness from his father James: he liked men of singular ideal, and his favourite at this time was Thomas Wentworth, Earl of Strafford. Strafford was an opportunist, very strong in ideal and with great influence over Charles, and particularly his Catholic Queen, the headstrong Henrietta-Maria. With negotiations with the Scots under way, Parliament began to look at their own security and how to preserve themselves from the King. Strafford, seeing the mood of Pym and his followers turning away from that of dutiful subjects, urged Charles to Arrest John Pym and other anti-court members in the Parliament on grounds of high treason, namely for entering into correspondence with the Scots against the nation's interest. In any other circumstances Strafford would have been correct in assuming that the removal of the the ringleaders would cause the assembly to flounder nervously and destroy itself, but he totally misunderstood Pym, underestimated John Hampden, and hardly took the strength of Hesilrige into consideration at all. These men were not careless enough to fall into the hands of the King, let alone those of the King's puppet-master Strafford. Like a cornered animal, Parliament, and chiefly the Commons House, bared its teeth and fought back against this move to cage it. John Pym opened a debate and moved for the impeachment of Thomas Wentworth, Earl of Strafford on grounds of high treason, thus catching him in his own net.

At the outbreak of the Scottish or 'Bishops War', Strafford had suggested that the Anglo-Irish army which maintained a rough and often brutal peace in that unfortunate country should be brought to England as a hard core to the English army engaging the Scots. Pym and his followers had been guilty of treason in the Earl's eyes when they refused to grant money to the King for his war and as a conse-quence the Irish forces could not sail. The puritans, on the other hand, knew that any troops brought into England to quell a Scottish puritan cause, could also be used to beat them—and this was treason to them.[19]

On the fateful day—11 November 1640—John Hampden was appointed to draw up the article for impeachment of the Earl of Strafford. The task was quickly carried out and the charges read. Legally there were no charges Strafford's enemies could press to cost him his life, but despite this the trial opened on 22 March 1641 at Westminster Hall. The leader of the Presbyterian puritans, Denzil Holles, was by unfortunate chance also the brother-in-law of Strafford and took little part in the ritual. Holles was a colleague of Hesilrige, but never a friend or even close to him, there being things neither man could tolerate in the other, and certainly Sir Arthur's part in Strafford's current position did little to recommend him to Holles. In his writings, Clarendon says it was 'Sir Gilbert Gerard, the lord Digby, Strowd, Hasilrigg and the northern gentlemen who were most angry with the earl'.[20] Hesilrige was certainly no friend of the 'Court Party', which included Clarendon, and was rapidly becoming infamous for the way the likes of Pym used him for their own ends.

Eventually the defence case for Strafford began to inch ahead in the trial, but news of a plot to march the parts of the army loyal to the King against London and seize the Tower brought forth a deadly proposal from Hesilrige. On the afternoon of 12 April, 'Sir Arthur Hesilrige drew out of his pocket a Bill, supposed to have been prepared before that day, for the Earl's attainer, and was with much ado kept from being read again the same afternoon.'[21] Hesilrige's bill called for the death of Strafford by that barbaric form of execution, hanging, drawing and quartering. Pym and Hampden were against the attainer, for it was death without trial, and must involve the King for he alone could sign the death warrant. The use of the attainer was however the only course left open if Strafford was not to escape. To avoid a quarrel with the Lords, of whom Strafford was one, John Hampden moved that the attainer should be argued alongside the act of impeachment. Parliament accepted this compromise, which said a good deal for the respect shown for Hampden by both sides. This middle path was not held to, however, and only a week later, on 19 April, the Commons, guided by Oliver St John, declared Strafford a traitor, and only ten days later the Earl's guilt was passed by 204 votes to 59 in the attainer. It is interesting to note that in this vote Pym joined with Hesilrige and St John, while Hampden abstained.[22]

Arrested at almost the same time as Strafford was William Laud, Archbishop of Canterbury, who was seen by the puritans and others to be all that was evil in the Church of England. On 18 December 1640 he was impeached for high treason; on 24 February 1641 the act was passed; and on 1 March the old man was imprisoned in the Tower.[23] It would appear that Hesilrige took his part against Laud with a personal joy, for he was totally opposed to the form of worship encouraged by the Archbishop.[24] In a speech made over a decade later Hesilrige said of William Laud:

> Our souls and consciences were put on the rack by the Archbishop, we might not speak of Scripture, or repeat a sermon at our tables. Many godly ministers were sent to find their bed in the wilderness. The oppression was little less in the lower courts and in the special courts. Altars were set up, and bowing to them enjoyed, pictures were placed in Church-windowes, and images set up at Durham and elsewhere; with many other exorbitancies introduced, both in Church and State. The Archbishop would not only impose on England, but on Scotland, to bring in the Book of Common Prayer upon them. They liked it not, and, as luck would have it, they would not bear it. He prevailed with the king to raise an army to suppress them.[25]

In this speech Sir Arthur told the complete history of the period as he saw it, and it is the only surviving statement concerning his overall view of those times and says more of his feelings than any other papers.[26]

These then were the crimes of Archbishop Laud, which were serious to the puritan but, not so easy to press in a mixed religion Parliament; therefore, unlike Strafford, he could be left in the Tower without pressing an attainer or even to enforcing the death penalty through the impeachment.

The bill against Strafford quickly passed from Commons to Lords, who, even though he was one of them, were so fearful of future events that they too passed it. The final dilemma rested with the King. Would he or would he not sign the 'Death Warrant'? Claims quickly spread in London that Queen Henrietta-Maria was urging the King to use force to release Strafford and arrest certain leading Parliamentarians. The Earl himself pleaded with the King for his life. In a move of utter madness, the Court Party attempted to bribe Balfour, the Lieutenant of the Tower, but he would have none of it. Hearing this, Newport, the Tower Constable, threatened to execute Strafford if a further attempt be made. With a howling mob crying for blood and

threatening the Queen—this 'Papist Whore'—the King, his conscience in turmoil, gave way and signed the death warrant on 10 May.
On his way to the block, Strafford looked to Archbishop Laud at his
window in the Tower; the Archbishop, raising his hand in one final
blessing, stepped back and fainted at the thought of the Earl's fate. So,
on 12 May 1641, the Commons avenged themselves on the life of
Strafford, the Earl's final words asking 'if it was well that the beginning of the people's happiness should be written in letters of bloud'.[27]
If Sir Arthur Hesilrige's persecution of Strafford, 'whose death he
fought perhaps more than any other member of the house', was the
gate to the people's freedom, they still needed to pass through it.[28]

During the same year, Hesilrige began a campaign against the clergy
of the English Church, and members of the Roman Church in
England because of Henrietta-Maria. Sir Arthur was 'a zealous pro-
moter of the bill for extirpating episcopacy'.[29] Like in previous
dynasties, the result of religious changes under the Stuarts was a general lust for blood by those opposing these changes and desiring changes
of their own; the Christ, being born of blood and suffering, taking
unto himself the suffering of his interpreters.

On 26 October, the House of Commons debated the crimes of
certain bishops and priests, this being the next stage in the search for
the puritan heaven. Edward Hyde, a staunch royalist and a well-
educated man, moved against the puritan view that 'seeing wee had
not thought it fitt to name it treason before wee could not do it
now', to which Hesilrige replied, 'as long as our accusation was no
condemnation wee might proceede to accuse them'.[30] This was the
measured double talk of a lawyer, learned in his youth. A month
later, on 30 November, Sir Arthur moved in the Commons against
thirteen other bishops, the 'lawyers of the House being required to
attend the following morning at ten o'clock'.[31] This period of only a
few months was perhaps the least creditable time of Hesilrige's career.

Even more important than the religious questions being argued
over in Parliament was the major constitutional bill brought forward
by Sir Arthur on 7 December 1641. The 'militia bill' was drawn up
by Oliver St John following discussions led by William Strode and a
yeoman farmer from East Anglia, Oliver Cromwell MP. It was however left to Hesilrige to introduce the highly controversial document
into the House of Commons. It was the desire of Parliament, or the
puritan faction, that the 'Trayned Bands' and militia that constituted

the vast majority of the armed forces in England, should be under
their control for King and Kingdom, rather than be the power of the
King and Court. The bill brought forward by Hesilrige, moved the
control of the army from the King, as captain-general, to a lord
general appointed by Parliament for the King. It was common gossip
that Robert Earl of Essex was to hold this position, and Essex was a
Parliament man.[32] If the militia was in the control of a lord general, it
could not be used against the liberty of Parliament without being
involved in an action of treason, the position being that they, the
King's servants in arms, would be acting against the role of the throne
and committing treason through a breach of parliamentary law, even
if the King himself ordered them to march. The militia bill, a masterly
document, if the King would stand for it, was at a time when
Parliament was in dire straits and fighting for its own survival.

Sir Symonds D'Ewes, a timid member of the Commons, sat each
day, and during debates kept a diary of events. He noted that Sir
Arthur Heslerige usually sat in the Gallery during session. For a small
man this could be an advantage, because should he wish to speak he
would tower above his fellow members sitting in the main arena
below. At a glance it would be possible to see all assembled, which
was the military tactic of the period: see your enemy and gain higher
ground than he. On the occasion of the militia bill, Sir Symonds
records that Sir John Culpepper, looking up at Hesilrige said 'that he
wondered that the gentleman in the gallerie should bring such a bill,
having soe often complained of the exorbitant power of the Deputy
lieftenants in his country'. This was a valid point, and Culpepper
knew Sir Arthur could not argue to the contrary. D'Ewes himself,
heartened by this, summoned up enough courage to add, tongue in
cheek, 'we have passed the Billes for the pressing of soldiers and
marriners and for the granting of Tonnage and Poundage all of which
actions are in themselves against the fundamental lawes of the Realm'.
For the mouth of D'Ewes to pronounce such lines is a wonder, for
although he was a pedantic journal keeper he was not one to risk too
much.

Although Charles was still trying to keep his country at peace, the
actions of this rebel Parliament were becoming all too much for him.
Pym and his fellows were scoring far too many points against him, his
Queen was criticizing his lack of power and his people his lack of foresight. On Monday 3 January 1642, his patience finally broke and the

floodgates of his temper burst, releasing a torrent of ill-advised action. The attorney-general, the newly appointed Sir Edward Herbert, addressed the House of Peers, accusing of high treason the Lord Mandeville and 'Five Members' of the House of Commons, namely John Pym, John Hampden, Denzil Holles, William Strode and Sir Arthur Hesilrige.

The same day, Sir William Killigrew and Sir William Fleming with a guard sealed up the chambers, studies and trunks of the 'Five' by royal warrant, this being a breach of the King's privilege to do such a thing. Then by royal warrant the King's serjeant-at-arms, a Sergeant Francis, made a bold demand in the Commons that the accused members should be delivered unto him that he might arrest them on charges of high treason.[33] One hundred years earlier, that powerful monarch Henry VIII may have risked and even succeeded in such a move. The charismatic majesty of Queen Elizabeth might have taken this step without danger. However, it is unlikely either would have dared attempt to do so in the House itself. But Charles Stuart lived at the very end of such times and had not come to terms with this new England of traders and Parliament of commerce. These people would not submit like the Tudor gentry, and the result of the King's action was almost forewritten. The next day Hesilrige takes up the story:

> ... the King demanded five members, by his Attorney-Generall. He then came personally to the house, with five hundred men at his heels, and sat in your chair (the Speakers) it pleased God to hide those members, I shall never forget the kindness of that great Lady Carlisle that gave timely notice. Yet some of them were in the House, after the notice came. It was questioned if, for the safety of the House, they should be gone; but the debate was shortened, and it was thought fit for them in discreation to withdraw. Mr Hampden and myself being then in the House, withdrew. Away we went. The king immediately came in, and was in the House before we got to the water.[34]

Had the King taken either man there can be little doubt that the London mob would have rioted, the mood of the people having reached boiling point. Sitting in the Speaker's chair, the King demanded 'the Five', again a breach of privilege, because he was sitting in the chair of the common-man, demanding the members of that House. Again Charles asked, this time directing his question at the Speaker, William Lenthall. The Speaker, relying upon all his privilege, replied:

> May it please your Majesty, I have neither eyes to see nor tongue to speak
> in this place, but as the House is pleased to direct me whose servant I am
> here; and humbly beg your majesty's pardon that I cannot give any other
> answer than this to what your Majesty is pleased to demand of me.[35]

The King, seeing there was no point in asking further, said, 'I see the
birds have flown,' and growing impatient, strode from the House a
frustrated man. The sight of armed men in their assembly both angered
and frightened the members, and D'Ewes, reverting to character,
made out his will.

While Charles questioned the Speaker, the accused members made
their escaped via the river and took refuge in a house in Coleman
Street in the city, which was loyal to Parliament.

The following day, 5 January, the King went to the city and,
finding no satisfaction, left London not to return for six years, when
matters had taken their course. On 11 January, Pym, Hampden,
Holles, Strode and Hesilrige made a triumphant return by the river, as
Clarendon describes in detail:

> The accused members, about two of the clock in the afternoon on the
> eleventh day of January, came from their lodgings in the city to
> Westminster, guarded by the shrieves and Train-bands of London and
> Westminster and attended by a conflux of many thousands of people
> besides, making a great clamour against bishops and popish lords and of
> the privileges of Parliament; some of them as they passed Whitehall asking
> with much contempt, what was become of the king and his cavalleers?
> and whither he was gone?[36]

From this the triumphant return can be viewed as a victory, but a
hollow one, for the King had gone to Hampton Court and could
not see it. One can just imagine Haslerig's elation at the support of
the city, as he marched in triumph to Westminster. Sir Arthur said of
the events during the next few months:

> Thereupon he (the king) left the parliament and went from step to step,
> till he came to York, and set up his standard at Nottingham, and declared
> the militia was in him. The House of Lords then sent down to declare
> that the king had broken his trust. The word of the king, seduced by evil
> counsel, lost us forty lords. The House declared the militia to be in them.
> That was the great question. Commissioners were then sent out in the
> name of the king and Parliament. Then was there the king against the
> Parliament, and the Parliament against him.[37]

With the 'Banner Royale' flying in the wind of change, the question of who controlled the militia was simply one for the lawyers to

argue. Against the royal standard, many hundreds of parliamentarians would raise their own, with them Sir Arthur Hesilrige.

NOTES

1. Collins, *Peerage of England* (1812), pp. 350-51.
2. DNB (Grevill, Robert Lord Brooke).
3. CSP Dom, 1631–33, pp. 445-46.
4. (E. Hyde) Earl of Clarendon, *History of the Rebellion* (ed. W. Dunn Macray; 6 vols.; Oxford, 1888), I, p. 300.
5. Early interpretations of Clarendon's works can be misleading.
6. Bradford, *History of Plymouth Plantation* (1912 edn), pp. 175-80; main secondary source, A.P. Newton, *The Colonizing Activities of the English Puritans* (New Haven, 1954), p. 176n.
7. Newton, *Colonizing*, p. 177.
8. CSP Dom, 1635, p. 199.
9. CSP Dom, 1635, p. 604.
10. *Massachusetts Historical Collections*, 5th series, pp. 223, 482; DNB (George Fenwick); J. Winthrop, *History of New England*, I, p. 306.
11. *Transactions of the Leicestershire Archaeological Society*, 12 (1917), pp. 262-64.
12. John Hesilrige named a son Arthur (b. 1633), and it is important not to confuse the three.
13. C.V. Wedgwood, *The King's Peace* (London: Collins, 1955), p. 155.
14. Rushworth, *Historical Collections*, III, p. 213.
15. DNB (John Hampden); also see J. Adair, *John Hampden the Patriot* (London, 1975), the best modern biography of Hampden to deal with the pre-Parliament life of the great statesman.
16. DNB (George Fenwick).
17. Nichols, *Leicestershire*, I, pt ii, p. 456.
18. Nichols, *Leicestershire*, II, pt ii, p. 743.
19. DNB (Wentworth, Thomas Earl of Strafford).
20. Clarendon, *History of the Rebellions*, I, p. 249.
21. CSP Dom, 1640–41, p. 540.
22. J. Rushworth, *Trial of Strafford*; DNB (Hampden).
23. DNB (William Laud).
24. CSP Dom, 1641–43, p. 547.
25. *The Diary of Thomas Burton* (ed. T. Rutt; 4 vols.; London, 1828), III, pp. 89-90.
26. Further extracts from this speech are used throughout this work.
27. DNB (Wentworth).
28. Nichols, *Leicestershire*, II, pt ii, p. 743.
29. Nichols, *Leicestershire*, II, pt ii, p. 743.
30. *The Journal of Sir Symonds D'Ewes* (ed. W.H. Coates; New Haven, 1942), p. 39.

31. *Sir D'Ewes's Journal*, p. 217.

32. *Sir D'Ewes's Journal*, pp. 244-45; Wedgwood, *The King's War*, p. 41.

33. Wedgwood, *The King's War*, p. 55; S.R. Gardiner (ed.), *Constitutional Documents of the Puritan Revolution, 1628–1660* (Oxford, 1889); CSP Dom, 1641–43, p. 236; CJ, II, p. 367.

34. *Burton's Diary*, III, pp. 92-93.

35. Rushworth, *Historical Collections*, IV, p. 478.

36. Clarendon, *History of the Rebellion*, I, pp. 508-10.

37. *Burton's Diary*, III, pp. 94-95.

∞ 3 ∞

Civil War

Beat your plowshares into swords, and your pruninghooks into spears: let the weak say, I am strong.

(Joel 3.10)

The political turmoil of the spring of 1642 turned swiftly to military conflict with the oncoming of summer. Sir Arthur Hesilrige was now at the forefront of the rebellion, having become 'one foremost to decide the cause between king and his parliament with the sword, throwing away the scabbard, without a wish ever to take it again, early falling into a scheme to ruin the king, to set aside monarchy'.[1] This is probably an overstatement. In fact at this time he, like Cromwell and Pym, appears to favour the reform of monarchy rather than abolition, and only later supports a Commonwealth republic.

Hesilrige had in June spent some time at Noseley, at the same time recruiting a troop of horse made up principally of his friends and neighbours in Leicestershire. This troop was commissioned on 1 September, with Hesilrige receiving the appointment 'to attend the Charge of a Captain of Horse'.[2] The following day he was ordered to see the county militia exercised and to continue at the head of a committee for raising troops, confiscation of property and assisting the lord lieutenant and sheriff on occasions that required his aid.[3]

Many of Hesilrige's earliest troopers were raised around Noseley. He had been a captain of trained bands from 1624, which made him ideal to recruit troopers for the army of the Earl of Essex. The officers of Hesilrige's troop were himself as Captain, Lieutenant Jervis Brakey, Cornet Thomas Horton, and Quartermaster Zachariah Walker.[4] Of these the cornet, Thomas Horton, is the most interesting. Horton's life before his military career is vague, but he was a man to whom the rebellion gave an opportunity to improve his social and economic position—indeed, the nation's misery boosted the personal fortunes of many of 'the middling sort' of people. Thomas he was part of a fairly large Leicestershire family living at Gumley, Saddington, Noseley, Mowsley and elsewhere. He is mentioned on deeds to a small number of Hesilrige transactions, where Horton is described as 'of Noseley'. The family clearly had a strong link with the Hesilriges over a number of years, two other Hortons, John Horton junior of Noseley and John Horton of Gumley, being parties to deeds in 1664, 1685 and 1698.[5] It is said that before 1642 Thomas Horton was Sir Arthur Hesilrige's falconer and servant, but this seems unlikely due to land transactions and his commission as cornet.[6] Horton might well have been practised at falconry, since it was a highly prized pastime, but he was literate and numerate and certainly no country yokel.

With the phoney war gaining pace, Sir Arthur, being forewarned that the King's forces were to make a lightning raid into Leicestershire, rode with his troop to Northampton, where Essex's army was assembling.[7]

On 3 September, Nehemiah Wharton a sergeant in the parliamentarian army quartered around Northampton, wrote to his master in London that 'this day came Sir Arthur Hasilriggs and other troops into our town'.[8] Discipline in the army at Northampton was poor, and the longer it quartered there the more social disquiet crept into daily life. Hesilrige therefore rode towards the Earl of Essex, who was on the march, in a bid to hasten the rendezvous. The lord general reached Northampton on the afternoon of 9 September, and with Hesilrige and John Hampden in support, quickly restored military order. On Wednesday 13 September, a great review of the army was made before the eyes of Essex, and that evening the whole force marched away in the direction of Rugby, marching eventually to Worcester where Mr Morton, 'a very worthy man', who was one of the Devines at the Westminster Assembly, 'was in attendance on Sir Arthur Hasleriges troop'.[9]

There is no evidence to suggest that Hesilrige's troop was among the horse chastised by the royalist Prince Rupert on 23 September at Powick Bridge. It had taken the slow-moving parliamentary army from 13 to 26 September to reach Worcester, where it stayed twenty-three days before again marching on 19 October. Meanwhile the King and his army were manoeuvring around the Vale of the Red Horse after leaving Shrewsbury on 12 October.

On 22 October the main body of the parliamentary army was in and around Kineton. The Earl of Essex firmly believed that the King proposed an attack upon Banbury, and had resolved to follow and thwart this action. By now, Hesilrige's troop had been placed in a regiment commanded by Sir William Balfour, the lieutenant general of horse, although the formation of permanent regiments was somewhat irregular at this time.

Late on the evening of the 22nd, the King received vital intelligence that Essex was quartered nearby, and in response the royalist commanders drew up their order of battle. Essex was left with no option than to follow the King, but the question remained would he be allowed such luxury. The official Parliamentary Account supplies the answer:

> In the Morning (23 October), when we were going to Church, we had news brought us that the Enemy was 2 Miles from us, upon a high Hill, called *Edgehill*; whereupon we presently marched forth into a great broad Field, under the Hill, called, *The Vale of the Red Horse*, and made a stand some half a Mile from the Foot of the Hill, and there drew into Battalia, where we saw their Forces come down the Hill; and drew likewise into Battel in the Bottom; a great broad Company.

Hesilrige's troop was held in reserve with Balfour's regiment behind the massed ranks of pike and musket towards the centre. This reserve numbered as many as 700 horse, made up of Balfour's regiment and a regiment under Sir Phillip Stapleton.[10] It was now afternoon, and before vision was restricted by clouds of smoke, which would hang in the damp autumn air like grey ghosts, Hesilrige must have had a good view from his position of the King's forces manoeuvring before them. Suddenly the quiet of the afternoon was broken by the crack of dragoon fire. With dragoons engaged along hedgerows in hot battle, the main advance began. The parliamentary field guns now began to play upon the royalist frontage.

On the King's right wing, Prince Rupert, the nephew of King Charles, spurred on his regiments of horse, and totally routed the parliamentary wing of horse commanded by Sir James Ramsey.[11] Equally triumphant, Lord Wilmot made his charge against the right wing of the parliamentary horse under Lord Feilding, whose troopers broke and fled with Wilmot and his reserve commanded by Lord Digby hot in pursuit.

As the royalist horse made their charges, the old royalist general, Sir

Jacob Astley, made his peace with God. 'Oh Lord,' prayed Astley, 'Thou knowest how busy I must be this day. If I forget thee do not Thou forget me.' Rising to his feet, he gave the command 'March on boys', at which the King's infantry, or foot, brigaded into large square bodies, began their advance down the hill. The waves of red, blue, green and white coated men swept forward at a steady measured pace, the drummers beating out their officers' commands, while ensigns waved and flourished their colours. By now Hesilrige could see the green colours of Sir William Pennyman pressing down towards them, the golden lion upon the red colour of the King's lifeguard almost immediately to his front. The main battle for the centre was about to be joined. As the muskets discharged on both sides, the story is taken up by Edward Hyde:

> The foot of both sides stood their ground with great courage; and though many of the King's soldiers were unarmed and had only cudgels, they kept their ranks, and took up the arms which their slaughtered neighbours left to them...the execution was great on both sides, but much greater on the earl of Essex's party.[12]

All this time Hesilrige sat behind the foot, watching the events through the mists from the musketry. News must have spread back along the lines that both Ramsey and Feilding were routed, so for all Hesilrige knew the enemy would attack their flank at any moment. Balfour had to make a move. With the two regiments under his command, he passed through the divisions of foot to the front of his own brigade and led his troopers forward. Hyde continues:

> ...their reserve, commanded by sir William Balfore, moved up and down the field in good order, and marching towards the King's foot pretended to be friends, till, observing no horse to be in readiness to charge them, brake in upon the foot, and did great execution.[13]

Sir Phillip Stapleton's regiment attacked the brigade of Sir Nicholas Byron and was gored by royalist pikes for their trouble. Balfour however was more fortunate with his charge against the edge of Sir Richard Feilding's brigade, breaking through a regiment with green colours.[14] Balfour rode on:

> ...beat them to their Cannon, where they threw down their Arms, and ran away; he laid his hand upon the Cannon, and called for Nails to nail them up, especially the two biggest, which were Demy-Cannon; but finding none, he cut the ropes belonging to them, and his Troopers killed the Canoneers; then he pursued the Fliers half a Mile upon Execution.[15]

The attack by Balfour and Stapleton had thrown the royalist foot into a state of disorder. The King himself now entered the centre, resolving to join the foot in an attempt to restore morale following the cavalry attack. He rode forward to join the regiments of Gerard and Belasyse, sending the young princes Charles and James, who were with him that day, to the rear under the escort of Sir William Howard and the gentleman pensioners.

At least one troop from Balfour's regiment now divided from the main body and rode hard towards the pensioners, mistaking them for royalist horse. The young Prince James saw this body approaching 'from the left hand of the kings foot'.[16] Being to the rear of the main action, and believing Balfour's horse to be part of their own forces, the princes, with their guards, Mr Edward Hyde and Sir John Hinton, made towards them in greeting. Hinton takes up the story:

> ...seeing the sudden and quick march of the Enemie towards you, I did with all earnestness, most humbly, but at last somewhat rudely, impertune your Highnesse to avoid this present and apparent danger of being killed or taken prisoner, for their horse was by this time come up within half a musket shott in full body, att which your Highnesse was pleased to tell mee, you feared them not, and drawing a pistoll out of one of your holsters, and spanning it, resolved to charge them, but I did prevail with your Highnesse to quit the place, and ride from them, in some haste, but one of their troopers being excellently mounted, broke his rank, and coming full careere towards your Highnesse, I received his charge, and having spent a pistoll or two on each other, I dismounted him in the closing, but being armed *cap-a-pe*, I could doe no execution upon him with my sword, att which instant, one Mr Matthewes, a Gentleman Pensioner, rides in, and with a pole-axe immediately decides the businesse, and then overtaking your Highnesse, you got safe to the Royal Army...[17]

Balfour had lost the chance of making the princes prisoner. Returning to the battle, it was now only left for Balfour to join with Stapleton's regiment in renewed support of the foot, a task carried out with some success. The two sides fought on till nightfall, fighting themselves to a standstill. The result was a bloody draw.

Hesilrige had been in the thick of the battle. His greatest critic, Denzil Holles, describes the euphoric state of Hesilrige's mind after his return to London:

> ...he thought himself invincible, and absolutely stick free and shott free having had the good fortune to be in a gallant regiment under Sir William Balfore at Kineton Field, and so not run away, but (as himself did

afterwards relate it), to wink and strike, and bear down all before him. This made him so absolute a soldier, that he thought Christendom had not his fellow.[18]

Holles is more than a little biased against Hesilrige, who in reality was only a politician playing soldiers. Years later, Sir Arthur himself summed up the Edgehill campaign:

> ...we met at Edgehill. The King went to Oxford, and gave thanks for the victory, and we at London gave thanks for the victory, and so it was in many other battles.[19]

Although the battle honours were almost equally divided, the tactical advantage lay with the King. Within three months of the battle of Edgehill, the military positions of the rival forces had reached stalemate. Both sides now needed to consolidate what they had and open new fronts in order to stretch the resources of the opposition. In November, the display of parliamentary loyalty by Philip Skippon and the London trained bands at Turnham Green had to all intents and purposes proven that the King could not regain his capital by a simple strike towards it. Any further hostilities would be protracted and decided as much by logistics and economics as by military prowess. This fact being begrudgingly accepted by the King, he withdrew to Oxford (29 November) and quickly established his headquarters and court.

In December 1642, Sir Arthur Hesilrige was commissioned the colonel of a small regiment of horse in a regional command under Sir William Waller. The regiment numbered no more than three troops, at the most two hundred men, but was certainly the best in Waller's army.

Lord Grandison occupied the old Wiltshire town of Marlborough for the King on 5 December. By this simple action the trade route from London to Bristol and the western counties was threatened. Waller's army was ordered to Marlborough and eventually forced Grandison into nearby Winchester, where Sir William Ogle had declared for the King.[20] Wasting no time, Waller attacked the ancient city on Tuesday 13 December, and, being unable to defend himself in a street-to-street confrontation, Grandison retreated into Winchester castle. The castle was surrounded and some of Waller's forces began to loot the suburbs. Bundles of faggots soaked in pitch were prepared for use in storming the castle, but Grandison's forces were in no condition to withstand a siege, and he capitulated.[21]

From Winchester, Waller's forces marched to Southampton, where they received pay and fresh orders to march on Chichester, arriving before the walls on 21 December, having secured Arundel Castle on the way. At Chichester the local 'cavaliers' had opened the gates to a force led by Sir Edward Ford, the High Sheriff of Sussex, after the city had initially declared for Parliament. Upon seeing the roundhead army approaching, the royalists greeted them with a fanfare of artillery, followed by a sally forth by the garrison, who 'was immediately beaten into port, one of ther men being slaine, and another taken prisoner, without losse or hurt of any man on our side only one horse was shott from the port'.[22]

Waller now took up position at a place called 'The Broils' with his own army and some Kent horse under Sir Michael Livesey, plus a few horse and dragoons commanded by Colonel Morley. The first day of the siege was occupied with mounting a battery of artillery, while the heavier guns in the city played upon the besiegers. Before ordering the assault, Waller, Hesilrige and their officers summoned the town by trumpet, offering Ford a treaty 'to save an effusion of blood'. Under this agreement, hostages were exchanged to uphold the peace. Subsequently Waller sent into Chichester Major Horatio Carey of his own regiment and Captain William Carre of Hesilrige's.[23] The parliamentarian commanders now offered terms, but all were refused except for one, the handing over of any papists who could be found.

The truce ended, the parliamentary guns began to fire on Chichester. No sooner had the siege opened but news reached Waller that Prince Rupert was advancing towards him. Despite this threat, the siege continued, and after a fortnight Rupert had still not arrived. Waller was by then ready to increase pressure upon the royalists, having made advances into the suburbs. After further negotiation, Ford accepted defeat rather than subject the place to the full horror of being stormed. On 5 January 1643, the gates swung open, and the defeated royalists and Ford passed into imprisonment in London.

In an attempt to buy off the parliamentary army, the MP for the city, Mr William Cawley, a prominent Sussex man, collected plate and coin to give the soldiers a month's pay.[24]

A service of thanksgiving was held in the ancient Chichester Cathedral, and after the sermon the victorious troops decided the terms of surrender could not possibly cover such a place. The Dean, Dr Bruno Rives wrote of the occasion:

...as men not inspired by the holy spirit, of which they so much boast, but possessed and transported by a Bacchanalian fury, they ran up and down the Church, with their swords drawn, defacing the monuments of the dead, hacking and hewing the seats, scratching and scraping the walls, Sir William Waller and the rest of the commanders standing by as spectators, and approvers of these barbarous iniquities.[25]

Following this behaviour by his men, Waller left for London, leaving Hesilrige to command the army. These extra few days in Chichester cemented a friendship between Hesilrige and William Cawley. Apart from Carre, Horton and himself, Hesilrige's regiment at Chichester probably included the troop of Captain Lieutenant Clarke.

On 11 or 12 January, Hesilrige made a return visit to the cathedral, where Dr Rives takes up the story:

About five or six days after, Sir Arthur Hesilrige demanded the keys to the Chapter House; being entered the place, and having intelligence by a treacherous officer of the Church, where the remainder of the Church plate was, he commanded his servants to break down the wainscot, round the room, which was quickly done, they having brought Crows of Iron for that purpose, along with them; while they were knocking down the wainscot, Sir Arthur's tongue was not enough to express his joy, it was operative at his very heels, for dancing and skipping (pray remark what music that is to which it is lawful for a puritan to dance) he cried out, 'there boys, there boys, hark hark, it rattles, it rattles'; and being much importuned by some members of that Church, to leave the Church but a cup for the administration of the blessed Sacrament, answer was returned by a Scotsman, standing by, that they should take a wooden dish ...[26]

It was not uncommon for Hesilrige to be overtaken by fits of pure joy, the passion of victory affecting all men differently. A man highly strung by the events engulfing his life might relieve tension by either tears or laughter, and Hesilrige was here taken by boyish humour.

Sir Arthur Hesilrige was certainly not quickly forgotten in Chichester; indeed, one story which although interesting is little more than folklore, tells how in 1647 on the invitation of William Cawley he returned to finish the destruction of the walls. The tale alleges that Hesilrige was only too willing.

NOTES

1. Nichols, *Leicestershire*, II, pt ii, p 743.
2. CJ, II, p. 743.
3. LJ, V, p. 147.

4.   E. Peacock, *Army Lists* (London, 1874), p. 53.

5.   Leicestershire Record Office.

6.   DNB (Thomas Horton).

7.   Wedgwood, *The King's War*, p. 117.

8.   CSP Dom, 1641–43, pp. 383-85.

9.   *Memoirs of the Life of Mr Ambrose Barnes* (London, 1867), p. 128.

10.   Brigadier P. Young, *Edgehill 1642: The Campaign and the Battle* (Kineton, 1967), p. 100.

11.   J. Adair, *Roundhead General* (London, 1969), p. 48.

12.   Clarendon, *History of the Rebellion*, II p. 353.

13.   Clarendon, *History of the Rebellion*, II, p. 353.

14.   Possibly Sir William Pennyman's regiment. The author spent many hours discussing Edgehill with Brig. P. Young, and now believes Balfour's regiment struck only the flank of Feilding's brigade, overlapping into Charles Belasyse's, cutting through the gap left by Pennyman's musketeers when sheltering amid their pike.

15.   Rushworth, *Historical Collections*, III, pt ii, pp. 35-39.

16.   T.S. Clarke (ed.), *Life of James II* (3 vols.; London, 1816), I, pp. 9-18.

17.   Young, *Edgehill 1642*, pp. 300-302.

18.   *Memoirs of Denzil Lord Holles* (1699), p. 11.

19.   *Burton's Diary*, III, pp. 95-96.

20.   J. Adair, *Roundhead General*, pp. 50-51.

21.   'Truth in two letters, 9–17 December', TTE 83 (11); 'The latest printed newes from Chichester, Windsor, etc.', TTE 83 (8).

22.   'A True Relation', reprinted in *The History of Western Sussex* (2 vols.; Dallaway & Cartwright, 1815), I. Although this volume is now difficult to obtain, it is invaluable in studying Chichester. The author is grateful for the assistance of the University of Durham for this material.

23.   William Carre is often confused with Sergeant Major General James Carre, who later served with Waller.

24.   J. Webb and T.W. Webb (eds.), *Military Memoirs of Colonel John Birch* (London, 1873), pp. 202-203.

25.   *Mercurius Rusticus* (1685), p. 243.

26.   *Mercurius Rusticus*, p. 243, possibly William Carre.

∽ 4 ∾

The Army of the West

And under their hand was an army, three hundred thousand and seven thousand and five hundred, that made war with mighty power, to help the king against the enemy.

(2 Chron. 26.13)

After a most eventful year, Sir Arthur returned to the political battle-field of the Commons in January 1643. Hesilrige returned to the chamber a champion of Parliament's cause. John Vicars, the pamph-leteer, called Sir Arthur: 'A most pious patriot of his country, a most worthie member of the House of Commons and a most valiant and courageous commander in the late famous battel at Keinton.'[1]

Hesilrige, having tasted the thrill of battle, at once set about preparing for the spring campaign of 1643. Of special interest was the finding of suitable horseflesh for military needs. Throughout January and February, Sir Arthur bought and seized horses for Sir William Waller's army. Where horses were not for sale, parliamentary warrants made them so, until the army's needs were filled.[2]

Despite his obvious political abilities, Sir Arthur failed to obtain a place on the newly formed Committee of Safety. If he had not been so deeply involved with the war in the field, he would probably have sat, for he would lead and attend numerous committees and councils throughout the conflict.[3]

By February 1643, things were not going too well for Parliament. In Cornwall the royalist knight Ralph Hopton had beaten the Devonshire forces loyal to Parliament, and on 2 February the town of Cirencester fell to Prince Rupert. Neither action was vital to the cause, but it worried the Earl of Essex into taking measures against any further threat. On 11 February, Waller was appointed major general in the west, and set up his headquarters at Farnham Castle.

Farnham was well placed to cover the western approaches to London, and for actions along the Bristol, Gloucester and Welsh border along the River Severn and the central drover's routes often used by seventeenth-century travellers. It is well to remember that where cattle can be driven, so can armies.

With Waller established at Farnham, it was left to Hesilrige to complete the raising of his regiment of horse and ride to Farnham with haste. The regiment was urgently needed with Prince Rupert in the field. Sir Arthur never had difficulty raising men. This may be due to two factors: first, Sir Arthur was a wealthy man and could afford to treat his men well, and, second, he played the military man well. Hesilrige joined Waller on the road to Dorset, where they turned to enter Somerset, reaching Bristol on 15 March.[4] The governor of Bristol was Colonel Nathaniel Fiennes, second son of Lord Saye and Sele, an old friend of Sir Arthur's from the Saybrooke Company and those happy days at Fawsley. But Nathaniel Fiennes, despite his pedigree, was not a good soldier, and was perhaps better suited to garrison duty than field warfare. This is not to say Bristol was an easy garrison life, for it was not, the people being in favour of the King and therefore hostile to Fiennes. The royalist forces soon received intelligence of Waller's movements and realized they needed to draw the parliamentarians into the open. Sir William did however have more wit than to march blindly into an engagement to suit the cavaliers. Instead, by cover of night on 23 March, the parliamentarians marched from Bristol with a view of attacking royalist-held Malmesbury with a surprise move.

Riding through the night, the Parliament men arrived before the town around noon, with as many as 2,000 men.[5] Malmesbury was well protected by dry-stone walls along its outer defences. As the parliamentarians went forward, royalist guns and musketeers opened up on them, but the attack flowed forward and Waller's men soon reached the defences. With pikes stabbing across the stone walls, the royalists fell back, allowing Waller's soldiers to enter the suburbs of the town. There followed an attack on the west port, where the parliamentarian musketeers entered into hot street fights, exchanging fire as they fought from house to house at very close quarters. Such was the confusion that Sir William ordered his men to fall back to allow him to assess the position before the next stage of the battle.

Suddenly news reached the parliamentarians that between seven and ten troops of royalist horse were approaching. It was time for Sir Arthur to enter the battle. Sending him from Malmesbury, Sir William Waller required Hesilrige to break this force before it cut him off between the town and the outer areas. Charging forward 'Sir Arthur Haselrig fell out upon them with eight troops but upon his approach they retired speedily.'[6] John Vicars added 'that most godly and gallant gentleman sir Arthur Hesilrige, a man of undaunted courage and bold as a lion, particularly distinguished himself'.[7]

The attack in Malmesbury was now rejoined, but after an hour of 'very hot fight' the parliamentarians were running low on powder, a situation that could cause victory to become defeat. Drums and trumpets again called the ceasefire and the attackers withdrew. Yet Waller was not beaten, for he again drew up his forces in the streets and made as if to storm the town.[8] At the sight of this quite magnificent bluff the royalist garrison surrendered.

From Malmesbury the victors marched towards that natural barrier between England and South Wales, the Severn. A pontoon bridge made with boats floated down from the Gloucester garrison greeted them at the crossing point, and with assistance from Sir Robert Cooke, the army marched to Mitcheldean where it rested on Friday 26 March.[9] After defeating 1,500 Welsh foot, 2 troops of horse and taking 5 guns at Higham House, Sir William and Sir Arthur rode back to the peace of Gloucester. At Gloucester rooms were in poor supply and Hesilrige and Waller were forced to share a house. At this time the two knights were colleagues in war, but it may be too strong to call them friends. In the words of John Vicars, Sir Arthur was Waller's 'fidus Achates', following the major general and faithfully supporting him in the pursuit of their joint cause. Yet the two men appear to have little in common in politics or personally. Politically Sir William was far more moderate than Hesilrige, and in personality, whereas Sir Arthur would rant and rave to achieve his point, Waller was much calmer and had a far sweeter approach to life. Unfortunately, neither man recorded his views of the other, but during the period 1643–44 no general had a more loyal or conscientious assistant. They stayed at Gloucester for ten days, planning the campaign and generally resting after the rigours of the march. Although a puritan, Sir Arthur would take pleasure in well-prepared meals, seeing nothing ungodly in a carefully roasted capon served with a highly spiced sauce and perhaps pieces of fruit and marzipan to sweeten the mouth to follow.

Gentlemen of Hesilrige and Waller's quality would enjoy fine wine with spoonfuls of sugar before sinking into a warm bed of swan feathers to dream of the peaceful days before the war.

While the parliamentarians were quartered at Gloucester, news of Prince Rupert reached them. By 22 March, the Prince had retaken Malmesbury, for Waller was unable to garrison it properly. At this time the sides were taking towns and then handing them back, under-lining the fact that wars were won in the field.[10] It was like a game of musical chairs.

During the ten-day rest at Gloucester, Sir Arthur met Captain Walter Parry, whose troop was part of the Gloucester garrison. Such men as he were vital to Parliament, and Hesilrige lost no opportunity in knowing them.

Their rest completed, the parliamentarians marched from Gloucester on 4 April to surprise the town of Monmouth. As they neared the town, their scouts brought word that the royalists had fled to Raglan Castle. There was no way this small mobile army could besiege the strong walls, and Waller decided to make for the fortified town of Chepstow on the Welsh border. Reaching their goal on 6 April, they found the royalist ship *The Dragon of Bristol* in the harbour. This particular Welsh dragon had little fire in its fat belly and was quickly made a pet of the parliamentary cause. That same day Lord Herbert was appointed the King's lieutenant general in South Wales, which accounted for the lack of resistance to the parliamentarians' march. Herbert fully understood the potential of Waller's army, and was drawing together the small garrisons from Newnham and Ross-on-Wye to form a small field army with which to hamper their advance. Also on this busy day, the parliamentarians received reliable intelligence that the younger of the Palatine princes, Maurice, had joined with Lord Grandison at Tewkesbury and crossed the Severn, thereby successfully cutting them off from the base at Gloucester. If Maurice could now join with Lord Herbert, the two together could attack the outflanked parliamentarians. However, perhaps lacking the military skills of his brother, the young prince failed to join with Herbert, choosing instead to cover the retreating parliamentarians. It was a mistake the older and wiser Sir William took full advantage of. On the night of 10 April, the parliamentarians marched quickly from Chepstow towards Maurice and the Gloucester lines. The foot did not, however, march with the horse and dragoons, but were sent with the baggage and small guns over the River Wye to escape the Severn crossing and the prince. By nightfall, Waller, Hesilrige and the horse were entering the Forest of Dean, where Sir William found himself separated from the main body of horse with less than a hundred troopers with him.[11] Hesilrige did not rejoin Waller until the morning and Waller must have been highly relieved to see him rather than Maurice's cavalier troopers. The parliamentarian horse having rejoined, they steadily moved towards Little Dean, where they viewed before them the prince with not less than two regiments of horse, and one each of foot and dragoons.[12] The Parliament men had no foot of course, but did have a small number of dragoons, and at least some of Hesilrige's regiment had carbines. The greatest weapon this force had, however, was mobility, having no carts or guns to slow it down. The two armies looked at each other, the royalist musketeers firing a round in the usual opening greeting. They stayed in this position for nearly three hours, each commander waiting for the other side to make the first and perhaps fatal move. Suddenly Waller struck, the parliamentary horse charging sharply at the ranks before them. A confused skirmish settled the matter and the road to Gloucester was open once more.

The war the western army was fighting was arduous, with forced marches and desperate skirmishing, so it is not too surprising to find Hesilrige and Waller once again resting their men in the lush pastures of Gloucester. Meanwhile, Edward Massey the governor of Gloucester, was ordered to seize Tewkesbury, which Lord Grandison had seriously weakened by joining with Maurice in the field. This was probably an excellent military move in lengthening the parliamentary line of communication, but by so doing Waller was obviously at risk of spreading his forces too thinly. Massey succeeded in his orders on the morning of 12 April, and Waller and Hesilrige rode to him very late that evening to discuss the next stage of the campaign. Sir Arthur was always joyful in victory, and had a bad habit of believing that each victory had won the campaign. This nevertheless was not a view shared by Prince Maurice.

The prince sent forward his horse that night to secure Upton Bridge, where, after a skirmish with Waller's advance guard, they allowed the main royalist force to cross the next morning.

The parliamentary brigades quickly answered Maurice's move. They advanced from Tewkesbury that morning, heading north towards

Upton over 'King Johns Bridge, which spans the River Avon, up the steep slope of Mythe Hill, and with the Severne on their left followed the old road on towards Worcester'.[13] Arriving at Ripple, three and a half miles from Tewkesbury, the parliamentarians could see Maurice's army deployed. The force with Waller was again mainly horse, although this time Edward Massey had sent a number of his own 'Bluecoat' companies to give the army around 100 foot. The horse numbered 1,300, well above the number with the prince. Yet Maurice had strength of foot and fielded near 2,000 soldiers.

To the roundheads' dismay, their field guns could not find suitable ground and their ball and case-shot did little to restrict royalist movements. If this was not enough, Waller had the added problem of what to do with Massey's bluecoats, for a standing battle would give such an advantage to Maurice that defeat would be certain, yet to run would leave the weaker foot dead or taken. A 'Forlorne Hope' of horse was sent from the parliamentary lines but quickly fell back upon receiving fire from the royalist musketeers lining the thick hedgerows around Ripple. Seeing the position was hopeless for his troopers, Waller decided to retire to Tewkesbury. Maurice could not allow this and ordered an advance. Slowly the parliamentarians made their confused way along the rough tracks, the tall hedges casting giant shadows and in places cutting out the light of day to an eerie amount. Dragoons held the rear, their short muskets ready to fill the narrow lane with deadly flying shot. Massey's now nervous foot plodded their way along the lanes, half expecting attack.[14] All at once a cry went up and the sound of dragoon fire spread along the lane as the royalist troopers charged towards them. The dragoons broke, diving into the hedges and throwing the poor Bluecoats into disorder. It is unlikely that Massey's men had even enough time to draw themselves into a defensive wall of pikes. In a last ditch effort to save the luckless foot, Sir Arthur thundered back along the lane with his own troop of fifty or sixty men. A sharp melee followed, with Hesilrige's small force managing the work of a regiment.[15] The parliamentarians finally struggled into the old town of Tewkesbury and safety.

If the parliamentarians had lost the battle, they had undoubtedly won the spring campaign in the west, and Vicars's description of Sir Arthur as Waller's 'fidus Achates' was no overstatement, for he had served him very well indeed. On 15 April, the Earl of Essex besieged Reading, and the King called upon the small garrisons of Cirencester,

Malmesbury and other loyal west country towns to relieve it. The roundheads had stretched the cavalier forces to their limit, forcing much-needed men away from the King's own Oxford army in order to control only part of the Severn Valley.

With this Sir Arthur Hesilrige hastened to London, leaving Waller to take Hereford in his absence. Hesilrige arrived in London sometime before 18 April, for that day he addressed the House of Commons, telling them of the campaign, after which he received public thanks for his good service.[16]

Since Sir Arthur had joined Waller on the road to Dorset, events at home had taken another tragic turn, and there was even more work to be done.

NOTES

1. *Birch's Memoirs*, p. 52.
2. CJ, II, pp. 949, 957.
3. In his biography of Sir William Waller (*Roundhead General*, p. 57), Dr Adair suggests Hesilrige failed to be voted on to the Committee of Safety because his personality or politics were not trusted by his more moderate colleagues.
4. J. Vicars, *Jehovah-Jireh*, p. 277.
5. Clarendon, *History of the Rebellion*, VI, p. 292.
6. 'A letter from Sir William Waller to the Earl of Essex of a great victory he obtained at Malmesbury', TTE 94 (12).
7. *Jehovah-Jireh*, p. 1292.
8. TTE 94 (12).
9. Adair, *Roundhead General*, p. 61.
10. This applies to the seventeenth century. With the introduction of air warfare in the twentieth century, war was changed to abuse the civil population. This type of strategy by politicians would have totally shocked Hesilrige.
11. Adair, *Roundhead General*, p. 65.
12. Adair, *Roundhead General*, p. 65.
13. P. Young and R. Holmes, *The English Civil War* (London, 1975), p. 120.
14. In recent years many farmers have stopped cutting hedgerows along their fields. It is therefore possible to imagine the countryside in its far wilder state in 1643. In many parts of the country, lanes appear almost boxed in by hedges and trees, and a heavy skirmish under such circumstances must have been horrific.
15. It would appear that only two contemporary accounts of Ripple Field exist: John Corbet, *Bibliotheca Gloucesthensis* (London, 1645); *Mercurius Aulicus*, 8–15 April 1643, reprinted in *The Oxford Newsletters*; of these *Bibliotheca Gloucesthensis* is most interesting.
16. CJ, III, p. 51.

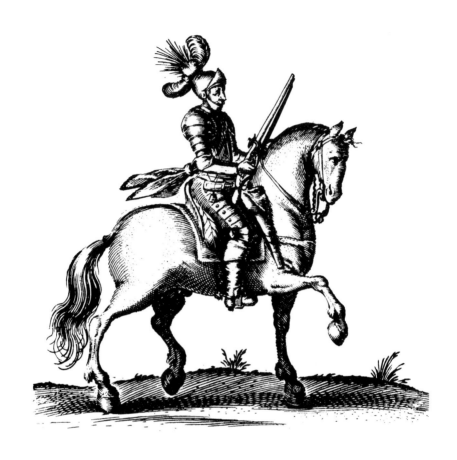

A cuirassier preparing to 'give fire' from John Cruso,
Militarie Instructions for the Cavallrie (1632).

∞ 5 ∞

The Lobsters

And he sent again a captain of the third fifty with his fifty. And the third
captain of fifty went up, and came and fell on his knees before Elijah, and
besought him, and said unto him, O man of God, I pray thee, let my life,
and the life of these fifty thy servants, be precious in thy sight.

(2 Kgs 1.13)

If Hesilrige's own military career was gaining momentum, that of his
brother-in-law Lord Brooke had come to an abrupt end in early
March. Although Brooke had arrived too late to participate at Kineton
Field, he had served Parliament with determined loyalty and was at the
forefront of the struggle. On 7 January 1643, Brooke had been
appointed general and commander-in-chief to the counties of
Warwick, Stafford, Leicester and Derby. His forces took Stratford-
upon-Avon in February and secured Warwickshire. Brooke then
turned into Staffordshire and attacked the royalist garrison at Lichfield,
but with victory almost within its grasp the parliamentary forces were
shattered when a ball from a royalist sniper struck Brooke in the eye
while directing the assault on 2 March.[1] Lord Brooke left a widow
and young children, Sir Arthur and Dorothy Hesilrige—Brooke's
sister—would now take some part in the care of these, for Hesilrige
was a compassionate man to distressed friends and even fallen enemies.

Where Dorothy Hesilrige stayed during 1643 is uncertain. Being
used to both town and country life, it is possible she moved to London,
where her husband spent most of his non-fighting hours. However,
if the words of Denzil Holles are true, Dorothy was in some degree
of safety while at Noseley. The civil war was not completely devoid
of civilities, and a lady and her children were invariably safe from a
passing enemy. Holles does, nevertheless, give an interesting if somewhat pointed description of Noseley during the hostilities:

> ... if his neighbours in Leicestershire say true, that his grounds have con-
> tinued full stocked all the while better than ever they were before, so safe
> and well protected (as I have heard) that his neighbours when there was
> danger, would send their cattle thither.[2]

Holles of course writes with a bitter tongue in cheek, but it is characteristic of Hesilrige to protect his own interests, and surely good farm
management is no crime—it being pure folly to plant seed for birds to
steal, or raise cattle for 'cavaleers' to feed upon.

As previously stated, Lord Brooke left a widow and children, but
what is more important to this story he left uncommanded some of
the finest officers and men to be found in the whole parliamentary
army. These men were ideal for Hesilrige's purpose, and turned to
him for advice. A short biographical examination of the names of
these officers is required in order to fill in the picture of Hesilrige's
soon to be famous new regiment.

Captain John Okey (or Okee): Quartermaster to Lord Brooke in
1642, he was captain of fifty reformadoes by March 1643.[3] Okey is
described by his contemporaries to have been a drayman and then a
poor chandler in London before the war. Yet despite these humble
origins, Okey is one of the best-remembered names from the whole
revolutionary and restoration period.

Many of Okey's troopers that took part in the attack on Lichfield
left there on 23 April to march to Lord Grey of Groby at Leicester.
Okey was by now a captain of foot in Brooke's own regiment.
Before joining Hesilrige, Okey spent a short time in Colonel Richard
Browne's dragoons, a role he would hold in the New Model Army.[4]
From his military record, it is clear that John Okey was a good solid
officer, not totally inspired like Cromwell or many of the future
grandees, but reliable and loyal with a systematic and workmanlike
military brain. John Okey was obviously an asset to any regiment.

Captain Edward Foley: Sometimes called Captain Flower, he was also
late of Brooke's regiment as captain-lieutenant of horse. Who Flower
or Foley was is vague, but an Edward Foley is recorded as matricu-
lating from Clare College, Cambridge, at Easter 1631, and other
Foleys are mentioned as 'of Stourbridge Worcester'.[5] The assumption
that Foley was a Worcesterian is no wild conjecture, for another of
Brooke's officers also came from the area. Foley's troop under
Hesilrige was partly raised in London, a further part coming from
Warwickshire and Staffordshire, Brooke's own areas.[6]

Captain Samuel Gardiner: A Worcestershire man, he fought at

Stafford and Lichfield under Brooke almost as an independent officer, having raised and equipped his own men. Samuel Gardiner was the son of Philip Gardiner, a past mayor of Evesham, who served in 1607 and 1616. Samuel was himself serving as mayor for the third time at the outbreak of civil war. Although he did not take part in the Edgehill campaign, Gardiner received many of those wounded in the battle at Evesham, Parliament paying him an allowance of £160 for the relief of those injured on both sides. For his sympathies towards Parliament, Mayor Gardiner was to become increasingly unpopular with the predominantly pro-royalist members of Evesham corporation, and was eventually removed from office because of his continued absence. It would seem Gardiner was a fairly well-to-do and even wealthy man, having forwarded Brooke and the Parliament sums of money for the war. It would appear alas that the repayment of these loans was rather slow and extremely difficult to acquire in happier days. In fact it is not certain that the good Samuel ever received payment.[7] Gardiner joined Hesilrige 'at ye Swan in ye Strand' on 15 May 1643.[8] The pay books show that Captain Samuel Gardiner, his officers and 56 troopers were paid £134 4s 6d for 14 days ending 19 June.[9]

Captain Walter Parry (or Perry): His probable meeting with Hesilrige was dealt with in the previous chapter. Parry's troop was still at Gloucester on 25 May 1643, for his cornet Nathaniel Hill drew pay for them. Parry himself received £25 on 12 April. By 4 June 1643, Cornet Hill was cashiered and petitioned with Cornet Will Bayley (cornet to Captain Thomas Talbot) for pay and expenses, being 'assured by old soldiers this is according to the ancient and usual disapline of war'. Waller agreed to pay them on 4 June under the military tradition of the 'troops which march are paid'.[10]

Captain-Lieutenant Thomas Horton: While Hesilrige was away in London, Thomas Horton was left for some considerable lengths of time in command of Hesilrige's own troop of horse. At Gloucester on 9 May 1643, Horton drew pay of £45 10s 0d for Sir Arthur Hesilrige's own troop.[11] In a previous chapter it is said that the early career of Thomas Horton is confused. The article in the Dictionary of National Biography would certainly appear to bear little resemblance to the life of Thomas Horton of Sir Arthur Hesilrige's regiment and New Model Army. The dictionary does state that Thomas Horton should not be confused with Jeremy Horton, but then itself confuses Thomas with another Thomas Horton known to Sir Thomas

Fairfax in the north. The dictionary says: 'He joined the army of Sir Thomas Fairfax, and by May 1643 had become a colonel. On 24 June of that year the Parliament resolved that he be recommended to Lord Inchiquin to have the command which Sir William Ogle formerly had in Ireland.' All this is incorrect for Thomas Horton of Noseley, for in May 1643 he was at Gloucester with Hesilrige's regiment and served with it throughout 1644 and 1645 up to its inclusion into the New Model. There were certainly Hortons from Leicestershire up to Yorkshire, for they appear in numerous pamphlets and papers for this period, but the Thomas Horton under Fairfax in 1643 is not the same man.

Other officers said to have served under Hesilrige in the pre-New Model Horse are named as Captain Mason, Captain Thomas Pennyfeather or Pennyfather, Captain Clarke, Captain Carr, Major Nicholas Battersby.[12] Some of those named not holding their appointment during the summer of 1643 and others disappearing from records after Roundway Down.[13] The New Model Army's Colonel John Butler was in the regiment during 1643 as a captain, and even the memoirist Edmund Ludlow claims to have been offered a commission in the regiment. It is quite extraordinary, the number of notable seventeenth-century political and noted personalities who were at some stage in Hesilrige's regiments. It was certainly not a disadvantageous move to be associated with Sir Arthur during the heady days of the early rebellion.

Before continuing with the summer campaign of 1643, a brief description of a 'Lobster', or cuirassier to use the correct term, is required. It is an unfortunate fact that since the last century historians have singled out 'Sir Arthur Hesilriges Lobsters' as an anachronism wholly befitting Hesilrige's character. More recently, Dr John Adair says in his biography of Sir William Waller:

> Politically his connections lay with that extreme wing of the House of Commons, distinguishable from the majority by their suspicion of all peace negotiations and militant desire to win the war, Hesilrige exemplified this latter characteristic by his extravagance in outfitting the troops...[14]

It should nevertheless be remembered that the first reference to Hesilrige's Lobsters is not found until just before the opening battle of the coming campaign. Up to this time Sir Arthur had undoubtedly equipped his men in the conservatively conventional buff coat and single or triple bar helmet. Therefore, why should the Lobsters be attributed to a personal whim, a rather expensive whim, when the whole concept of very heavy cavalry was introduced midway through 1643.

In his cavalry manual published in 1632, John Cruso included a chapter devoted to the military function of the cuirassier. Although by the civil war Cruso's manual was already outdated, it was possibly the only manual available to the cavalry officer in 1642 and the lifeblood of the rare English troopers:

> The Cuirassier is to be armed at all points, and accoated with a buffe coat under his arms, like the Launce. (a) His horse not inferiour in stature and strenth though, not so swift. He must have two cases with good firelocks, pistols hanging at his saddle, having the barrel of 18 inches long and the bore of 20 bullets in the pound (or 24 rowling in) a good sword stiff and sharp pointed like the Lancier. This sort of Cavallrie is of late (b) invention: for when the Lanciers proved hard to be gotten, first by (c) reason is their horses, which must be very good and exceeding well exercised: secondly, by reason their pay was abated through scarcitie of money: thirdly, and principally because of the scarcitie of such as were practised and exercised to use the lance, it being a thing of much labour and industry to learn: the Curassier was invented, onely by discharging the lancier of his lance. He is to have a boy and a nagge (as is otherwhere said) to carry his spare arms, and oat sack, and to get him forrage. His saddle and bit must be strong, and made after the best manner. He is also to weare a scarf, as hath been shewed cap. 20. He is to have his bridle made with a chain, to prevent cutting; and he must be very carefull to have all his furniture strong and usefull.
>
> a. By the Edict for musters published by the States, neither cuirassier, nor harquebusier is allowed to have his horse under 15 hand high.
> b. Namely by the Germans.
> c. Another if not the chief reason why the Lances were left is because they are of no effect, or use but in a straight line, and where they may have leisure and room for their careers: whereas the Cuirassier is not subject to either of these inconveniences.[15]

Cruso's textbook cuirassier would have been difficult to find, if not impossible, in the England of the 1640s. It is unlikely that every member of Hesilrige's regiment had a boy and nagge for example, although officers usually had a servant, and Sir Arthur himself certainly did. Any man so completely armed would require assistance in his arming to fasten the buckles which hold each of the closely fitting plates and hinges in the correct place. The lancer had almost died a natural death by evolution in England, but a few light Scottish lancers could be found in the north within a year, and indeed did good service at Preston in 1648.

Sir Arthur Hesilrige had trained as a cavalry officer long before Cruso wrote his manual and probably already had firm ideas on the use of the horse in battle. More important than that, Sir William Waller had served during the Thirty Years War, undoubtedly seeing the massed squadrons of European cuirassiers outweigh the lighter-armed buff-coated troopers—a good sound military reason for introducing men so armed into the present conflict. If by 1642, regiments of very heavy cavalry were unfashionable, a few cuirassiers armed 'cap-a-pe' could be found on both sides at Edgehill, mainly gentlemen in their personal arms. It is said that cuirassiers required heavier horses than the typical civil war troopers. The same theory maintains that the 'Greate Horse' of the Middle Ages, or the great Tudor charger, had by this time become increasingly rare, heralding the demise of the cuirassier. Nonetheless, during the reign of Henry VIII the English 'demi-launce' in their full armour found mounts enough for the purpose of carrying man and sustaining the 'shock' of a lance attack. The conclusion from this is not one of 'horse breeding' but of finance. It is far more likely that the cuirassier died a financial death, through the cost of equipping a man so. Throughout the war, no regiment under Hesilrige was ever poorly mounted.

The army under Waller frequently faced the King's cavalry under Prince Maurice. Maurice in many respects had greater overall military success than his brother Rupert, and if he was overshadowed by Rupert, it was because Rupert was a romantic, dashing figure with noble features and long dark hair, all anyone could desire in a hero.

Prince Maurice was a continual threat to Waller, and Rupert was rarely more than a few days away ride, so why did Waller not conclude that a shock force of cuirassiers could be useful against superior forces? Hesilrige raised this regiment during spring 1643, adding the experienced and trustworthy officers of Brooke to his small regiment to enable him to field a regiment capable of standing against the best of the royalist horse.

The arming of a cuirassier was truly an economic burden, the full equipment being:

    A breast of pistol proofe
    A backe
    A close caske (helmet)
    A payre of pouldrons
    A payre of vambraces
    A payre of guissets

A payre of gauntlets gloved
A cullet or guarderine
A gorget lined[16]

A surviving example of a Hesilrige suit of cuirassier armour has all
these parts, lined in buff leather, and with breeches of leather to protect the back of the legs and buttocks. It is too convenient to assume
the regiment of cuirassiers were merely a whim of a rich lieutenant
general of horse. The difficulty of obtaining arms of all descriptions
makes the sudden appearance of a complete regiment of cuirassiers
improbable, but nevertheless historically correct. Equipping the
Lobsters must have taken time and planning. As the war progressed,
the armour would have been modified, a triple or single barred helmet
replacing the close casque for better vision and comfort. Indeed, by
the summer of 1644 the cuirassier had possibly died out in Waller's
army too. There is little to suggest that following 1643 Hesilrige's
troopers wore full armour, indeed there is evidence to the contrary.
The actual replacement or repair of broken pieces of armour would
be difficult in an army almost continually marching, even if the cost
of replacing a battered pouldron or bent tasset was met out of private
funds. The armies of Henry V or the Rose Wars could afford the
luxury of a score of armourers with the army, but that kind of warfare
had been eliminated by the appearance of the musketeer. Armies
during the seventeenth century did include 'The Gentilmen of the
Armes' being responsible for the general care of the soldiers' weapons,
but to make a full suit of armour takes time, time a fast moving army
simply has not got.

Waller, awaiting Hesilrige's return, also lacked time. The Journal of
the House of Commons, 25 April 1643:

> For Mr. Wm. Lenthall, Speaker of the House of Commons, The Lords
> and Commons assembled in Parliament, having received information by
> Sir Arthur Hesilrig, a member of the House of Commons, that there is
> great Need of a present Supply, both of Horse and Foote, to be sent, to
> Sir Wm. Waller, the better to enable him to keep the Field, the Enemy
> being very strong; they do hereby declare that all such as shall assist for
> the promoting this great work now in hand, and to the End shall lend to
> Sir Wm. Waller, or to Sir Arthur Hesilrige either Horse or men, fitted and
> prepared for the war, or Money for the carrying on the Work, shall not
> only manifest their being well affected to the Publick, but shall do an
> acceptable Service to the kingdom; And further, the Lords and Commons
> do hereby give order, and declare that what Money shall be by any

disbursed and lent, or other Charge undertaken in this Behalf, upon just Accompt, shall be repaid with interest, out of the publick Stock of the Kingdom; for which, they do engage the publick Faith: And likewise the said Lords and Commons do authorize all such Persons, as shall be appointed by Sir Arthur Hesilrige to receive the monies, Horse, Arms, and other Provisions; as aforesaid, so to have full Power and Authority to give Receipt and Certificate for the same.[17]

Although in theory and practice an active soldier, Hesilrige was still and would remain primarily a politician. While in London, Sir Arthur fulfilled his post with the pedantic vigour associated with his political style. On 12 May, Parliament gave order:

> That the Deputy Lieutenants of the neighbouring Counties of Herts, Middlesex, Essex, Serrey, Suffolk, Cambridge, Sussex and Hantshire, do most urgently meet this Afternoon, and give unto Sir Arthur Heselrig a List of Malignants and ill-affected in their several Counties; to the end that he may, according to my Lord Generals Warrant, seize such Malignants Horses for furnishing his Troops.[18]

During his career Sir Arthur made a speciality of persecuting malignants, because to him a malignant who supported the King was the same as a man fighting in the war for personal gain.

Again on 29 May 1643, Parliament made order in favour of strengthening the army under Waller. His situation in the west was slowly becoming desperate and help was urgently required. The latest order read:

> That a Thousand Pounds be forthwith paid to Sir Arth. Haselrig, upon Account, out of the monies that shall come in upon the Ordinance of Sequestrations to be employed for the Service of the Forces under the Command of Sir. Wm. Waller.[19]

More money was ordered for Waller's forces by sequestration by Hesilrige on 7 June, and Sir Arthur Hesilrige left London with several carts of armour, the sequestered money and the ideal of his new regiment ready to join battle in the west.

NOTES

1. DNB (Robert Greville).
2. *Holles's Memoirs*, p. 135.
3. SP 28/7, fol. 540. The best life of Okey is by H.G. Tibbutt, 'Colonel John Okey, 1606–62', *Bedfordshire Historical Record Society*, 35.

4. H.G. Tibbutt, *Colonel John Okey* (Streatley, 1955), pp. 3-4; DNB (John Okey).

5. Venn and Venn, *Alumni Cantabrigenses*, II, pt i, p. 154.

6. J. Adair, *Cheriton, 1644*, p. 174.

7. *Evesham Notes and Queries* 3 (1973) (with thanks to Worcester and Hereford Record Office for drawing my attention to this material).

8. SP 28/147: 'Account of Samuel Gardiner giving an outline of his career 21 January–15 May 1643'.

9. SP 28/7, fol. 540.

10. SP 28/299.

11. SP 28/299.

12. SP 28/29, Mason: a receipt of Capt. Mason 1643; Pennyfeather: BM Add. MSS 5247; Clarke: Adair, *Cheriton*, p. 174; Carr: BM Add. MS 5247; Battersby: Adair, *Cheriton*, p. 174; BM Add. MSS 5247.

13. For the later careers of these officers, see C.H. Firth and G. Davies, *Regimental History of Cromwell's Army* (2 vols.; Oxford, 1940).

14. Adair, *Roundhead General*, p. 57.

15. J. Cruso, *Millitarie Instructions for the Cavallrie, 1632* (ed. Brig. P. Young; Kineton, 1972). Included here by kind permission of Roundwood Press.

16. W.J. Emberton, *Love Loyalty: The Siege of Basing House* (published privately), p. 117. Mr Emberton assesses the price for a cuirassier's armour to be £3 10s 0d.

17. CJ, III, p. 61.

18. CJ, III, p. 81.

19. CJ, III, p. 109.

∞ 6 ∞

The Invincible Roman

And Saul armed David with his armour, and he put an helmet of brass
upon his head; also he armed him with a coat of mail.

(1 Sam. 17.38)

Sir William Waller had not been idle in Hesilrige's absence, having
made the royalists certain of that by a series of moves. On 16 May,
the royalist army, under Sir Ralph Hopton, Sir William's old friend
but now adversary, gave a defeat to the embryonic Western Association
forces of the Earl of Stamford at Stratton, subsequently making an
advance into Devon. In this 'tussel' at Stratton, the men of Cornwall,
led by their natural leader, Sir Bevill Grenville, fought with distinction. Their loyalty to the Cornish gentry made them a force to note
during that period. To add to Parliament's displeasure, Hopton then
received reinforcements of horse, these being the quality regiments of
the command of the Marquis of Hertford and Prince Maurice, whom
Waller's horse had faced before to some considerable disadvantage.
With this stronger force at his disposal, Hopton continued his advance
to the alarm of the Parliament. By 22 May, Waller was at Bath, aiming
to concentrate a force for the Western Association of Parliament large
enough to meet Hopton in the field. On the march to Bath, Waller
asked the governor of Bristol for six companies of Colonel Alexander
Popham's regiment and they were duly sent. Seeing the problem Waller
faced in assembling a field force of sufficient size to stand against
Hopton, Alexander Popham wrote to Nathaniel Fiennes, governor of
Bristol, requesting his remaining two companies of foot, plus Fiennes's
own regiment of horse and other troops and money, lastly requesting
arms for their use.[1] Colonel Fiennes's regiment duly arrived at Bath on
26 May. Three days later Sir William Waller reached Worcester in an
attempt to take the city before moving to renew the field campaign.
Waller's attempt was abruptly cut short when intelligence reported

that a large brigade of Oxford horse had set out to cut off his army from the western bases. The short siege was ended and Waller marched to Gloucester, arriving on 30 May.

On the return to Gloucester, the pre-New Model disease set in, much of Sir William's force refusing to march unless pay was forthcoming. Eventually only four or five troops of horse failed to march with the army and would still join it once paid.[2]

Meanwhile the royalists had joined forces at Chard on 4 June, their army now numbering some 2,000 horse, 4,000 foot and 300 dragoons, with an added strength of some sixteen field pieces—an army to be faced with some caution.[3] The royalists marched to Taunton, which local horse and Edward Popham's foot gave up. The Marquis of Hertford remained in Taunton and Prince Maurice advanced against Waller. On 8 June the forces under Waller entered Bath, the final move before the main action of the summer. The following day, eight troops of horse and the regiment of dragoons were sent from Bath to shepherd home the retreating forces from Taunton. A small scouting body sent by Waller was surprised by a party of the Earl of Carnarvon, which fell on their rearguard and broke it just south of Chewton Menduip (Mendip). Next day, after a chase, Waller's regiments stumbled upon the bulk of Prince Maurice's horse near Chewton, and after a day of skirmishing the royalists returned to Wells and Waller's troopers to Bath.

Sometime during the next two weeks, Hesilrige rode into Bath with the equipment for his regiment and chests of much needed money.[4] Many thousands of pounds were handed to the soldiers from those noble men in London—on paper, that is. Unfortunately, little actual hard cash ever reached the troops.

Clarendon perhaps gives the best description of Hesilrige's now expanded regiment, although it is extremely doubtful that he ever saw it. He wrote:

> Sir William Waller having received from London a fresh regiment of 500 horse, under the command of Sir Arthur Haslerigge, which were so prodigiously armed that they were called by the other side the regiment of lobsters, because of their bright iron shells with which they were covered, being perfect cuirassiers; and were the first seen so armed on either side, and the first that made any impression upon the king's horse, who being unarmed, were not able to bear a shock with them; besides that they were secure from hurts of the sword, which were almost the only weapons the other were furnished with.[5]

For Clarendon's estimated regimental strength of 500, one must reckon that Hesilrige had six or seven troops. Hesilrige's own troop had not been to London. It had stayed at Gloucester and marched with Waller to Bath. If Walter Parry's troop is included in the number of Clarendon's figure, they too must have marched from Gloucester with the main army. Therefore Hesilrige's entry into Bath was with no more than 360 troopers.

A further large string of bought and sequestered horses must have arrived at Bath with Sir Arthur as first chargers and replacements—a regiment of 500 men require far more mounts than that number, many officers having three or more mounts and quite often with different characteristics. For general transportation, a sturdy horse with stamina for long periods of marching is ideal, but for battle a strong animal with a touch of 'turk' or 'barb' for added speed is desired.

Each of Hesilrige's new troops of horse had a new standard or cornett, each of these small fringed banners having a regimental field of green, and carrying upon it the choice of picture and motto of each troop commander. In all probability, Hesilrige's own standard now changed from the bold anchor device bearing the motto 'only in heaven' to a plain green colonel's standard.[6]

Even with the money and promises of more to come from Hesilrige's appointed friends in London, there was never enough to pay every man his due, eventually local militia units would insist on returning home and desertion would become commonplace. With this in mind Hesilrige and Waller wrote to Speaker Lenthall:

> Wee have a bodie of horse by God's blessinge able to doe the Kingdome good service. The enimie lies still att Wells. That part of the countrie is altogether unfitt for horse. It greeves our soules wee dare not attempt what wee desire. Wee must not hazard your trust like fooles, neither can wee stay heare and starve. Wee have longe and often supplycated you for money. Find us but a way to live without it, or else wee humblie begge a present supply, if not this horse will certainly disband, which thought makes our hearts to bleed.[7]

The parliamentary horse with Waller and commanded by Hesilrige as lieutenant general now totalled as many as 2,500, a force large enough to match Prince Maurice, or even face Rupert if fate deemed it so. To lose any of this magnificent assembly would be a catastrophe, but lose them they would if pay was not forthcoming.

The army assembled at Bath was truly rich in horse, but it lacked sufficient foot. There was an incomplete regiment commanded once by Colonel Horatio Carey, who, having first served with Waller, turned coat just before the skirmish at Chewton. Added to these was Popham's eight companies, plus two weak companies of Sir Edward Popham's and further weak regiments under Colonel Strode and Thomas Essex. A small number of foot from the defeated Earl of Stamford's army were at Waller's disposal, such as they were. All the foot drawn into a single body would not have made a brigade up to Edgehill strength, for even counting Nathaniel Fiennes hurriedly sent party from Bristol, the foote numbered no more than 1,500—the royalists numbering almost three times this. Nathaniel Fiennes had been loath to send any troops to Waller, and it had taken all the pleading of both Waller and Hesilrige to obtain as few as 500 men from him. It has already been stated that Fiennes was in a difficult situation at Bristol, this making him over-cautious in his approach to Waller's field army and meagre with his supply of reinforcements.

During this time letters passed between both sides, arranging for exchanged prisoners, and exchanging the civilities of gentlemen. A proposal that the old friendship between Waller and Hopton should not be spoiled by the simple fact that soon they would be facing each other on a smoke-covered hill, and that despite their obvious differences the two should meet, came from Hopton while Waller was at Bath. Sir William answered in the tone of a friend but declined the invitation.[8] Waller's letter is dated 'Bath 16th June 1643', possibly just before Hesilrige's return.

In due course, for Lieutenant Colonel Herbert Lunsford the royalists exchanged the Scottish professional James Carre, who was taken at Cirencester on 2 February. Carre was appointed sergeant-major general to the foot and dragoons with the rank of full colonel, an obvious reflection upon Waller's officers of foot.[9]

By the end of June, the royalists had advanced to Frome, where they were joined by more horse and dragoons under Major General of Horse Sir James Hamilton, who was no Rupert or Maurice, but with this force added to the royalist offensive things were getting more difficult for the parliamentarians day by day. These fresh royalist troops were billeted in villages between Frome and Bath, away from the main army's guard. Early one morning the royalists awoke to the sound of exploding grenades, and to the total surprise of Hamilton's sleepy troopers, the whole regiment was captured by 250 parliamentarians under the Frenchman, Major Duet.[10]

On 2 July, the royalists moved to Bradford-upon-Avon, securing the bridge over the river. Waller countered the move by drawing upon Claverton Down, two miles west of Bath. From there the parliamentarians could match the royalist movements. The following day, a Monday, saw little in the way of decisive action, only manoeuvring and scouting by both sides. A regiment of horse under the roundhead Colonel Burghill or Burrill, advanced to Monkton Farleigh to wait in nearby woods. The next morning Burghill beat up the outguards of the royalist army, at which the royalists counterattacked and after a time beat him from his position, forcing a fighting retreat to the main army upon Claverton Down. With the aid of the main army's foot and extra horse, Burghill now stood to face the oncoming royalists, fighting a fierce battle with the King's Cornishmen. The bulk of Waller's army retreated back into Bath. The King's forces now found themselves on Lansdown and quickly withdrew for the night rather than risk a night attack. Just before dawn on Tuesday 4 July, an advance guard of royalists approached the southern side of Lansdown Hill. In the early light of morning they saw to their utter surprise the whole of Waller's army deployed above them. Sir William had lived up to his name—the night owl—yet again and stolen the march on the royalists, his army having marched to the top of the hill just before dawn.

There is no evidence to suggest that the royalists saw 'Hesilrige's Lobsters' before the fight at Lansdown, indeed, it was tactically important that the first meeting should be a complete surprise. A full regiment of cuirassiers would be a bitter pill to swallow. However, on 4 July the Lobsters had no part to play. Such was their advantage with the high ground that the parliamentarians simply watched the enemy below struggling to handle teams of horses half maddened by the roundhead guns that played on them from the safety of the hill. Falling back the royalist advance guard found the main body of their army on Banner Hill, in sight of Lansdown, but considering they had lost the surprise, or rather had it taken from them, the royalist commanders decided to retreat to Marshfield to the north-west. The royalists easily accomplished their retreat after beating off a roundhead 'forlorn hope' and reached Marshfield without great hardship.

The parliamentarians moved to the western edge of Lansdown on the 5th, advancing along an old Roman road until they reached the ridge appropriately called Hanging Hill. None of the ground around

Bath was ideally suited to the cumbersome heavy cuirassier, but if Hesilrige was to prove the worth of his heavy troopers, it must be today and not when flat cavalry ground with wide long charges and sweeping movements presented itself. As usual Sir Arthur Hesilrige was probably confident of victory.

Waller had chosen his ground so that any advance of foot would have to be made uphill, a hard contest for even the finest pikes. Breastworks were thrown up by the parliamentarians at the highest point of the position on the hill—Waller would not be thrown from these defensive lines without a bitter fight.

The royalists were advancing. Leaving Marshfield they deployed for battle upon Tog Hill, a position fifty feet lower than Lansdown.

Both sides advanced their dragoons to clear and hold hedgerows between the hills, like the opening gambit of a chess game establishing a pattern of play before committing the main pieces of the game. The dragoons fought hard on the plateau of Freezing Hill. In support rode a troop under Captain John Butler, possibly of the conventional horse in Waller's army, although he claimed to be a Lobster, and after four or more hours the royalists were pushed steadily back to the foot of Tog Hill. The royalists were by this time running low on ammunition. It had been a hot skirmish and another retreat to Marshfield was becoming increasingly likely. Realizing this, and not wishing to lose the advantage of his early morning ploy, Waller ordered a body of 200 horse and a further 200 dragoons to join the attack. The horse were led by the already famous Major Duet, the dragoons by Colonel James Carre. The royalist Captain Richard Atkyns, to whom historians are most grateful, takes up the story in a detailed style:

> ...they sent down a strong party of horse, commanded by Colonel (Robert) Burell, Major (Jonas) Vandruske and others; not less than 300 and five or six hundred dragoons on both sides of the hedges, to make way for their advance, and make good their retreat. And this was the boldest thing that I ever saw the enemy do; for a party of less than a 1,000 to charge an army of 6,000 horse, foot and cannon, in their own ground, at least a mile and a half from their body.[11]

The royalist troopers attempting to cover their retreating foot received galling fire from the nearby roundhead dragoons, and panic and disorder spread to the foot, the royalist mounts bucking and kicking as the dragoons emptied their weapons into the ranks of the enemy. The parliamentarian horse charged forward after the fleeing

royalists, scattering to bodies of royalist horse before they were finally
halted by the Cornishmen and the horse under the Earl of Carnarvon.
Moreover, more of the royalists now turned to fight, and, suffering
from the fire of royalist field guns, Duet, Carre and their brave little
band fell back towards Waller's position on Lansdown. To support the
retreat, Waller ordered Burghill's regiment to cover them. A confused
and dangerous melee followed with the opposing horse charging and
counter-charging fiercely, dragoons and musketeers adding support
from fire power. So far, Duet and Carre had made their mark, while
Burghill had held the ground before the parliamentarian position.
But what of Hesilrige and his metal men? Here is Clarendon's description of what happened when the royalists decided to fall back on
Marshfield:

> As great a mind as the King's forces had to cope with the enemy, when
> they had drawn into battalia and found the enemy fixed on top of the hill
> they resolved not to attack them upon so great disadvantage and so
> retired again towards their old quarters: which Sir William Waller per-
> ceiving, sent his whole body of horse and dragoons down the hill to
> charge the rear and flank of the King's forces; which they thoroughly, the
> regiment of cuirassiers so amating the horse they charged that they totally
> routed them, and standing firm and unshaken themselves, gave so great
> terror to the King's horse, who had never before turned from an enemy,
> that no example of their officers, who did their parts with invincible
> courage, could make them charge with the same confidence and in the
> same manner they had done.[12]

The regiment of cuirassiers described by Clarendon was obviously
part of the main body, which does not fit well with the claims by
Atkyns. Nevertheless, Richard Atkyns was only a small part of that
royalist army and may not have known of the main cavalry action at
Cold Ashton, where the Lobsters, with the element of surprise, forced
a setback to Hopton's plans that day.[13] Clarendon continues:

> ... three hundred musketeers, had fallen upon and beaten their reserve of
> dragooners, Prince Morrice and the Earl of Carnarvon rallying their horse
> and winging them with the Cornish Musketeers, charged the enemy's
> horse again and totally routed them, and in the same manner received
> two bodies more, and routed and chased them to the hill: where they
> stood in a place almost inaccessible.[14]

Of course the reserve of dragooners were those of Carre aided by
John Butler and later Duet, the two bodies later received and routed
being Burghill's covering force. But again, where was Hesilrige and

the main body of horse? Clarendon calls the turn of the royalist horse a rally, but if indeed Hesilrige's forces did rout a goodly number of the royalist cavalry, it would have taken time to halt the rout and redress the ranks, enough time for the Lobsters to redeploy on Lansdown Hill ready to stand against a royalist counterattack or make the general advance. The only other explanation is that the Lobsters were themselves routed after their opening success, but this does not agree with Clarendon's earlier statements.

With the return of his army to the hillside fortifications, Sir William Waller feigned a wholehearted retreat. Powder was dramatically blown up, implying that the parliamentarian army was on the move. Waller planned to draw the royalists on. The royalist foot on Freezing Hill were under fire from the guns above them, and rather than stay there cried to their officers to advance. The foot began a do or die frontal attack with flanking movements to east and west of the hill, while Sir William watched the advance from his position on Lansdown. Waller had strong parties of horse and foot in the wooded areas either side of the main parliamentarian body. The Cornishmen led the assault, with musketeers to their left and a body of horse to their right. The ground on which these brave Cornish pikemen were forced to advance was almost impossible, steep and broken by hedges and other natural obstacles, making the frontal attack arduous. Upon reaching the top of the hill the royalist foot was greeted by a blast of case-shot from Waller's artillery and volley after volley from musketeers—they halted. By attacking the breastworks to their front the royalists had met a real baptism of fire, but the hardest fighting was still to come.

Hesilrige now led his regiment in three desperate charges, Sir Arthur himself charging with great courage. John Vicars describes his exploits:

> Sir Arthur, like another Roman Marcellus charged so magnanimously, and was himself so far engaged that, had he not most invincibly beshired himself, he had been taken prisoner more than once or twice; in which terrible bickerings he received a wound in the thigh with a push of a pike, and after that another in his arm; but not mortal or dangerous, but only as cicatrices or scars and badges of honour.[15]

It must be stressed that John Vicars was the closest thing Sir Arthur Hesilrige had to a fan club, and the above glowing report of his hero's behaviour may be somewhat biased. The tale of the 'invincible

Roman' is nonetheless a superb if overstated case.

Many of the Lobsters received pike wounds in the thighs, their mounts suffering even more.[16] At the third charge, the royalist colonel of the brave men of Cornwall, Sir Bevil Grenville, collapsed mortally wounded, his captain lieutenant falling dead beside him. At this point, the shock of losing their commander could have swung the battle into a total royalist rout, but, seeing his father fall, the young son of Sir Bevill cried heroically for the Cornishmen to fight on, the men attacking even more fiercely in response. Waller now led a further four charges, but despite this the royalists were edging ever closer to the parliamentarian breastworks. Richard Atkyns relates: 'When I came to the top of the hill I saw Sir Bevill Grenvill's stand of pikes, which certainly preserved our army from a total rout.'[17]

The air grew thick and stale with smoke and shot. Royalist field guns were dragged up, their fire adding to the slaughter. Eventually, under considerable pressure, the parliamentarians fell back to a stone wall a hundred yards to the rear of the breastworks. The royalists moved their musketeers through the woods the parliamentarians had used for a defence, but the cavalier army had fought itself to a stand-still and Waller's men held the wall. With the night the sounds of battle died away, the darkness swallowing up both armies until peace was once more the delight of Lansdown Hill.[18] Waller withdrew his army to Bath, and safety. He took all his guns from the bloody hill, leaving clumps of flickering light, yards of burning match and clumps of pikes to represent his army to tired royalist eyes. Unknown to the parliamentarians, the King's men had also partly withdrawn to Tog Hill and one swift advance would have settled the matter.

In a letter to the Speaker dated 'Roundway this 12 Juli 1643' Waller and Hesilrige told of Lansdown Fight:

> Sir,
>
> We cannot but give you a short account of some fast passages amongst us...we had a weary and dangerous days fight the night partinge us and soe well did we knocke each other that in the night we both retreated many of their Cheife Commanders and officers were slayne or hurt we lost only one Sergeant Major of the Dragoons and two Cornetts and not twentie common soldiers. We had the advantage of the ground but the Cornish Hedgers beate us from it though they bought it att a deare rate when our foote left it wee mayntayned it with our horse, and those Sr Arthur Hesilrige brought from London did most exelent service. Upon Fryday followinge hearinge the enemie drew towards the Devizes wee

resolved to attend him not doubting but his bulke of plunder would something Retard his journy upon Saturday about foure in the afternoone we undertooke that the enimie was att Chipnum about 3 miles from us whereupon taking a playne we drew up with a body & sent out our scoutes & stronge parties and faced the enimie expectinge a battaile in the playne. But the enimie drew up in a moore close by the towne side and there stood that night and the next day beinge the Lords day til about 12 of the clocke and then began to draw of towards the Devizes wch we understandinge advanced and about 3 miles from the Devizes we fel upon there rear...[19]

The foot of Lord Mohun's regiment took the weight of the parliamentary attack, losing some forty dead and a further seventeen wounded The royalists were beaten into Devizes, and that night three troops of parliamentarian horse rode to secure the high ground called Roundway Hill.

Royalist morale was not high. Ralph Hopton had been terribly burned the day after Lansdown when a powder cart exploded near him. Sir William Waller had been distressed at this news, and Hesilrige was never a man to receive pleasure from such a disaster.

On Monday 10 July 1643, the two armies skirmished near Devizes, but once more the royalists retreated to safety in the town before a full battle could be joined. That evening, a strong party of royalist horse under Prince Maurice and Hertford broke out of Devizes in a dramatic attempt to ride for Oxford and reinforcements. 'Over Salisbury playne they rid very fast yet all cried halt, halt, but noe man stood.'[20]

The 11th saw the parliamentarians capture five wagons containing ammunition much needed by Hopton, fresh royalist horse from Oxford under Lord Crawford also being chased off by Waller's troopers. By now Waller had before Devizes his whole army, which was at least as strong as at Lansdown and undoubtedly in high spirits. With the parliamentarians before this important royalist garrison town, Ralph Hopton sent forth a trumpeter requesting a truce, which was agreed. The royalist commander used his time well: on hearing of a shortage of match for the musketeers, he ordered that a collection of all the bed cords in the town should be made. Amazingly, from Hopton's sequestered bed cords the musketeers were provided with fifteen hundredweight of match, after preparation, that is.

The parliamentarians made their assault upon Devizes on Wednesday 12 July, the streets of the town having shot fired into them. However, in a town so heavily and well defended, a siege would take considerable time—time Waller quite simply had not got. The next day news was received of a great body of royalist horse advancing swiftly from the direction of Marlborough, the besiegers withdrew to Roundway Down.

The ground at Roundway was no better suited to the Lobsters than the hills around Bath, being high and impossible in places. Hesilrige must have been confident. Eight days after Lansdown his wounds would still be sore, but would be healing, and his cuirassiers were invincible—were they not?

By early afternoon the roundheads could see massed ranks of royalist horse on Morgan's Hill. Prince Maurice had achieved his aim, returning with three brigades of horse, perhaps 2,000 men, under Lords Wilmot, Crawford and Sir John Byron. From Morgan's Hill the royalists fired light guns, the signal for Hopton to break out of Devizes and advance upon the 'enemie'. Hopton urged his officers to march, but the safety of the town was too great an attraction and the foot refused.

The parliamentarians had meanwhile drawn up with their foot in the centre, their horse upon each wing and cannon before the foot. Of the Lobsters, Captain Richard Atkyns, who charged that day in the regiment of Prince Maurice to the right of Wilmot's brigade, gives by far the best account: '...their right wing of horse being cuirassiers, were I'm sure five, if not six deep, in so close order, that Punchinello himself had been there, could not have gotten into them.'[21]

From this, it would appear Atkyns had not seen the cuirassiers before. With the royalist horse coming on, Sir Arthur Hesilrige led his cuirassiers forward, not with any pace at first, the object of the exercise being to keep good order, to deny Punchinello, or Richard Atkyns for that matter, any access. No doubt Hesilrige had it in mind to force the regiment through the royalist ranks and to sweep both left and right to attack the rear and exposed flanks—not unlike the old naval ploy during Drake's time. But the English success over the Armada would not be reconstructed on Roundway Down. Sweeping up the steep hill, the Lobsters struck the looser ranks of Lord Wilmot's brigade, the shock being heavy on both sides, but to their horror the cuirassiers had not broken through. The next few moments must have been a nightmare, as, instead of being on the far side of the royalist line, the Lobsters themselves were caught in the flanks by the extended royalist brigades and thrown into complete disorder. Hesilrige rallied his men once and recovered four pieces of artillery, but the Lobsters fled at the sight of a second brigade advancing in support of Wilmot. Clarendon says of the parliamentary horse: '...more perished by falls and bruises from their horses, down the precipices, than by the sword'.[22]

Hesilrige's tin men could not cope with the ground upon that steep slippery Down in their heavy cuirassier arms, and their fate was sealed. Of Sir Arthur himself, Atkyns has left a dramatic account:

> Twas my fortune in a direct line to charge their general of horse (Sir Arthur Hesilrige), which I suppose to be so by his place; he discharged his carbine first, but at a distance not to hurt us, and afterwards one of his pistols, before I came up to him and missed with both: I then immediately struck into him, and touched him before I discharged mine: and I'm shure I hit him, for he staggered and presently wheeled off from his party and ran. When he wheeled off, I persued him, and had not gone twenty yards after him, but I hear a voice saying, 'Tis Sir Arthur Haslerigge follow him' but from which party the voice came I knew not they being joined.

Atkyns would have little difficulty chasing Hesilrige, the heavy armour slowing him down:

> And in six score yards I came up to him, and discharged the other pistol at him, and I'm sure I hit his head, for I touched it before I gave fire, and it amazed him at that present, but he was too well armed all over for a pistol bullet to do him any hurt, having a coat of mail over his arms and a head piece (I am confident) musket proof, his sword had two edges and a ridge in the middle.'

If Atkyns is to be believed, Hesilrige was wearing a normal suit of clothes under his cuirassier armour lined with buff leather at every joint, with chain-mail over all this. Atkyns surely does not describe a seventeenth-century cuirassier, for mail was not normally worn over plate armour. Indeed, the sixteenth-century noble 'Gendarme' would have been proud of the armour described by Atkyns that day. Down a hill rode Sir Arthur, fighting his way clear of the royalist captain— but within 120 yards Atkyns was up to him again, having the swifter mount:

> I stuck by him a good while, and tried him from head to the saddle and could not penetrate him, not do him any hurt; but in this attempt he cut my horses nose, that you might put your finger in the wound, and gave me such a blow in the inside of my arm amongst the veins that I could hardly hold my sword.

Once again Sir Arthur escaped, but within 'eight score yards' Atkyns caught up to him and the desperate melee continued. Atkyns attacked Hesilrige's horse, running it through the belly, to which the parliamentarian replied by striking his enemy's mount upon the cheek. By now the running battle had taken its toll on both men, and at this point a second royalist, Robert Holmes, later an admiral, entered upon the conflict:

> In this nick of time came up Mr. Holmes to my assistance, and went up to him with great resolution and felt him before he discharged his pistol, and though I saw him hitt him twas but a flea biting to him; whilst he charged him I employed myself in killing his horse, and ran him into several places and upon the faultering upon his horse his headpiece opened behind, and I gave him a prick in the neck, and I had run him through the head if my horse had not stumbled at the same place: then came in Captain Buck a gentleman of my troop, and discharged his pistol upon him also, but with the same success as before, and being a very strong man, and charging him with a mighty hanger, stormed him and amazed him but fell off again: by this time his horse began to faint from bleeding, and fell off from his rate, and which said Sir Arthur, 'What good will it do if you kill a poor man?' said I 'take quarter then' with that he stopped his horse, and I came upto him, and bid him deliver his sword, which he was loathe to do; and being tied twice about his wrist, he was fumbling a great while before he would part with it...[23]

But Hesilrige was not to fall captive, for at that moment a runaway troop of parliamentary horse saw him in dire distress and made the rescue. With Hesilrige's Lobsters totally routed the rest of Waller's army soon broke, leaving the foot to the mercy of the enemy. For over an hour the roundhead foot beat off repeated royalist charges, but at the sight of the Cornishmen, who were at last coming from Devizes, the parliamentary foot were forced to fall back under such great pressure that they were put to flight.[24] The royalists claimed to have killed 600 and taken 800 prisoner.

On the same evening as the Roundway disaster, much to the astonishment of Nathaniel Fiennes, Waller and Hesilrige, with the 'shattered remains of the lobsters, rode through the gates' of Bristol.[25] Denzil Holles puts the blame for the parliamentarian defeat squarely on the shoulders of Hesilrige, saying:

> When their Army was beaten through Sir Arthur Haslerig's default one of their invincible Champions. First by his ignorant fool hardiness; and afterwards, by his baseness and cowardice; who then found himself to be

mortal; and finding that resistance which he did not expect, ran away as
basely with all him horse, leaving the foot engaged.[26]

It is a fact that Holles accuses almost all his enemies of cowardice,
and up to this time Sir Arthur had been a model of dash and fearless
spirit. To say Hesilrige lost his nerve at Roundway Down is far too
convenient. He had every reason to believe his heavily armed troopers
could punch their way through the royalist brigades, for eight days
earlier, according to Clarendon, the royalist horse had suffered at the
hands of the Lobsters. Holles neither takes into consideration the flair
for success of Prince Maurice, nor the uphill attack which slowed the
roundhead horse and decreased the shock along the line. If Hesilrige
ran, so did the rest of Waller's horse. If Richard Atkyns was correct in
assuming hand-to-hand combat with Sir Arthur, the mounted fighting
had carried them both at least half a mile from the main position. The
fact that troopers on both sides were still with them signifies above all
else a confused and sprawling cavalry action split into many groups.
Holles also declares: 'He would not be governed by his Commander
in Chief, in that Western Brigade, (a gallant and discreet gentleman;)
but would charge contrary to order without sence or reason'.[27]

If the Lobster's charge had broken Lord Wilmot's brigade, the battle
was won, but by waiting as at Lansdown the parliamentary army
would have been caught between horse and foot. What would
Denzil Holles have said then?

Whether or not Sir Arthur lost his nerve at Roundway Down, he
would never again lead his regiment with the same dashing style. The
wounds he received there must have left a lasting memory of battle.
An old story attributed to none other than King Charles tells how,
upon hearing of Hesilrige's narrow escape, the King turned to one of
his officers and remarked that had Sir Arthur 'been supplied as well as
fortified, he would have withstood a siege'. The jest was one that
Hesilrige would not have enjoyed. It was also taken up in royalist
song, as the soldiers sang their verses of the 'Ballad of Runnaway
Down', telling of how Hesilrige was 'armed from his head to his arse,
in a hundredweight of iron'. Had Richard Atkyns taken Hesilrige
prisoner, Oxford would probably have been witness to a great political trial of the kind Strafford had suffered at the hands of the puritans.
No quick escape would be given and no exchange for some royalist
officer would be forthcoming for such an enemy of the Court, just a
show trial followed by the noose, knife and axe of the executioner.

How badly Hesilrige was injured in the fighting is difficult to say. He had a wound in the neck and pistol shots to the body and head, plus attacks from two other royalists with pistol and the sword called a hanger. Head blows are serious, whether lessened by armour or not, and even with armour the body blows could cause severe bruising. Whatever the truth of his condition, he was at least sufficiently hurt to warrant 'publicke prayers' to be read in the London Churches.[28] Sir Arthur was not alone in his injuries or the only one to suffer hardship at Roundway. Young Edward Harley, the eldest son of Sir Robert Harley, was with a younger brother at Roundway, where he lost a horse that 'his anxious mother Lady Brilliana had given him, and narrowly escaped there with his life'.[29]

On 16 July, Waller's army, or rather the remains of it, marched from Bristol to Gloucester, leaving at Gloucester 200 troopers for the governor, Edward Massey. This garrison force of troopers included Walter Parry's troop. The army now marched back to London via the friendly Warwickshire countryside. Waller and Hesilrige rode into London beaten, Waller with about 100 troopers, Hesilrige with 20.[30] Considering the completeness of their defeat, Waller and Hesilrige must have been apprehensive at their welcome, but to their surprise Parliament received them in triumph.

NOTES

1. Alexander Popham to Nathaniel Fiennes, 24 May 1643, Bodl. Clarendon MSS 22, fol. 43.
2. Adair, *Roundhead General*, p. 72.
3. Adair, *Roundhead General*, p. 72.
4. *Weekly Intelligencer*, 13–20 June 1643, E 55 (8); Waller to Speaker, 26 June, Portland MS vol. I, p. 714.
5. Clarendon, *History of the Rebellion*, VII, p. 104.
6. A sketchbook of standards in the National Army Museum describes 'Sir Arthur Hesilrige's new Cornet, plaine greene damaske'.
7. Waller and Hesilrige to Speaker, 22 June 1643, Bodl. Tanner MSS 62 fol. 128.
8. The author believes this letter is famous enough not to be included herein. A copy is to be found in Dr Adair's *Roundhead General*, pp. 75-76, and M. Coate's *Cornwall in the Great Civil War and Interregnum 1642–1660* (Oxford, 2nd edn, 1963 [1953]), p. 77. Clarendon, MSS 22, fol. 113 is the original.
9. SP 28/7, fol. 535; SP 28/8, pt 1, fol. 63; SP 28/14, pt 1, fol. 70.
10. Adair, *Roundhead General*, p. 76.
11. *The Vindication of Richard Atkyns* (ed. Brig. P. Young), p. 18.

12. Clarendon, *History of the Rebellion*, VII, p. 106.

13. S.R. Gardiner, *The History of the Great Civil War, 1642–1649* (3 vols.; London, 1886), I, p. 170. This account can be most misleading but is nevertheless worthy of consideration.

14. Clarendon, *History of the Rebellion*, VII, p. 106.

15. Vicars, *Jehovah-Jireh*, pp. 379-80.

16. It is the author's experience that horses will only near levelled pikes under great urging and even then with the greatest reluctance. To charge the Cornish pikes, the Lobsters must have opened the ranks with their carbines and pistols.

17. *The Vindication of Richard Atkyns*, p. 19.

18. 'A True Relation of the greate Victory etc.', E 60 (12); Vicars, *Jehovah-Jireh*, pp. 376-80.

19. Waller and Hesilrige to Speaker, 12 July 1643, Tanner MSS 62, fol. 164.

20. Waller and Hesilrige to Speaker, 12 July 1643, Tanner MSS 62, fol. 164.

21. Young, *Richard Atkyns*, p. 23.

22. Clarendon, *History of the Rebellion*, VII, p. 118.

23. Young, *Richard Atkyns*, pp. 23-25.

24. *Mercurius Aulicus*, 9–15 July 1643, TTE 70 (80), repr. Oxford Newspapers; *Kingdomes Weekly Intelligencer*, 11–18 July 1643, E 61 (1).

25. *Birch's Memoirs*, p. 44.

26. *Holles's Memoirs*, p. 11.

27. *Holles's Memoirs*, p. 11.

28. *Bibliotheca Gloucesthensis*, p. 202.

29. *Birch's Memoirs*, p. 44n.

30. *Parliament Scout*, 20–27 July 1643; *Birch's Memoirs*, pp. 50-51n.

∽ 7 ∾

Colonel of Horse and Foot

And he found a new jawbone of an ass, and put forth his hand, and took it, and slew a thousand men therewith.

(Judg. 15.15)

That Hesilrige is said to have ridden into London gives little idea of the sad state of his health in the days following Roundway Down. The death of Sir Arthur would have been a severe blow to parliamentary morale, having already lost Brooke, and on 18 June their patriotic champion John Hampden had fallen at Chalgrove Field. In the north the Fairfax-led army had been soundly beaten at Aldwalton Moor on 30 June, and now the great hope of their cause in the west lay in ruin on the hills around Devizes. Add to this news that Nathaniel Fiennes had surrendered Bristol to Prince Rupert, and that the King marched even now on Gloucester, and the Parliament's cause was quite clearly at its lowest ebb. Fiennes was made the scapegoat for the surrender of Bristol, and tried for his life—which he almost lost.

At Gloucester, Colonel Massey put up a stout defence. During the siege, Captain Walter Parry joined the defenders, drawing saddles and pistols for a troop by order of the Commons.[1] Parry was like so many of the Officers, wealthy and able to lend money to Parliament to pay for the war.[2]

Even before the destruction of the Western Army at Roundway Down, the idea of a new standing army had been proposed by the radical war party in London. Upon his return, despite his defeat, Waller was elected to lead it. This idea of a 'New Army' was taken by the Earl of Essex to be a slight upon his position as lord general, the militia bill giving him the authority to appoint generals. Parliament had made a serious mistake in their privilege by overlooking Essex's authority over the militia. Even worse for Essex, he was not popular with many of his own army, and the men were flocking daily to the banners of the new force under Waller. On Friday 28 July, Essex reported to the Lords that, because of the 'New Armie', his own now numbered no more than 2,500 horse and 3,000 foot, and with biting jealousy he demanded an explanation be sought into the defeat of the old Western Army.[3] It was typical of Essex to complain that his own troubles were caused by others, but if his own soldiers wished to leave him, he failed to ask himself why. The Commons, not wishing for a rift between themselves and the Peers, voted the lord general some 4,000 recruits, but refused to hold an inquiry into the western disaster and pillory Waller.

For the period following Sir Arthur Hesilrige's return to London, nothing is heard of him. It seems likely that the pike wounds he received from the Cornishmen at Lansdown and the further blows from Atkyns during the frantic melee along Roundway Down were enough to keep him from public life for some weeks. During this period of rest and healing, the New Army was assembled, vastly reduced in size following Essex's objections. The petty jealousy of the lord general delayed the war effort by nearly three months.

Once again Hesilrige's horse were numbered in Waller's army. The old 'Lobster' captains being reappointed, strengthened by others and the regiment slowly brought up to the muster. The latest formula for Hesilrige's horse was possibly far less in the way of cuirassiers, the heavy armour having served them badly at Roundway, and was difficult to replace.

At Bristol earlier in the year, Hesilrige had met John Birch. Reunited in London during Sir Arthur's enforced rest, Birch was invited to hold the commission of lieutenant colonel in a newly raised regiment of foot commanded by Hesilrige.[4] The new infantry regiment never received the same love Sir Arthur felt for the horse. It was against Hesilrige's nature to suffer the self-discipline required of the foot officer, to allow for a steady, even orderly advance or to watch the enemy guns test his range, hot lead flying into the ranks. Although the massed blocks of pike and musket were the rigid backbone of the army, the charging horse, with their sweeping movements across the field of battle, were the decisive arm in the field—the winner. And above all things Sir Arthur considered himself a winner. It is hardly surprising then that Sir Arthur left the everyday administration of the foot to Birch, who was handed his commission on 2 September.

On the same day a warrant of Sir John Dingley to the hundreds of Kingston and Elmbridge in Surrey, ordered:

> Wheras the Committee for Sir Wm. Waller and Sir Arthur Haselrig for raising a force of horse and foote are informed that there are divers horse and arms belonging to the state left within your hundreds for the recovery of which the Committees have directed an order to me: these are to require you to make search and seize all such horses and arms as you shall find to be left, sold or pawned, and to bring the same to the sign of the Crane at Kingston on the 7th inst by 8 a.m., where I will be ready to receive them.[5]

From this order it is clear that Sir Arthur was second-in-command to Waller, but in reality he was far more than a lieutenant general of horse, for he commanded a place of high prestige in the Western Association itself and was governable by few outside of Parliament.

Unfortunately, the officers in Waller's new force did not please the more radical members of the war party of Independents the Commons was now breeding, who favoured more fiery zealots than Sir William gave consideration to. To placate these radicals, Waller appointed Sir Arthur as president of a council 'to examine the merits of every man that should stand to bear any office in that army, with power to cross all such out of the list as should be judged unfitt or unworthy to be employed'.[6] Sir Arthur himself was considered a radical, but was a friend of Pym and the old 1641 group that was so trusted by all bar the ultra-moderate peace group of Presbyterians led by Denzil Holles. Even as Sir Arthur undertook this role of political St Peter, weighing and noting each sin of the chosen, war was raging in the green fields of England. Blinded by a case of reckless political dogma, the radicals were themselves causing the new army to bleed to death from their own savage cuts. Being unpaid and without service, the men of Waller's force began to seek service elsewhere. The second and third weeks of September, saw this army still around Staines and Windsor, with Hesilrige still in London.

Suddenly, without warning, the game was thrown wide open. On 23 September, Essex rode into London carrying news of a tactical victory at Newbury, having consequently opened the Gloucester road.[7] Yet again Essex was back in favour, and to present a unified picture Waller yielded to public opinion and surrendered his commission over the new force. There followed a short costly period for the western leader, when to build flagging morale he and Essex chose a cosmetic closing of the ranks. Things looked considerably brighter now than in mid-summer. To add to Parliament's joy, the Scottish Kirk had agreed to a Presbyterian army crossing the border in aid of their puritan brothers in England. There would be a delay before any Scottish covenant force was ready to join the war, but once joined the King would always have a superior force against him in the north.

In the second week of October, news reached London of a victory against the Lincolnshire cavaliers at Winceby, a victory brought about by the combination of the Eastern Association forces of the Earl of Manchester, and the Northern Army of Lord Ferdinando Fairfax and his son Sir Thomas. Also involved in this victory was the slowly emerging cavalry commander, Oliver Cromwell, whose name was just becoming known outside of his own East Anglia. It is interesting to note that, even towards the second winter of the war, Hesilrige was superior to Cromwell in both the debating chamber and military. Tactically, the judgement of Cromwell on the battlefield far surpassed that of Sir Arthur, but both men were merely learning the craft in the field. Whereas Hesilrige charged with the heart and God's grace upon his soul, Oliver fought with head and heart and full knowledge that God was his strength and saviour. Cromwell's attitude to the field of force was workmanlike, owing little to previous generations but much to a belief in good men and their place in the Kingdom of Heaven. During this baptism of Oliver Cromwell, further victories came at Gainsborough and Lincoln, and Newark was once more put under threat.

In late September the Western Association's old adversary, Ralph Hopton, attended a meeting at Oxford, where he was ordered to renew the campaign by regaining control of Wiltshire, Hampshire and Dorset, and press as far as possible towards London—no small feat. Before Waller could make ready an army for the Western Association, which was formerly to have been part of the 'New Army'—Ralph Hopton would have to play the poacher and bag what choice morsels he could before he was caught. By mid-October, the royalist army under Hopton was assembled around Bristol, and a quick attempt was made on Wardour Castle before falling on Lyme and Poole. News reached London of Hopton's whereabouts soon after, and Essex marched in a counter-move not south-west but north and Newport Pagnell, threatening Oxford. Meanwhile the Western Army was to gather at Farnham by 1 November to march against Hopton.

For once this Western force included a strong number of foot in the guise of 'The London Trayned Bands', and the newly raised regiment of Sir Arthur Hesilrige in their 'blewcoats', under the careful eye of John Birch. Only two troops of Hesilrige's horse set out at this time, but they included the old, experienced 'Lobster' Samuel Gardiner, who had recently been relieved of his position as mayor of Evesham by the pro-royalist corporation. In reality the removal of Gardiner by those paper tigers was but a token of their feelings, for he had only a few days left to serve as mayor and had been absent for most of the year. The rest of Hesilrige's horse mustered near London on 17 November and joined the army at Farnham Castle four days later.

The London trained band's own travelling amateur historian, Elias Archer, noted the arrival of 'five Companies of foote, under the command of Sir Arthur Haselrig' on the morning of Monday 27 November. However it is unlikely that Sir Arthur was with his men; indeed, it is unlikely that he took an active part in this final 1643 military move at all.

For their part Hesilrige's horse took part in the skirmish at Alton on 18 December, when they blocked the eastern road from Alton, forcing the retreating royalist horse of Lord Cranford to gallop back from where they came.[8] A lieutenant under Hesilrige lost a leg at Alton, the Commons ordering him to receive 'Twenty-fix Pounds, for which the Raw Hides going to the Mayor of Reading was fold'.[9] The foot under Birch must have received numerous wounds, perhaps in the hot firefight around Alton Church, for again on 23 December the Commons ordered:

> That Mr. Trenchard do forthwith pay unto the Surgeon, and his two mates, of Sir Arthur Haselrig's Regiment of foot, Twenty-three Pounds Eight Shillings, upon Account, for the speedy sending down of the said Surgeons to Sir Arth. Haselrig's Regiment.[10]

A wounded soldier during the seventeenth century was a pitiful object, with wounds so easily infected and fever, gangrene and death quickly ending his suffering. Death was often the happiest of releases, the loss of a leg being far worse than the loss of life itself.

Of all the setbacks suffered by Parliament in 1643, the most tragic came on 8 December with the death of John Pym, who had been ill for some time with an internal growth of which no cure was possible with the 'quack' doctors of the time. In the early years of Hesilrige's career, Pym had introduced him to the cut and thrust of the debate.

At the hands of Pym, the political virgin of 1640 had grown into the fully experienced parliamentary whore of 1643, leaving Hesilrige more than able to look after himself between the dirty sheets of intrigue. Any tricks learned by Sir Arthur in the early days of the Long Parliament were learned from John Pym. Although of the old radicals in the Commons, the emergence of a new breed of republican radical had left Pym in a far more centre position. Hesilrige was himself in a stance between Pym and these new hot-bloods, but was not however in 1643 a republican. It can be argued that at his death John Pym was a fading light: that summer a howling mob of peace seeking London women had called for the radical members of the Commons, and chiefly Pym, to be thrown into the river, a bath Sir Arthur would have no doubt shared.

The war was very finely balanced when in January 1644 the Scottish Presbyterian army crossed into England in support of their brother puritans. They believed that by so doing the English Parliament, when victorious, would help with the foundation of a Presbyterian church-state in Scotland. While assisting with the English war, the Scots required representation in army affairs, this being undertaken by the 'Committee of Both Kingdoms' by an ordinance of 16 February 1644. The members appointed for both kingdoms differed very much in temperament from member to member, but overall it was better balanced than many of the previous councils and committees.[11] The first Committee of Both Kingdoms was ordered to sit for three months and no longer, which was long enough to settle a work pattern without the members forming a politically dangerous junta of their own. Sir Arthur Hesilrige and Oliver Cromwell were both chosen to sit on the committee, and they quickly became friends. Sir Arthur probably knew Cromwell from before the war, when they had of course worked together on the militia bill, and the slightly hearty, ribald nature of Cromwell may well have been a good match for Hesilrige's fire.

With Pym's death the Commons fell prey to the young Henry Vane and Solicitor-General Oliver St John, who could rule the House by their influence with the radicals. Although lacking the eloquence of Harry Vane and the legal style of St John, when present Hesilrige could command respect through his pre-war notoriety, military experience and fiery tongue—noise being a great asset in political debate.

Another army for Waller was needed if Ralph Hopton was not to overrun the west and, even more vital, join with the King's Oxford forces. If Hopton could do this, London itself would be threatened. Waller's army changed very little towards spring 1644, but for added strength Sir William Balfour's horse were loaned to the west, from Essex's main force. Hesilrige knew Balfour well, having served under him at Kineton Field. He knew him to be a very reliable soldier, but a moderate like Essex. In Essex's army, the role of Balfour was the same as Hesilrige in Waller's. With Sir Arthur so often in committees, it was useful to have Balfour, if only for a short time.

Soon after 4 March, Sir William Waller's army marched forth, consisting of 5,000 foot, 3,000 horse and 600 dragoons, plus Balfour's brigade. Sir Arthur did not march with the army, but stayed in London. On 7 March the Committee of Both Kingdoms sent Hesilrige to the Commons, recommending the speedy dispatch of Sir William Bereton and Sir Thomas Middleton to the war zones, where they were needed. Middleton was yet another of the able Scottish officers employed by the cause. In future years, Waller would write of his liking for that race, but this could not be said of Hesilrige, who would for diplomacy's sake call the Scots his brothers, but in reality had little in common with the Presbyterian Scots.[12] Even on 19 March, Hesilrige was still at the Derby House–Committee of Both Kingdoms, where he began the administration of money supply for the Western Association forces, the trained bands and Balfour's horse. Who should pay the Londoners and Balfour's horsemen was a matter of some argument. They were not serving their own areas and the people of London were therefore against paying soldiers not in their employ. It is an interesting conjecture that, had the 'Pied Piper of Hamlyn' been hired by the Committee of Both Kingdoms, just how many area subcommittees would have haggled over his pay. Hesilrige duly raised the problem in the Commons.[13] The Piper being paid his due, soon after 19 March, Sir Arthur sported his thick buff-coat, strapped on his double-edged sword, no doubt thrusting a pistol in his belt, and rode to the Western Association. It is highly probable that Hesilrige had not seen action since Roundway Down, and how much he looked forward to the smoke and leaden rain is uncertain.

The roundhead opponent for the spring campaign was in theory the 76-year-old General Patrick Ruthven, Earl of Forth, but through age and a severe bout of gout, the practical control of the army was once more the responsibility of Ralph Hopton.

The 25th of March saw the two opposing forces facing each other near Winchester. Like two great 'praying mantis' they stood eyeing each other's every move, awaiting the moment to strike and deliver the fatal blow. For two days this game went on, both armies within cannon shot and moving back and forth to redress the ranks and test the other's nerves. Each pikeman stood in order watching his alter ego on the other side look back at him. The tension in the ranks would build until self-control was almost at breaking point. This tension is mentioned by Roe, the secretary to John Birch, for Birch was eager to fight and the waiting was playing upon him:

> On the 25th March following you had sight of marching on the plain towards you in batalia: upon which you drew up by Sir William Waller and Sir William Balfour's command: while the army was at that posture a council of warr was called, at which it was resolved, as I have heard (upon the defeat of the Parliaments forces at Newark and in the North,) to make fiers and retreat; which being sore against your minde, whoe then was Captain of the watch, you used these words to Sir Arthur Haselrieg, (publiquely) that surely wee did feare whither that were Gods cause wee had in hand: for did wee assuredly beleeve it, when he called us to fight with his eneimies, wee should not run from them; for mans extremitie is Gods opportunitie.[14]

A reluctance to risk defeat at the hands of Hopton would be high on the minds of the parliamentarians. After his terrible crushing at Roundway, Waller could not afford a setback so early in 1644. But the royalist army could not simply be allowed to wander the lanes of Hampshire unchecked, and sooner or later a stand would have to be made. Sir Arthur knew of course that a royalist victory would leave London open.

Hesilrige's horse now numbered seven troops under command of Major Nicholas Battersby, Captains Edward Foley, John Okey, Thomas Pennyfeather, Clarke and the ever-faithful Samuel Gardiner. Hesilrige's own troop was still being commanded for much of the time by Thomas Horton.[15] It is surprising that Gardiner had not raised his own regiment, because he was of a good social level and had been a parliamentary hero the previous year when his troop captured Lord Salter, the King's ambassador, upon his return from the Court of France with a baggage train containing money estimated to be between £300 and £6,000.

Following the two nerve racking days watching each other, Waller decided upon action. During the night a party of 1,000 musketeers commanded by the foul-mouthed Lieutenant Colonel Walter Leighton, occupied Cheriton Wood.[16] The language of this rough soldier was offensive to Birch's ears, for he 'did sweare too hard to have God with him', but the command of a body of musketeers must have demanded considerable spirit.

The night of 28–29 March was cold, the soldiers in the open fields would have felt it even more with the chill of a fight turning their bellies. The musketeers would pray between snatches of sleep that when the call came they would be able to keep their matches burning, and that cold fingers would not lead to mistakes in the firing process. They would also hope that if battle came it would be in late morning to prevent the damp of a spring dawn causing too many misfires. Some officers like Birch would be going from rank to rank making warlike speech to steady their men, the soldiers making themselves as comfortable as they could and what peace with God they could in the lonely hours before dawn.

Needless to say the following morning saw a thousand roundhead musketeers deployed in Cheriton Wood, about to defend this flank with steady continuous fire from their matchlock pieces. A strong body of foot and dragoons lined the hedgerows towards Hinton Ampner, awaiting a move from Hopton. That morning, however, it would appear that God had risen early, spotted Walter Leighton in the wood, weighed his sins in his great hands and judged him a sinner. Looking across at the royalist army, the Lord, it would seem, found Colonel Matthew Appleyard upon the field, and, seeing an opportunity to punish Leighton, put it in Ralph Hopton's heart to send Appleyard to Cheriton Wood. Within half an hour the roundheads were beaten from the Wood, Leighton's men running as fast as their heels could carry them. Had the royalist horse been waiting for the flying parliamentarians, their heels would have offered scant protection.

The battle had not even really begun, and the opening gambit had been won by the royalists.

At this point, Roe makes a claim concerning Hesilrige's opinion on fighting. He says that Hesilrige said to Birch, 'Now Collonel have you fighting enough?', to which Birch replied, 'Sir this is but a rub; wee shall yet win the cast'.[17] Secretary Roe, in his writing, relays the impression that John Birch was totally fearless, carrying the shield of heaven into battle like a latter-day Samson who marched forth to smite the hordes of Hopton's 'Philistines' armed with a 'Jawbone of a Ass'. With permission from Waller, the magnificent Birch led Hesilrige's foot forward to stabilize the right wing. This would secure the safety of Leighton's fleeing men and stop the advance of Appleyard. Meanwhile, with or without orders, the young Sir Henry Bard made a march on Hinton Ampner with his own foot, where he came face to face with Colonel Carre's foot and dragoons. A volley came from the roundheads, the muskets of Bard's Greycoats replying as they came on. The battle at Hinton Ampner was joined, and powder smoke spoilt the sweet fresh air of an early spring morning.

Before another shot is fired, a claim by Denzil Holles on Sir Arthur Hesilrige's conduct at Cheriton must be examined. In his memoirs, written many years later, Holles accuses Sir Arthur of 'crying under a hedge', saying he cried out,

> 'Ah woe is me, all is lost! we are all undone'—in so much that a great officer, a Scotchman, finding him in that tune, wished him to go off the field, and not stand—'gudding there to dishearten the soldiers'.[18]

Over the years this statement made by Holles with such pleasure has gained more respect than perhaps it should or even deserves. Hesilrige was a political enemy of Denzil Holles, and the Presbyterian moderates in the Commons. It is doubtful that Holles ever liked Hesilrige, even in the first months of the Long Parliament. It is even less likely Holles thought well of Sir Arthur after the attainer against his kin, the doomed Strafford. The memoir was published some 30 years after Hesilrige's death, when Holles was thought of kindly by a new Court and Hesilrige was long dead. It is true that his nerve may have deserted him after his wounds at Roundway Down, but Hesilrige was to be involved in other military situations where his nerve held, and Holles writes with far too much spite and political malice for us to accept this story without question.

But Holles's memoirs had yet to be written and meanwhile the fight around Hinton Ampner was reaching a critical stage. Seeing that young Bard had led his men too far on, the troopers in Hesilrige's horse charged the royalists repeatedly. Attacked in front and flank, perhaps the officers in Bard's regiment just had time to form the defensive 'hedgehog', their pikes jutting from a great ring of men and musketeers firing from under the long wooden shafts. Round and round this trapped body rode the horse, discharging pistols and carbines into the luckless hulk. Bard's men tried desperately to hold their position. Suddenly the horse broke in, 150 falling to the charges, a further 120 taken prisoner. Those who were lucky enough to escape the fire and steel of Hesilrige's charges fled helter-skelter through the woods nearby until they were captured or free.

Birch, in the meantime, had found himself in a hot fight along the Hinton Ampner–Cheriton Wood line, the hardest of the infantry action upon the field. For three hours the pikes and muskets dealt their fatal blows. Sir Michael Livesey joined Birch with a few troops of Kent horse, eventually causing the royalists to give ground.

Seeing Bard's plight, the old Earl of Forth resolved to draw up the horse and try a last ditch charge upon the swarming mass of the parliamentary army. By the time the royalist horse had gathered into anything remotely like a body, the parliamentarian horse had deployed 'in nine faire bodyes' and met the charge at great advantage. The royalists advanced down a single lane and were caught by a round-head net of troopers, which soon found them at a disadvantage when they could not charge in number or manoeuvre from danger.[19] The hedgerows of East Down had been lined with royalist musketeers, and it was only heavy fire from these stout-hearts that prevented the loss of Down once the horse were broken. During this fight, one of Hesilrige's troopers administered a mortal wound to the royalist hero Major General Sir John Smith, who had been knighted for his valour in rescuing the Banner Royale at Kineton Field eighteen months earlier.

As the battle raged on, old Forth, realizing his army was in dire straits and not allowing Hopton the freedom he needed, committed the last reserves of royalist foot to join the fearful pike and shot battle on Waller's left flank. Again a frantic hedge fight developed, and again the parliamentarians pushed the royalists back. It is only justice that Secretary Roe should tell the rest of the story, considering he attributes its success to John Birch, who was it seems still smiting joyfully with his 'Asses Jawbone' and slaying all before him:

> At which time twoe thousand musketeers were drawne out at your request; one thousand whereof on the left wing were commanded by Colonel Rea; who did very gallantly, the rest by yourselfe on the right wing; all the rest of the army being to second them. Those twoe great parties went on with such success, that in one houre the enemies army was between them, all our horse and foote comeing on in the front of them. The first thing that I could perceive, they puld off their collours, thrust them in their breeches, threw down their arms, and fled confused.

Your selfe and others, hot in pursute had not followed them above 100 paces into their own ground, before one, whome I shall not name, overtook you, commanded you to stand; but for what end I never yet could tell, except it was to give the enimy leave to runn away, and carry away their cannon; shure as you stood there 3 quarters of an houre, untill the enimy was far enough.

Thus was that dayes victory gayned: unto which I make bould to add, that it was indeed a victory, but the worst prosecuted of any I ever sawe.[20]

Little more needs to be said, the royalist army in that corner of England was bruised and unfit to fight again if needed for some weeks. The fliers, as the broken soldiers are called, fled to Alton, Winchester and the brave garrison at Basing House, leaving the nearby village of Alresford ablaze.[21]

The battle over, Sir Arthur Hesilrige rode hard for Winchester at the head of a body of horse. The gates of the old walled city were flung wide, but the royalists had sealed themselves tight behind the strong defences of the ancient castle. The day after the battle of Cheriton, the Committee of Both Kingdoms wrote in praise of the victorious army and God's blessings, ordering Waller to keep the army in the field rather than risk defeat in sieges.[22] With this Hesilrige rode to London with the intention of relaying the general's views on this matter to the Committee and Commons.

With Sir Arthur and his guard troop was carried the badly injured young royalist knight, Sir Henry Bard. During the fight with Hesilrige's horse, Bard had received a wound to the arm, and, whether by infection or simply the extent of the wound, the arm was amputated. For a man so ill-used by history, Sir Arthur treated Bard like a son or younger brother, personally making provision for his care in London—for a time at his own home—and generally showing great kindness to his stricken enemy.

Hesilrige stayed in London two weeks before the Committee of Both Kingdoms sent him back to Waller on the road to Farnham. The Committee recalled the Western Army to London to guard against a swift move by the King.[23] Within two days Sir Arthur was back in London, and the Committee ordered pay to enable a further Western Association army to be sent to the west.[24]

For the remainder of April, Sir Arthur found enough work at Derby House and the Commons to keep him from the army. For a man whose life was to say the least busy, this time in London was meant to be a holiday, but events would hardly leave it at that.

NOTES

1.   CJ, III, p. 295.
2.   CJ, III, p. 309.
3.   LJ, VI, p. 160.
4.   *Birch's Memoirs*, p. 55n.
5.   CSP Dom, 1641–43, p. 483.
6.   Adair, *Roundhead General*, p. 107.
7.   W. Money, *The First and Second Battles of Newbury* (Newbury, 1881), is the best if outdated account.
8.   Emberton, *Love Loyalty*, p. 50.
9.   CJ, III, p. 347.
10.   CJ, III, p. 350.
11.   Gardiner, *Constitutional Documents of the Puritan Revolution*, pp. 271-73.
12.   CSP Dom, 1644, p. 38.
13.   CSP Dom, 1644, p. 59.
14.   *Birch's Memoirs*, pp. 9-10.
15.   Adair, *Cheriton 1644*, p. 147. Dr Adair does not list Walter Parry in the battle of Cheriton, but he petitioned Parliament on 12 February for arrears and was at Cropredy Bridge. Captain Gwilliam was at Cheriton in Waller's regiment, having left the old regiment of Lobsters in 1643.
16.   *Birch's Memoirs*, p. 10.
17.   *Birch's Memoirs*, p.10.
18.   *Holles's Memoirs*, p. 28.
19.   Adair, *Cheriton 1644*. Dr Adair believes the royalist horse advanced along Bramdean Lane. Even today the lanes around Alresford/Cheriton are narrow and winding, giving some idea of the difficulty in deploying horse to any effect.
20.   *Birch's Memoirs*, p. 11.
21.   Accounts of Cheriton can be found in 'A Fuller Relation of the Victory obtained at Alsford 28 March', TTE 40 (1); Capt. Robert Harley to Col. Edward Harley, 12 April 1644, HMC Portland MSS, vol. 3, pp. 106-110; Bellum Civille: *Mercurius Aulicus*. The best modern account is by Adair cited above.
22.   CSP Dom, 1644, pp. 23-24.
23.   CSP Dom, 1644, pp. 117-18.
24.   CSP Dom, 1644, pp. 121-22.

❦ 8 ❧

Sacrifice in the West

And he said, Take now thy son, thine only son Isaac, whom thou lovest, and get thee into the land of Morish; and offer him there for a burnt offering upon one of the mountains which I will tell thee of.

(Gen. 22.2)

By May 1644 neither King nor Parliament had gained the upper hand, and Parliament's best hope of a peace settlement rested in a wayward cannonball carrying Charles to his heavenly court, leaving Parliament apologizing and negotiating some face saving solution with his heir.

The first week of May found Hesilrige with the Western Army. He had evidently become acquainted with Edmund Ludlow, a young republican some sixteen years his junior. Ludlow was a prolific writer, and mentions his earliest association with Sir Arthur:

Upon an invitation of Sr. Arthur Haslerig to be Major of his regiment of horse, in Sr. William Waller's army, which was designed for the service of the west, I accepted of it, and mounted my choicest of my old soldiers with me, Sir Arthur buying a hundred horse in Smithfield for that purpose.[1]

Hesilrige was known for his buying of quality horseflesh in the London markets. His own home counties of Northamptonshire and Leicestershire were good horse country, and Northampton during the Civil War and after was a leading horse market in England, supplying large numbers of quality mounts to the armies of Parliament.[2] Hesilrige was it would seem a good horseman; even in his advanced years he preferred the saddle to the coach, and was an excellent judge of a good horse. Yet even with Hesilrige's trip to Smithfield, it seems unlikely if Ludlow ever served under Sir Arthur, leaving to raise his own regiment.

On 25 May, Hesilrige was at Derby House, where the committee decided he should rejoin Waller to relate the next stage of the

Parliament's strategy. With Sir Arthur went Washbourne's Troop out of the newly raised regiment of Colonel Harvey.[3] This small body reached Waller before 31 May, and was present at a muster of the army at Newbridge on 1 June. Three days later on Tuesday 4 June, Waller and Hesilrige wrote a long detailed letter to Derby House relating the current situation in the Cotswolds where the army lay:

> Wee know you expect daily intelligence from us which cannot bee unlesse yor Messenger constantly attend the Armie. After our last letter from Abbington (sic) which was on ffriday the 31st of May wee received commande from his Excellency to march towards Woodstocke leaving Oxford on the right hand, his intelligence being that the kings force were drawing away towards Worcester whereupon on Saturday the first of June wee marched to Newbridge five miles from Abbington which was broken up by the Enemy and kept by one hundred Musquetiers in a short time wee gained the bridge not one being hurt, and tooke the Captain and Officers with sixtie foure Common souldiers. There wee received orders from his Excelency not to advance further till he had recoured his passe at Islip which was not effected upon monday morning but about twelve of the clocke wee heard it was taken and that the kings Armie was drawne back into Oxford. Thereupon wee sent out a party of three hundred horse to see if they could goe to his Excellencye and also for gaining Intelligence. That party is not yet returned neither have wee heard from them, and now it is Tewsday twelve a clock. Wee suppose they are whithe his Excellency. If any thing had happened a misse certainly wee should not have wanted one Messenger. Wee have him at Newbridge this foure days and are ready to obey Commands wee find no want of provisions nor affections from the Countrey yet wee cannot but by lying long in a place wast it sufficiently. God can bring mighty things to passe but wee apprehend the kings Armie defended by the Rivers neare Oxford will hold us in play the greatest part of this summer unless you please to command the Garrisons to draw out that as now yor affaires stand profit little and spend much or else to send us some considerable strength from the Cittie or Committee of Hertford, Northton (sic) Warwick & c, that may be able to make a Third quarter. If this way be taken their provisions will quickly faile and this worke may prove short and successful.[4]

That same evening, Hesilrige and Waller, having heard the King was again on the move, made to follow him and that night reached Witney. It is interesting to note that, despite continual strain in counter-marching against the King, Sir Arthur kept faith with the Committee of Both Kingdoms and wrote again that same day. The King was marching towards Bristol, with only musketeers, a few small guns and very little baggage to hinder him. On the night of 4 June, the King rested at Burford, within a 'mile & halfe of his Ex.quarter'.[5] Upon this march, the King received word that his loyal garrison at Tewkesbury had fallen to Massey's forces from Gloucester. To cover his advance, which was now threatened by Essex to his flank and Waller to his rear, the King marched at once to the pro-royalist market town of Evesham. Arriving during the afternoon of 5 June, King Charles took shelter at the home of Alderman William Martin, the man Samuel Gardiner had succeeded as mayor in 1642. While he was there, false information reached the King of Waller's movements and the royal army quickly marched on to Worcester. In the meantime Waller and Hesilrige marched on to Stow-on-the-Wold, where they once more wrote to the Committee of Both Kingdoms on 5 June. In this letter Hesilrige and Waller wrote of the danger to the west and principally Lyme Regis. Essex had decided upon a plan to march into the west to prevent this. In the same letter Hesilrige and Waller had said the royalists were at Burford, which was already outdated, for the King lay at Evesham and his troops split into bodies at Stowe and nearby Bourton-on-the-Water. The King's army was not in good spirit, and being in divided quarters gave the parliamentarians hope of picking off stragglers.

The weather that spring and early summer was cold and wet, and the soldiers lived wretchedly, huddled together in improvised tents, their uniforms mud-splattered and their footwear rain-soaked. Yet Hesilrige reported that the soldiers' morale was high, writing that 'the soldiers march cheerfully'.[6] The next day a meeting took place between Essex and Waller at Chipping Norton. Being the representative of Derby House, Hesilrige rode along with Sir William. Although Sir Arthur was inferior in appointment to Waller in the army, he was far more powerful than Waller in the Western Association, it being Hesilrige not Waller who administered the Association, and it was Sir Arthur who was referred to in Association business in both committee and Commons. It would seem that Hesilrige was the spokesman and representative, despite Waller being 'the Generalle'. It is difficult to ascertain who was the dog and who the flea in this army.

On 7 June, the day following the Chipping Norton meeting, Waller and Hesilrige wrote yet again from Stow, explaining the decision of the lord general which would ultimately lead to his ruin at the hands of the King and the Committee of Both Kingdoms:

On the morning of the 6th instant we attended the Lord General, who staid for the night at Chipping Norton, and the next day marched back to Burford. His resolution is for relieving Lyme Regis and the west. Being thus put out of our way, and his Excellency commanding that an eye should be had which way the King takes, we resolve to follow the king wherever an army can march. Our reasons are, we believe the war can never end if the King be in any part of the land and not at the Parliament, for break his army never so often his person will raise another; all the histories of England and our experience at Shrewsbury, will manifest that sufficiently. And the king has no other hope but that delay in time may bring changes, and we know there is no season which, when God offers, wisdom embraces. If he go to Prince Rupert, by the blessing of God and the assistance of the country's forces, we may take him out of his armies. But if you conceive this not to be the best course we readily submit to be directed as you please; fear not our breaking with any Association upon points of honour. We know that if the king go northward our commissions fail; yet for the public good, we will leave it to Parliament that seldom wants mercy. We fear lest this army consisting of several forces, City, Association and Waller's, they should not be paid, and so for want dissolve.[7]

The army was in very bad condition despite being in good spirit. It had taken to plundering local royalist populations in the pro-King area of the Cotswolds, causing the towns and villages to turn against them and endangering supplies. There had also been a skirmish near Evesham between a body of parliamentary horse and the royalists in which they took a lieutenant, three cornets and 50 men.

Essex had ruined any chance of totally defeating the King by the dividing of the two armies. Together Essex and Waller could have crushed the King's Oxford army, ending the war in 1644. It was a vital statement in the letter of 7 June, when Hesilrige and Waller had asked if they could actually attempt to take the King out of his armies. At no time before this date did the capture of the King enter into their strategy. The idea was revolutionary, and they knew that associations who would wage war upon cavaliers like Rupert would turn aside from it.

The letter of 7 June was so vital that Hesilrige himself rode hard to London with it. With Sir Arthur reporting to Derby House, the committee, seeing Essex's folly, commanded him to return. Considering that the meeting at Chipping Norton was held on 6 June, that Hesilrige had waited four days before returning to London, then a further three days had passed before the message was sent to Essex, it was far too late.

While Sir Arthur had been with the army, the first term of the Committee of Both Kingdoms had ended. Instead of simply reappointing the assembly, Parliament played a rather futile game by demanding some changes in those sitting. With the King in the field, the merchants and men of commerce who controlled the city and therefore the purse strings petitioned for the committee to resume, but the Lords still requested changes in those attending the assembly, which held up the second committee of Both Kingdoms until 22 May. Despite this utter nonsense from the so-called Peace Party, the new committee was very much the same rabid beast it was before.[8]

Towards the end of June, Hesilrige left London with the army's pay. By 1 July the convoy had reached Leighton Buzzard, where to his horror Sir Arthur received news that Waller's army had been severely mauled by the King in the fields around Cropredy. Hesilrige's horse had been in the thickest of the fighting and had received a number of casualties in a very confused cavalry action across Cropredy Bridge.[9] Fearing the worst, Sir Arthur immediately sent the money he guarded to Aylesbury for safety. At Leighton a meeting took place between Hesilrige and Major General Browne, who had a small army with him and could call upon the local militia regiments if danger was at hand. Sir Arthur immediately drew up plans to defend the area from the King and hopefully cover Waller's retreat. It had been three days since the battle at Cropredy, and the King, who was still at large, could head in any direction he chose. Forces needed to be able to move quickly, and the security of the area depended on mobility and the careful use of what troops were available. At this time Hesilrige saw so unusual a sight that it is worthy of mention—mounted Pikemen:

> ...such a sight as pikes to march mounted I never saw, and should we have had an alarm our mounted pikes would have made rout sufficient. To dismount the pikes and not musketeers would discontent the pikes, which caused Major-Generall Brown to send back all their horses.[10]

The sight of poor Pikemen gripping on to rough, hairy 'nagges' must have been comic, and although it was perfectly normal to mount the infantry for rough marches if the horses were available, Hesilrige gives the impression that Browne's pikemen were expected to carry their pikes instead of them being carried on carts, which was the normal practice.

Waller's defeated army made its steady retreat from Cropredy without further mishap, arranging a rendezvous with Hesilrige and Browne
at Northampton. There is some evidence that Sir Arthur left Browne
on the road to Northampton, meeting with Waller near Towcester,
where he could inform Sir William of the mutinous state of Browne's
army and lead the parliamentarians through those Northamptonshire
lanes of his youth. Sir Arthur knew the Towcester to Northampton
route well, because it had been a regular ride when he lived at
Alderton.

Browne's troops were the additional force Sir William needed to
strengthen his beaten army, but these troops were in an even worse
condition than Waller's own. Mutiny was a daily blight upon
Browne's badly paid men, something the Western Army had not
suffered even during the bad days of 1643 and the defeat at Cropredy.
Waller's men had always been of good heart, a strong vintage which
could be ruined by the addition of low spirit. Waller had no option
but to enter Northampton, whatever the cost.

Now rejoined, Heslerige and Waller wrote to Derby House,
informing the committee, 'We have certain Intelligence that the King
lay last night at Evesham. He is (bent) for the North, but we do not
hear of any foot with him...'[11] Charles, however, would not head
north, for within a day or two the news would arrive that Prince
Rupert and the northern royalists under the Marquis of Newcastle
had suffered a terrible defeat on the moors around York at the hands
of the tri-party forces of the Northern Army of the Fairfaxes, Earl
Manchester's Eastern Association and Lord Leven's Scots. It was now
too late for the King to join Rupert, and he turned west instead to
where the Earl of Essex lay like the sacrificial lamb.

Believing the King marched north, Waller and Browne parted
their forces at Northampton, and Sir William resolved to chase the
Royalists. Whether the state of Browne's army influenced them or
not, the city forces of the trained bands, which made up most of
Waller's foot, refused to march, and worst of all decided to return
home. Of course this was the problem that concerned Hesilrige and
Waller before Cropredy Bridge. Sir William's fortunes were at their
lowest ebb, far more desperate than even after Roundway. Then the
Western Army had risen like a phoenix from the ashes, but Waller's
flame was burning out both militarily and politically.

By 8 July, Waller and Hesilrige had reached the old village of

Fawsley, the estate of Sir Arthur's friends the Knightley family, where he had spent so many happy hours with his wife Dorothy. The deer that ran wild around Fawsley would have made a handsome meal for a hungry soldier's belly, but provisions were high they having just left Northampton. It was nevertheless another deer that worried the two generals, the old stag the Earl of Essex.[12] From Fawsley they marched steadily to Towcester, where, on 13 July, Sir Arthur was sent back to the Committee of Both Kingdoms with an urgent message:

> I have received several intelligences that his Majesty is marched towards Bristol. The order I received from your lordships commended me to attend his march and I am ready with all humbleness to obey it, but there be something which stick with me upon the motion of the king westward, which I have desired Sir Arthur Haslerigg to communicate to you, therein I humbly crave further directions.[13]

There was obviously something on Waller's mind which he did not trust to paper. He surely realized that, if the King marched westwards, the army of the Earl of Essex would be caught between the victorious Oxford army and the army with Prince Maurice already there. Therefore, what was Waller thinking when Sir Arthur rode for London on 14 July? Sir William had already weakened his force of horse by sending the five troops of Colonel Norton to join Browne. Hesilrige was at the committee with Waller's message two days later, quickly covering the 60 miles on horseback and going immediately to Derby House, where the committee quite incredibly decided not to send Waller in relief of the cut-off Essex.[14] By their action the committee had given the King a human sacrifice in the west, in the meaty shape of the main parliamentary army. They had long disliked Essex, favouring their darling Waller, whom they could command through Hesilrige. Now they could seal Essex's fate with the decision to throw him to the kingly lion of England. It is interesting to note that in the north, where the Fairfaxes were not controlled to the same degree, and where the armies worked in unison, the war was slowly turning in Parliament's favour.

Hesilrige now rode to Major General Browne ordering him to again join with Waller to make a better force, Browne replying to Derby House that his men would not march for want of pay.

Time was running out for Essex. Instead of being the saviour of the west and wearing Waller's crown, he found himself surrounded and deserted at Fowey near Lostwithiel, his army demoralized and lost. On 4 August, the Earl wrote to the committee for aid by land and sea. He blamed Waller for his plight in not stopping the royal advance, which was a very valid point if one believes political jealousy is the ground on which to fight wars. Two days later, King Charles, watching yet another tasty morsel dropping upon his plate, sent the roundhead lord general terms which amounted to changing sides. The King knew Essex to be a moderate, but he was no turncoat, and, despite his burning anger over Waller, a loyal Parliament man.

Cut off by the King, Maurice, Ralph Hopton and George Goring, with rumours that Prince Rupert was galloping west with the remnants of his horse from Marston Moor, the Earl of Essex pleaded one last time to Derby House. Strangely, this time the committee acted, commanding the Eastern Association under the Earl of Manchester to march to his aid. The committee knew only too well it was far too late for Manchester to carry out a rescue, even if Oliver Cromwell's highly mobile force of horse and dragoons rode hard in front of the slow trail of the foot. Rather than lose his regiments of horse, which consisted of some of the best in any army, the Earl of Essex, on the night of 31 August, ordered Sir William Balfour to cut his way through the royalist lines. Essex himself left the foot in command of that dependable soldier Philip Skippon, and was rowed to a waiting ship and safety.[15] The foot desired to fight and leave a taste of their pikes in the royalist mouths, a policy favoured by Skippon, but he was overruled and forced to seek terms. The King being in no position to hold prisoners allowed Skippon to march his troops away, having left behind, 'Thirty six cannon, ten thousand muskets and pistolls, and severall wagon loads of powder and match.'[16]

Was this the problem foreseen by Waller and Hesilrige at Towcester? The answer may never be known. But it is a certainty that Sir Arthur would lose no sleep through the defeat of the lord general, a man whom he had after all helped to bring to power.

NOTES

1.   *The Memoirs of Edmund Ludlow* (ed C.H. Firth; London, 1894), I.
2.   A Lieutenant Russell 'payed' £500 for about 80 horses for the Eastern Association at Northampton horsemarket in April 1644. The old place names of 'Horsemarket' and 'Marefare' survive in Northampton.
3.   CSP Dom, 1644, pp. 168-69.
4.   BM Harleian MSS 166, ff. 83-84v.

5.   BM Harleian MSS 166, ff. 83v-84.

6.   CSP Dom, 1644, p. 206.

7.   CSP Dom, 1644, pp. 214-15.

8.   CJ, III, p. 504.

9.   'The Account of Thomas Ellis', TTE 53 (18).

10. CSP Dom, 1644, pp. 296-97.

11. CSP Dom, 1644, pp. 307-308.

12. The arms of Robert Earl of Essex were a stag's head.

13. CSP Dom, 1644, p. 347.

14. CSP Dom, 1644, p. 358.

15. CSP Ven, 1643–47: Clarendon, *History of the Rebellion*, III, pp. 109, 116; Rushworth, *Historical Collections*, V, pp. 704-705.

16. Wedgwood, *The King's War*, p. 360.

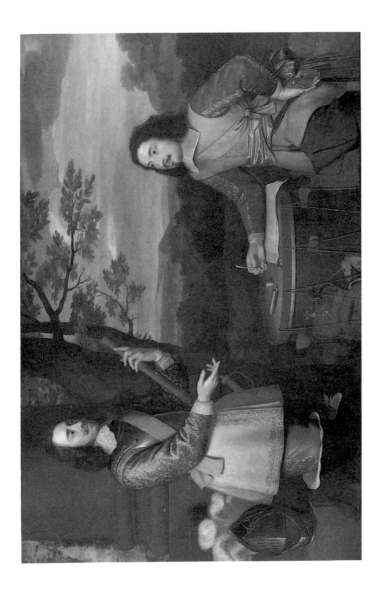

Charles I with Sir Edward Walker, by an unknown artist. By courtesy of the National Portrait Gallery, London.

∽ 9 ∽

The Bloody Fellow

For I said, Hear me, lest otherwise they should rejoice over me: when my
foot slippeth, they magnify themselves against me.

(Ps. 38.16)

The news of Skippon's surrender reached London on 7 September,
and rather surprisingly—or perhaps not so considering parliamentary
affection for fallen idolism—a letter was drawn up thanking the lord
general for his conduct and also assuring him that help in the guise of
Waller and Manchester was being sent. In the Commons, unlike the
Committee of Both Kingdoms, the Essex supporters still held the
majority. Instead of blaming Essex for losing an army its arms and
therefore rendering it useless until it could be re-equipped, they turned
their wraith upon the innocent Middleton, who, they claimed, had
failed to reach Essex in time. If anyone was to blame and deserved
severe admonishment, it was the members at Derby House. However,
by early autumn 1644 it is debatable who was the greater force, the
free Parliament or the radical junta ruling by consent of the city. The
city's power during this time was a forceful representation of grandee
capitalism. The ruling powers of the trade and money supply were
playing an important part in the structure of the war. They were not
in favour of a return to a monarchic rule, and supported the junta
rather than the Commons. If and as the economic growth fluctuated
during the war, the city grandees would bend in the capitalist wind,
but in 1644 their sails were set to catch the prevailing tide held by the
junta.

When the letter to Essex was read in the Commons, a burst of
laughter came from Hesilrige which gave general offence to his fellow
members.[1] But was Sir Arthur so bad-mannered in his cynicism? The
civil war was fast becoming a sick joke, and in fact the general con-

sensus felt the Earl of Manchester for one was finding the thought of actually defeating the King frightening. Manchester was in open disagreement with Oliver Cromwell, the rising star of the Eastern Association, and within a few short weeks the conflict between them would boil and lead to the drastic change the war required to break the deadlock. Cromwell was far blunter in character than the more timid aristocracy represented by Manchester, and to Oliver a war that was simply letting blood stain the fields of England was an insult to the common man and an affront to God's cause on earth, for which he was fighting. Cromwell knew that to fight a battle without the heart or desire for a victory was a defeat in itself, and every time the royalist army marched from the field it was free to defeat Parliament at a later date.

Following the outburst from the heart of Sir Arthur's contempt for Essex, he was not in favour in London, and it was an opportune time to rejoin Waller for what was to be Heselrige's last taste of the true battlefield. On 12 September, the two old comrades wrote to Derby House, relating their position:

> The Lord General (Essex's) horse lie about Dorchester and those under Lieut. Genl. Middleton about Sherborne, at least ten miles distant. We fear that unless Sir Wm. Balfoure command or the now commander-in-chief be called off for a time the horse will scarce join as they ought to do; something must be done in this without delay; if we fight devided both are lost.[2]

The experience at Cropredy and Lostwithiel signified the need for joint action against the royalists, but to control three armies in one body was difficult owing to the different associations to which the armies owed allegiance. The whole system of area associations had been the major drawback in moving armies to battle zones from the outbreak of the war. The Western Association under Waller had long suffered in this respect, being a smaller force than the landowning Eastern Association, or the rich grandees who controlled the midlands and London markets. If the King was to be given any setback in the field, a degree of unity was needed between generals who could hardly agree on anything.

By the middle of September, Waller and Hesilrige were at Weymouth, where their latest despatch on the 18th informed the committee that Colonel Birch had sailed with his regiment for Plymouth, and stated their concern that latest intelligence put Charles Stuart at

Exeter, thus endangering Birch should the siege be raised. For the rest of September, Sir Arthur remained with the army, riding from town to town and constantly writing to London for money to pay the troops. During this month the army began to suffer mutiny and desertion from the low morale known in other forces for some months, and there was even a hanging. Things with Waller's army were not well: the leaves on the trees were turning brown and yellow, nights were growing longer and the chill in the night air reminded soldiers that their homes and wives were sweeter than this endless wandering in search of nought but another town.

On 24 September, Waller and Hesilrige described the army as 'a gallant forlorn hope', continuing 'the extremely long marches our soldiers have had have drawn upon them such wants of clothes, and money to shoe their horses, that we cannot but cry out for the 5,000 *l*.[3] They had been requesting the £5,000 for some time, those at Derby House being like the Commons, that is, most generous on paper with vast sums of money for the maintenance of their armies, but being slow to convert their theoretical generosity into food and clothing. By the last day of September, Waller and Hesilrige were still writing to the committee, expressing the need to consolidate the armies of Earl Manchester and Essex's reforming army with their own. Writing that day from Shaftesbury:

> We have not heard that the king is removed from Chard. He calls in the country, yet we cannot learn that his army increases. A rendezvous is appointed at Kings Sedgmoor on Wednesday next. If the Earl of Manchesters forces advance to us and the Lord General (Essex's) foot, being armed, such of them at least as are fit for present service, be also sent up, you will not only grow upon the king in the west, but keep your armies on the enemy's (quarters) and preserve your Associations. If this be timely done we may most easily restrict the miseries of our (civil) war within a narrow space, if not bring it to an end. Some of the enemy's horse are come to Evell (Yeovill) four miles beyond Sherborne. Our party meet often, we have taken diverse prisoners, and upon Friday last the enemy killed Major Clutterbuck, he was religious and valliant we have cause to lament his loss. We shall not yield any ground but what we must needs.[4]

It would seem likely the major killed was Benedict Clutterbuck, who was at one time in the troop of Samuel Gardiner—the name Clutterbuck not being common.

At long last London felt threatened, and the Committee of Both

Kingdoms, seeing what appeared to be a move against London, ordered Manchester to join Waller at Shaftesbury. In his usual slow manner the Earl did not set forth at once and ten days later, on 10 October, Waller and Hesilrige wrote to Derby House imploring action be taken. They had held the King's advanced for far longer than had seemed possible and the royalists were only four miles from them. The royalist foot were at Sturminster and 'Prince Maurice with his horse was at Wincanton, and 500 horse came into Blandford on Wednesday morning'. They continued to explain that, although they were so close, to fight would mean certain disaster. That same morning they had received a letter from Manchester saying he intended sending his horse to Salisbury.[5] By the fact that the Earl was not hurrying himself, the King was secure to fill his ranks as he marched and Waller could do nothing but watch his flanks for attack and wait for Manchester.

That same day, at Winterbourne, Hesilrige set up his position, and two days later, while the royal army closed even more, he wrote a personal letter to the committee on behalf of Sir William in connexion with a business deal concerning a fellow MP:

> Mr Harvey, M.P. is to pay to Sir Wm. Waller 500 l. a year upon a lease for the prisage of wines in London and Sir William is to pay the king 400 l. The committee of Revenue forbids Harvey to pay this money to Sir Wm. Waller. This king has seized his estate and this is the only subsistance left for his lady and children. I beseech you to move Sir H. Vane senr, that the Committee of Revenue would take off their injunction laid upon Harvey so that the lady may receive her money. Letters are sent to Waller from London concerning this which troubles his thoughts. You are bound both in honour and wisdom to preserve your servants from suffering in their absence when your weighty employments hinder their presence. I humbly beg a return from your Lordships, and (that you will) not look upon this as that which concerns neither you nor me.[6]

Of course it was the Committee of Revenue's duty to help Waller in this matter, and Hesilrige's reminder of their 'honour and wisdom' was curt but timely. It is a remarkable war that leaves a man awaiting the alarm of battle time to write of wine and the state of conscience of the general in not paying his bills.

At long last, on 14 October, the reinforcements arrived in the shape of ten regular troops from Manchester's horse and two companies of dragoons riding into the roundhead lines at Winterbourne. It was expected the King would move to Salisbury the next day and so the three armies under Waller, Manchester and Essex needed to join without delay if a strike towards London was to be stopped in its tracks. With this in mind, Waller moved to Andover by the night of the 15th. If the King was to be taken on in the field, the horse with Waller and Manchester, plus Balfour's old band of roundhead troopers, would enjoy the sweeping gallops around the Vale of the White Horse. The disciplined troopers under Cromwell would enjoy the true cavalry ground of this horse country far better than the hedge fighting and broken footing of so much of England. A fight was coming, for the next day Waller and Hesilrige desired the committee to send their army 'immediately 500 backs, breasts and pots'. Men so armed found the armour too uncomfortable in the summer, and the marching of Waller's travelling circus during 1644 had made lightness all important. Even the hard-fighting pikeman may lose his helmet when his brain boils under the sun, but only a fool fights a battle half armed, so the request for arms was urgent.

Suddenly, while at Andover on the night of 18 October, a party of royalists burst into the roundhead lines, panic setting in almost immediately as they attempted to vacate their position. Colonel William Carr was taken by the skirmishing 'cavaliers' and a hot cavalry action ensued before Waller could withdraw to the area of Basingstoke. But with this move the armies of Parliament were joined, and at last the King could not expect to destroy the forces one at a time.

On the 19th, a detachment of 120 horse was drawn from Sir Arthur's regiment and, commanded by Major John Okee (or Okey), rode to scout the area. During this excursion Okee stumbled across a body of royalist horse near Alresford and took a lieutenant, quartermaster and four troopers. Major to Hesilrige's horse was the highest rank John Okee attained in Waller's army, but he was quite obviously a very capable officer.[7]

Now the armies were joined the officers sent a joint letter to the Committee of Both Kingdoms, informing them on the 20th: 'You may now look upon the forces as joined. We hope there will be a battle shortly; to our understanding it cannot be avoided...'[8]

With the armies once more were the trained bands of London, the extra foot that gave the armies a body from which the great arms of horse could extend in pincer movements. Waller's army was still in dire need of clothes and food, and Sir William knew well the dangers of an army bare-arsed and empty-bellied, and in the same letter he asked for '800 suits of clothes' and '10 loads of Cheese and Bread'.

The wet weather that replaces the warm, sweet English summer had been badly received by the lord general, who had caught a cold and retired to bed in Reading by the 25 October.[9] In the royalist ranks, much was made of the Earl's swift exit to bed, the common, and not so common, soldiers jesting that Essex preferred 'the fanny of a serving maid' to the taste of battle.

Saturday 26 October saw news of the royalist dispositions given to the generals by Sir John Urry, a man who had already changed sides twice. The royalist horse and foot occupied two fields between Donnington Castle, which they held, and Newbury. To the west of the King's forces stood the village of Speen and a little further there was a high heath, where, around the houses and at the foot of it, Prince Maurice's horse and a body of Cornish foot were deployed. An earthworks was cast up on the heath, and here the Cornishmen waited. The combined parliamentarian armies were in a position to strike at the enemy with great force, there being at least 8,000 horse, 11,000 foot and 24 guns in the field. The joint military capability of the roundhead army made victory quite possible. The army was now divided into two halves, Waller to lead one part against Speen, while Manchester assaulted Shaw House in the centre. That evening Waller led his army to Hermitage ready for the conflict next day.

The following morning, on the Lord's Day, the long-awaited battle began when Manchester's foot attacked along Lambourne River only to be driven back. This was by way of a false start, for the Earl's forces now waited for the sounds that would signal that Waller's army had launched itself at Speen, that is, the rumble of cannon and the firecracker sound of smoothbore musketry muffled by distance and air, and the smoke rising into the sky.

The accounts of the second battle of Newbury are many, but two letters to Derby House written by Sir A. Johnstone and John Crewe MP, on 27 and 28 October respectively, tell of Waller's action at Speen. They wrote on the 27th:

> The forces mentioned in our last letter came from Wickam Heath towards the place where the King's forces were drawn up between Donnington and Newbury, near the castle, having no way to pass but by a wood and through lanes. We met with works and fortifications crossing those lanes, which the enemy had thrown up during the night and planted ordnance therein; they had also other ordnance, two bodies of horse, and two brigades of foot at a little distance. They played also from the Castle

upon our men with great shot. These (works) were very hard to gain, yet it pleased God so to encourage the spirit (of our forces) among whom the Lord General's had a most special care, and so to bless their endeavour that about 5 o'clock, only an hour after their falling to work, our men took it by storm and got 4 pieces of ordnance; afterwards, beating the enemy off his ground, they got another five ordnance. The Lord General's foot took much contentment in regaining some of their ordnance. Our horse stood very gallantly under the view and danger of the cannon playing directly upon them, when they were drawing themselves together to secure the foot, and by charging the enemy put them to a retreat, taking the Earl of Cleveland, who commanded that brigade. All the general officers performed very resolutely their parts, and the Earl of Manchester fell upon the other pass in seasonable time.[10]

They took the works and ordnance of which six non-specified pieces had been taken at Fowey. What Johnstone and Crew fail to mention, however, is that Prince Maurice and Hopton's force about Speen threw back three regiments of the city militia before they too were pushed from the village. With Speen taken, Waller ordered the horse to advance north and south, while to the south Balfour pushed back troops under Sir Humphrey Bennet, and Cromwell did likewise to Cleveland. Eventually the royalists managed to check Balfour and Cromwell, driving the roundheads back in some confusion.

In another letter written on the 28th in case their first miscarried, Johnstone and Crewe added to their account:

> Upon the unexpected entrance into the works the (enemy's) foot which held them all ran, leaving the ordnance placed in and about the works. Major General Skippon hazarded himself too much, Sir William Balfour used great diligences there being but few field officers of horse, while Waller, Haselrigg, Harrington, Middleton, Cromwell, Crawford, Holborne, Col. Greeves and others did very good service. The Earl of Manchester about 4 o'clock endeavoured to force a passage through Shaw, a village on the other side of the field, where the king's forces lay. Prince Maurice was on that side, and many of the king's best foot, who maintained those passes although they were very bravely assaulted. For want of day light and by reason of the strength of the guard who held those passages the Earl was unable to take them, but his keeping so many of the king's forces engaged on that side was so great advantage to our other forces. The battle lasted about three hours being continued at least an hour by moonshine. The Earl and those on the other side were ignorant of each others success till the next morning. Skippon guesses the number slain on both sides at between two and three hundred. All our horse and dragoons, except 1,000 who stay with the Earl of Manchester, are gone in pursuit of the king's forces, which we hear are gone toward Wallingford.[11]

The King did indeed make for Wallingford, but after a short rest at Donnington Castle rode with 500 horse to Bath. Waller, Cromwell and Hesilrige followed the enemy as far as Blewbury, ten miles from Donnington, before returning to the Earl of Manchester at Newbury.[12]

The royalist army had marched from Wallingford to Woodstock to rendezvous with the King, who had brought Prince Rupert and a rumour of 2,000 more horse. Even so the royalist army of 15,000 men were matched by the parliamentarians if battle was joined. The royalists intended to relieve Donnington Castle and rescue their ordnance. By 10 November, the parliamentarians found the King's army in battle order, after skirmishing the previous day. That morning the roundhead army marched forth from Newbury to Shaw's open field, but before battle could begin a 'Council of War' (sic) was held in a nearby cottage. If the third battle of Newbury had been joined and fought with subsequent malice, the King's war would have been lost.

Amazingly, the Earl of Manchester urged against another battle, to which a boiling Hesilrige disagreed violently. 'Thou art a Bloody Fellow,' cried Manchester at Sir Arthur's desire to fight.[13] The Earl continued:

> Gentlemen, I beseech you lets consider what we do. The king need not care how oft he fights, but it concerns us to be wary for in fighting we venture all to nothing. If we fight 100 times and beat him 99 he will be king still, but if he beats us but once, or the last time, we shall be hanged, we shall lose our estates, and our posterities be undone.

At this Cromwell flared and turning to Manchester replied:

> My lord, if this be so, why did we take up arms at first? This is against fighting ever hereafter. If so let us make peace, be it never so base.[14]

The Earl's argument must have turned the stomachs of the likes of Cromwell and Sir Arthur Hesilrige. Those who lay slain at Speen and Shaw must have surely rejoiced at preserving Manchester's estates, and was this what Skippon's boys had fought for? What Birch had led his men for at Cheriton, or Cromwell at Marston Moor? No! Waller, Hesilrige, Skippon and Cromwell wished to fight, but despite this Manchester carried the day aided by Crawford and Balfour, and the King was allowed to march off. It is interesting to note how much of this story fits the tale told by Holles concerning Hesilrige, at Cheriton.

'Woe is me, we are undone' becomes in Manchester's case 'we shall be hanged, we shall lose our estates, and our posterities be undone'. The case against Hesilrige which was never mentioned during his lifetime, fits Manchester extremely well. In Birch's memoirs, Roe had claimed Sir Arthur was against fighting at Cheriton—'have you fighting enough?'—but were these not Manchester's views at Newbury? The similarities are astounding, but the reader must draw his or her own conclusions, for, like Holles, historians have used this story to blacken Sir Arthur's character for many years.

On 12 November, while still at Newbury, Waller, Manchester and Balfour wrote to Derby House:

> It is the desire of the chief officers in these armies that you should have a right understanding of this late action, of the kings advance towards us, and of his relieving Donnington Castle, and therefore they have thought it fitter that Sir Arthur Haselrigg, who was present here, should give you an account of it, than to make a relation of it by letter.[15]

With true reverence to the gods of drama, Hesilrige made his entrance into the Commons in style; of all people Holles tells the story:

> Therefore, the soldiers of that army, which had lost their arms in Cornwall, are presently armed again and two other armies joined to them, the Earl of Manchester's and Sir W. Waller's who gave the king's forces a ruffle at Donnington gaining some of the works. Yet when the king came with the remainder of his strength, they did not think it convenient to put it to the trial of a day, but suffered him to march away, when it had been a most easy thing to have prevented it. And Sir Arthur Haslerig could come up to London, and into the House of Commons, all in beaten buff, cross-girt with sword and pistols, as if he had been killing his thousands…and there like a great soldier, in that habit, he gave a relation of what had passed, highly extolling the gallantry and conduct of all the Commanders, and valour of the soldiers; saying, that no mortal men could do more, that the best soldiers in the world could not have hindered the king's marching off; and that it had been no-wisdom to have adventured to fight…[16]

For once Hesilrige's explanation was not entirely believed by the Commons and when Waller and Cromwell arrived in London nine days later, despite an attempt by Sir William to smooth things over, Oliver spoke in the House of Manchester's backwardness to all action. The quarrel which had smouldered for so long now burst into political flame, each accusing the other of the same charge, at which point Hesilrige relinquished his loyalty to Waller's stabilizing influence and sided with the hawkish Cromwell. Holles is somewhat cutting in his reference to this action, and in retrospect finds the fault for Manchester's position to be in Cromwell:

> ...this worthy knight forgot all he had said for it is, by Cromwell, laid as a crime to the Earl of Manchester's charge (whom then meant to lay-aside) that he was the cause they fought not with the king, and Sir Arthur is a principle witness...to make it good; But on the other side, the Earl of Manchester returns the Bill charging Cromwell, that it was his not obeying orders, who being commanded, Lieutenant-General of the horse, to be ready at such a place at such an hour, early in the morning, came not till the afternoon, and by many particulars, makes it clear to have been only his fault.[17]

The latter statement is inconsistent. Holles in fact appears to refer to the earlier battle when Manchester had been repulsed from Shaw by his own premature attack along the river line. A committee was eventually set up to receive evidence concerning the charges laid by Cromwell, each of the principal officers making a statement to the committee. The first examination of Sir Arthur Hesilrige took place on 6 December; in the chair sat Zouch Tate, MP for Northampton. Hesilrige said:

> That he was present at the Council of War when Parliaments army wars drawn out upon Shaw Field, and the king's upon Winterbourne Heath and marching away. That it was there urged as a motive for present fighting and engaging with the king's army, that if the king's were now beaten it would prevent the bringing over the French or of any foreign force which was the present design in hand where unto the Earl of Manchester answered, 'upon my credit you need not fear the coming of the French, I know there is no such thing'... These were the very words as this examinant remembereth, but he is sure words to this effect were there used by the Earl as a motive against present engaging...[18]

Hesilrige then told the story of Manchester's fear for his 'posterity' and Cromwell's reply. It was not impossible that European assistance could come to Charles. Indeed, very powerful foreign interests were involved in royalist arms supplies, and the Queen's influence abroad was a major factor never to be ignored. Remarkably, the King's foreign policy had prevented involvement in the Thirty Years War, although unofficial involvement by mercenaries and semi-official involvement with the French Huguenot cause during Charles's early years had not exactly endeared him to many courts. It can be reasonably argued that the English rebellion was merely the chain reaction to the continental wars that had brought political and economic chaos to European trade. The general unrest in the changing emancipational climate of the seventeenth century had started with the European conflict and would lend itself to evolutionary change for the next two hundred years or more. The religious and economic transformation of the pre-industrial revolution made the foundations for a trading community, of which the English puritan movement was part. In this movement, however, the semi-royalist landowners like the Earl of Manchester could see their involvement with this change removing the stability of the monarchy which had supported them. This fear was the root cause of Manchester's concern at Newbury.

During Hesilrige's second examination, on 28 December, he told of the period before Newbury Fight:

> That Sir Wm. Waller whilst he lay with his brigade about Shaftesbury, Dorchester, and those parts keeping back the king's army from advancing further from the west, sent several letters to the Earl of Manchester then with his forces at Reading, to desire his speedy advance towards him. That Waller lay about Dorchester 6 weeks before the Earl's forces came up to him. That the Lord General (Essex's) horse then joined Waller at Shaftesbury, and this examinant doth verily believe that if the Earl had marched thither likewise with his horse and foot the king's forces could not have advanced beyond that place but that the forces of the Parliament might in all probability have safely fought with the king's army, or com-pelled them to have remained in those parts about Serborne. That 1,000 men might have safely come from Reading to Shaftesbury, the enemy being further westward, and Waller's army lying betwixt Reading and the King's army. That by reason no forces came he was enforced to retreat to Winterbourne Stoke in Wilts. The King's army then coming to Salisbury, Waller retreated to Andover, and after an engagement retired to Basing, where this examinant then found the Earl of Manchester to have drawn forth all his horse and foot, intending to retreat towards Odiham in Hants, but upon consulting the Earl consented to stay at Basing if until the Lord General's foot and the City brigade came up to them. Whilst the two armies were joined this examinant never remembers the Earl to have declared any opinion in favour of fighting, but often to have declared opposition to it at the Council of War. That Waller commanded and being advanced 5 miles from Newbury in pursuit of the King's army, the Earl sent to him and this examinant desiring them to halt as the enemy was gone another way, and to attend a Council of War.[19]

That the Earl was slow in joining Waller when ordered was perfectly true, but he had friends and officers in Essex's army who were circulating rumours blaming Waller for Manchester's misdeeds. The whole situation was completely ridiculous. As things stood the armies were defeating themselves, with officers happily cutting each other's throats. The matter needed quick adjudication, and to save so many faces the great parliamentary universal whitewash was applied thickly to cover the visible cracks in the foundations of the cause without apportioning the blame.

The trouble with Manchester added to the disasters of 1644 with Essex and Waller and called for radical action, which was now to come.

NOTES

1. Gardiner, *Great Civil War*, II, pp. 28-29.
2. CSP Dom, 1644, pp. 495-96.
3. CSP Dom, 1644, p. 532.
4. CSP Dom, 1644, p. 545.
5. CSP Dom, 1644–45, pp. 28-29.
6. CSP Dom, 1644–45, p. 34.
7. Tibbutt, *John Okey*, p. 4.
8. CSP Dom, 1644–45, p. 60.
9. Adair, *Roundhead General*, p. 169.
10. CSP Dom, 1644–45, p. 75.
11. CSP Dom, 1644–45, pp. 76-77.
12. Accounts of Second Newbury can be found in 'A True Relation of the most chiefe occurrences at and since the Battell at Newbury etc.', TTE 22 (10); 'A Letter wherein is related the Victory obtained by the Parliamentary Army neer Newbury', E 14 (16); Walter Money's *The First and Second Battles of Newbury* is now very dated but still useful for reprint material and notes; main modern secondary source, P. Young and J. Adair, *Hastings to Culloden*, pp. 156-68.
13. C.E. Lucas-Phillips, *Cromwell's Captains* (London, 1938), p. 125.
14. CSP Dom, 1644–45, pp. 150-51.
15. CSP Dom, 1644–45, p. 116.
16. *Holles's Memoirs*, p. 28.
17. *Holles's Memoirs*, p. 28
18. CSP Dom, 1644–45, p. 151.
19. CSP Dom, 1644–45, pp. 156-57.

⧉ 10 ⧉

In Parliament's Name

If it had not been the Lord who was on our side, now may Israel say;

If it had not been the Lord who was on our side, when men rose up against us;

Then they had swallowed us up quick, when their wrath was kindled against us.

(Ps. 124.1-3)

When the militia bill had been introduced by Sir Arthur Hesilrige under the guidance of Cromwell and Strode, Parliament had believed the militia 'to be in them'. This mistaken assumption had cost the war-torn country most dearly in blood, no social class escaping the blade of the reaper. In two years of bitter conflict and stubborn negotiation the Parliament had failed to obtain a victory. The generals were so deeply divided that it was unlikely that the much-needed joint effort would be found of the battlefield. Added to these problems, the civil population was tired of war, and social discontent was stretching the people's patience beyond its limits. Looking for a solution to break this stalemate, the war party offered a plan to change the face of military life.

Probably designed by the fast-growing ideals of the young Henry Vane and Oliver St John, an army singular in stature and for service in 'all England' was proposed. As early as 23 November 1644, the Commons ordered the Committee of Both Kingdoms 'to consider the Frame or Model of the whole Militia', their findings to be reported to the House.[1] It is interesting that those at Derby House were to 'Frame or Model' this new army, for the war party held the majority there. It must also be considered that the case between Manchester and Cromwell was still being hotly argued on 23 November, although this was well and truly whitewashed over the winter. It is therefore possible to conclude that Parliament had pre-judged the situation and found the military wanting.

On 31 December and 1 January—not then New Year of course—the committee discussed in detail the construction of the new army.[2] Earlier in December, Oliver Cromwell had with great persuasion managed to introduce a plan that would exclude many of the old generals from seeking command of the new army. The self-denying ordinance (9 December 1644) forced members of both Houses to relinquish command, and, although brought in by Cromwell, it was really a stroke of pure genius by the war party. Gone from military power would be Manchester, Waller and the Lord General Essex. If Waller had been the darling of Derby House, the great romance was over and he was thrown aside like a worn-out paramour never to be wooed again. Essex, the chosen leader in 1642, would not do. He had failed and cost Parliament dear at Lostwithiel, so 'old Robin', as his soldiers called him, was pensioned off with grateful thanks and a huge sigh of relief. The Earl of Manchester returned to the Lords, which was a somewhat closely knit family, and he quickly became Speaker of that House.

The self-denying ordinance also robbed Hesilrige of his role in the Western Army, but this was perhaps no great disappointment to Sir Arthur, with his military activity being greatly reduced by his work at Derby House.

On 1 January 1645, Hesilrige's horse were at Petersfield in Hampshire, a week later riding west against a threat from the royalists.[3] This was their final action before inclusion into the New Model Army under the command of ex-Lobster John Butler. Thomas Horton was to be the new major, and Gardiner, Pennyfeather, Foley and Parry made up the six troops.

One vital question in forming the new army was the reaction of the Scots, but this was largely overcome by the inclusion of a large number of Presbyterian commanding officers to please them with equal numbers of Independent second-in-commands to please the war party members at Derby House. The New Model was designed by Parliament to remove the problems of area-controlled associations. A regiment of the New Model would serve anywhere in England, unlike the various association forces or trained bands.

While the new army took its first embryonic breath, another series of peace negotiations were under way. Organizing peace talks while devising a war machine has an air of the ridiculous about it, but it never seems to bother anyone involved. Like so many peace talks, the Uxbridge negotiations were a complete farce. Parliament proposed terms that would give them overall options and political power in the nation's affairs, leaving the monarchy as figurehead in a constitutional free state. They also demanded that certain royalist leaders should not be pardoned in an act of oblivion. These of course included the hated Palatine Princes Rupert and Maurice, but strangely also men of the honest calibre of Ralph Hopton. If men like Hopton had committed any crime against the people of England, it was a crime of conscience, not of malice. To include such men of honour, as Hopton most certainly was, in a list of war criminals was an insult to Parliament as much as the royalists. On the other hand, Parliament desired that certain members of their side should be rewarded. Perhaps the most controversial of these rewards was to Hesilrige, who was to be made a baron with lands worth £2,000 per year, if the negotiations succeeded. No doubt the King had other plans for his arch-traitor, for Sir Arthur still faced the impeachment from 1642 should he fall into royalist hands. This said, the two sides could never agree and the Treaty of Uxbridge was doomed before it began.[4]

The New Model Army bill and self-denying ordinance moved steadily through the chambers, albeit with some rough passages and hot debate. But at least progress was being made. A major hiccup then unfortunately occurred on 13 January when the Lords threw out the bill for self-denial which was the backbone of the new army. The Lords demanded that not all those barred from taking commissions should in fact be so. The bill was revised to allow for exceptions, and now pleasing to the Peers it passed, leaving only those who had outlived their useful service in the wilderness. In February 1645 the act passed to structure the New Model Army as

12 Regiments of Foote
11 Regiments of Horse
1 Regiment of Dragoons

In command as lord general was placed Sir Thomas Fairfax, the Yorkshire general whose Northern Army had defeated the King at Marston Moor. The new army was uniform in style of clothing, pay and organization. For the first time the army would be for the nation rather than any commander. The Army was dressed in new coats of 'Venetian Red', lined in contrasting colours to signify the regiment.

The coats of the lord general's foot marching out in their russet red coats lined in green. The regiment of dragoons was given to John Okey, who had served under both Lord Brooke and Hesilrige, and was a stout-hearted man in a fight, which suited dragoon service.

Many old officers from the associations applied for commissions in the New Model. Hesilrige, having so much influence upon the Committee of Both Kingdoms, was petitioned daily to speak on behalf of one of them or another. During this time Sir Arthur did write on behalf of Edmund Ludlow to Fairfax through his secretary John Rushworth:

> Mr. Rushworth,
>
> I entreat you to present this gentleman Colonel Ludlowe to Sir Thomas Fairfax. You may let him know what a good patriot his father was, and what honour this Colonel hath gayned by holding oute the siege at Wardour Castle after halfe of it was blowne up. I pray you do him what good offices you can. I present my services to yourself and so rest your loving friend and servant.
>
> Arthur Haslerig

Despite this Ludlow did not obtain a regiment, the committee for Wiltshire claiming they could not do without Edmund's services.[5]

With all his vast experience in the administration of military matters, it fell to Sir Arthur to prepare the New Model through the committees, to raise its pay from the 'Commiffioners of Exfise' and generally prepare this army for the field.[6] In the long speech made by Hesilrige years later, he told of the forming of the New Model:

> Thus the English pushed on both sides, and much precious English blood was spilt on the ground. Several propositions, at length, were tendered; but god hardened his heart. He would not accept. Then we came to make a new model, and a Self-Denying Ordinance. Thereupon this noble Lord was chosen the Parliaments General. The Commission as to him, was from the Parliament only; the name 'King' was left out. I appeal to all the world for the undeniable, the unquestionable victories after that. We had not one doubtful battle. The King after that never gave thanks. In process of time there were propositions, again and again, seven, eight, or nine times, at least seven times, sent to the King, desiring for ourselves, our ancient liberties with our ancient Government, but his heart was still hardened.[7]

It is clear from Hesilrige's words that the commission given to the New Model was in Parliament's name, the fight against the King rather than to fight in spite of him. Sir Arthur Hesilrige clearly believed the cause was to reclaim the old constitution of England. In the struggle

between King John and the upper nobility, the King is the bad
brother of good King Richard, and is firmly put in his place by the
champions of the people—the picture is black and white, the victory
of good over evil. Early in this speech, Sir Arthur outlined such
idealism in regard to the present conflict:

> Time was, this nation had seven Kings, and no doubt but the strongest
> put down the weakest, against the will of the rest. I never knew any single
> person to have power, willing to lay it down. After it was one single
> person, then came in the Conqueror. The English-men stood up for their
> liberties, and in some sort, preserved liberty to all the rest.
>
> Succeeding Kings, sons and others, began to grow very oppressive to
> the people's liberties. Then rose up the noble Barons who struggled so
> long till with their swords, they obtained our Magna Charta. That our
> Barons were men of great power, appears by what they compelled the
> King to grant; the whole estate being in them and the Bishops, Abbots
> and King. They were so great, and sensible of their greatness.
>
> The Government was then in King and Parliament, Lords and
> Commons sitting altogether. They withdrew and went into another
> House, to make a distinct jurisdiction. Thus the Lords had all but the
> power of the purse, which, to this day, preserved the liberties of the nation.
> Then the Government was enlarged into three estates, Kings, Lords and
> Commons, and continued thus above three hundred years.[8]

Obviously Hesilrige saw himself as one of those great barons saving
the liberty of the Englishmen through 'their swords'. It is a weakness
in the parliamentary cause that they so often identified their cause
with the Anglo-Saxons under the Norman yoke.

By his beliefs and subsequent actions, Sir Arthur had made himself
extremely unpopular with some very influential people on his own
side, and who were not beyond taking the law into their own hands,
or the sword even. On 21 May 1645, Hesilrige was ordered by the
Commons to relate the circumstances of an attack upon him by the
Earl of Stamford and his servants Henry Polton and Matthew Patfall
with a 'drawn sword and other offensive instruments'. Sir Arthur had
been riding to his house in Islington from the Commons, along the
highway from Peephole Lane to Clerkenwell, when the Earl and his
men attacked him. Luckily Sir Arthur's footboy, young Will Goode,
was with him, and Major Bridges and Captain Titus also came to his
aid. The Commons ordered that Sir Arthur should not receive or
issue a challenge to Stamford, and likewise the Lords to the Earl. Sir
Arthur at forty-five was hardly the meat duellists were made of,

although of course Bertin Hesilrige had died in a duel. The Commons insisted that Stamford was impeached for a high breach of privilege. The Lords kept the business in committee for almost a year to protect their man before it was settled with the usual coat of whitewash.[9] The Earl of Stamford had little love for Hesilrige because of the latter's influence at the Western Association, and in time would become a supporter of the monarchy. With this and other turmoils of conscience and jealousy the war was splitting Parliament open. The irony of being cut down by his own side would hardly have found Sir Arthur's sense of humour, and to add insult to injury Stamford was a neighbour of the Hesilriges in Leicestershire.

On 14 June 1645, the New Model Army had its baptism of fire, passing through the flames and emerging victorious on Naseby Field. The man who had all but fathered this precocious child, Oliver Cromwell, won the victory the Parliament so badly needed. Despite the self-denying ordinance, Cromwell had arrived on the eve of battle with troopers from the associations, took command of the right wing on the field and, when victory for the King looked certain, had turned the tide and won a resounding victory for the New Model. At the direct request of Fairfax, who could be denied nothing after such a success, Cromwell was appointed lieutenant general of horse, the clause which barred him from the new army being waved aside.

At Naseby, the King's cause suffered its death knell, his army being reduced to the state suffered by Essex the previous year. For Charles, however, the ultimate result was far more serious, for never again could his army offer 'le grande battalia'. The wandering of the King until his surrender to the Scots a year later are of no interest to this story. It is enough to say that Charles's cause in the military arena was over.

Hesilrige's temperament, brought forth another claim for a breach of privilege, against a man Sir Arthur clearly did not like. The man was the most famous English astrologer of the seventeenth century, William Lilly. It is strange that, at a time when poor people could be hung for witchcraft on the evidence of a jealous neighbour, the words of Lilly were regarded with respect as a science. The writings of William Lilly were a cult as well as occult, and his latest predictions would be discussed by educated men and poor troopers alike. Man's interest in the stars was not, however, Hesilrige's concern, and the charge he laid before Lilly was perhaps more serious than simple witchcraft. In July 1645, Hesilrige brought before the Commons a motion against Lilly for his publication 'The Starry Messenger—with an interpretation of three suns seen in London May 29 1644'. This astrological summary is interesting in its own witless right, but, obviously not foreseeing the trouble it would bring upon his head, Lilly had been far too outspoken concerning the committee of Leicestershire. Like an astrological Leo, with typical laurean bluster, Sir Arthur attacked Lilly:

> On this occasion sir Arthur Hasilrige, a knight for the county and a furious person made a motion in the House of Commons against Lilly, and the business was refered to the committee, whereof Baron Rigby was chairman, where by the good offices of Mr. Seldon, who stated sir Arthurs 'humour and malice towards Lilly, and that the charge was frivolous, and only presented by a choleric person to please a company of clowns', meaning the Committee of Leicester.[10]

The stargazer was acquitted, his influence in high places swaying the issue in his favour, no doubt assisted by some planetary conjunction. In all fairness to Lilly the charge was frivolous, probably brought about by the insult upon the committee of Leicester, upon which Sir Arthur's brother Thomas sat. To call the Leicestershire committee a 'company of clowns' was nevertheless a slur upon an honest profession—clowning.

By January 1646 the Civil War was all but over, only small pockets of futile resistance remaining in fortified houses and the great city of Oxford. Earlier in the war, it was noted how Sir Arthur had shown great kindness to young Sir Henry Bard after his wounds at Cheriton had caused him to lose an arm. When his wounds had healed, Bard had been exchanged, and was at the royalist storming of Leicester, leading the assault against the walls by climbing the ladder one-handed. At Naseby, Bard had commanded a tertia. However, in 1646 Sir Arthur's kindness to Bard had its rewards, when, on 26 February, a trumpeter from Oxford appeared at the door of the Commons with a letter to Hesilrige from Sir Henry.[11] This one act of kindness in 1644 now allowed the royalists in Oxford to negotiate with Parliament. Bard eventually received his discharge from all war crimes, perhaps because of his friendship with Hesilrige and the young man's disability.[12] Free to leave England, Bard joined the Prince of Wales at the Hague, where, as Baron Bard, he served the Prince loyally.

In Leicestershire it fell upon Sir Arthur Hesilrige to negotiate the surrender of the royalist stronghold at Ashby-de-la-Zouch, where Henry Hastings held out for the King. The Committee of Both Kingdoms and the Commons had failed to reach a negotiation with the Hastings family, and, because to attempt to storm such walls would have been so costly in men, Sir Arthur, who was known by Hastings and respected if not liked, opened talks with a letter on 13 February.[13] In this negotiation Hesilrige allowed Hastings to march out with what they would consider a moral victory.[14]

Another name from Sir Arthur's past had returned to England in 1645. George Fenwick, who was Sir Arthur's best friend and colleague from the Saybrooke adventure, had been governor of 'The Fort' at that colony, but things had gone badly in the New World when the war broke out in England. Following the death of his wife, Fenwick had little to bind him at Sayebrook, and, being known and trusted by parliamentarians like Lord Saye and Sele, and of course Sir Arthur Hesilrige, he was chosen MP for the vacant seat at Morpeth on 20 October 1645.[15] George Fenwick remained a close friend of Sir Arthur for the rest of their lives, giving support and advice when needed both politically and in family life.

In the Commons, the parties were becoming deeply divided, neither side trusting the other, and a slowly increasing hostility developed between Denzil Holles's moderate Presbyterians, and the Hesilrige, Vane, St John-led more radical Independents. The Independents were beginning to abstain from sitting and voting at the Committee of Both Kingdoms by mid 1646, Sir Henry Vane hardly attending at all. Sir Arthur Hesilrige, however, seemed to make a point of attending. It was his duty to do so, and, being a pedantic follower of duty, he would expect to attend. This absence of the Independents from the committee was in itself not vital, the work not having the same military importance, but the Presbyterians were thought to have plans alien to the Independent view, and it was becoming clear that a split would soon endanger the success of the New Model.

The Scots too were unhappy. They were an embarrassment to the English Parliament, no country enjoying having a military power in its sovereign land without control over it. In 1643 the Scots were needed to supply a firm rearguard between the King and the border, but now they were surplus to the military need. Charles also realized this, and, defeated, he chose to surrender himself to the Scots rather than the more hostile English. Riding to Newark-on-Trent, the King gave himself into the hands of the Scots who were besieging that fine old town. In good faith, the royalist commander at Newark also surrendered, after an epic defence of the area throughout the war, and with this act the English Civil War shuddered to a halt.[16] The cannons stopped 'a'Roaring and bulletts stopt flying',[17] the honour of the field gave way to the voice of politics.

NOTES

1. CJ, III, p. 703.
2. CSP Dom, 1644–45, pp. 204-205.
3. G.N. Godwin, *The Civil War in Hampshire* (London, 1882), p. 188.
4. See Gardiner, *Constitutional Documents of the Puritan Revolution*, pp. 273-87; Rushworth, *Historical Collections*, V, p. 858, LJ, VII, p. 54.
5. *Ludlow's Memoirs*, I, pp. 113, 127, 141; Nichols, *Leicestershire*, II, pt ii, p. 744.
6. CJ, IV, p. 119.
7. *Burton's Diary*, III, p. 96.
8. *Burton's Diary*, III, pp. 87-88.
9. CJ, IV, pp. 150-52, 188.
10. *Life of William Lilly* (1774 edn), p. 71.
11. CJ, IV, p. 455.
12. DNB (Sir Henry Bard).
13. CSP Dom, 1645–47, p. 342.
14. CSP Dom, 1645–47, p. 352.
15. Winthrop, *History of New England*, I, p. 306.
16. For a detailed account of the King and the Scots, see Wedgwood, *The King's War*. For highly detailed work on Scottish political history, there are a number of excellent works available written in recent years by Dr David Stevenson.
17. 'When Cannons are roaring, and bulletts are flying, he would that honour win, must not fear dying'—the chorus of a popular seventeenth-century soldier's song.

↪ 11 ↩

Cromwell's Nose

When thou sittest to eat with a ruler, consider diligently what is before thee:
²And put a knife to thy throat, if thou be a man given to appetite.

(Prov. 23.1-2)

A prisoner, the King was carried north to Newcastle-upon-Tyne, but what good was an English king to the Scots when it appeared the English did not want him? Within a few short months, the Scots, looking for a way out of this bloody rebellion, sold the King for a few pieces of silver, and for the first time in five years Charles was in English puritan hands. The Scots had tried to convert the King to a Presbyterian style of church, and Charles had played his usual games. Yet in reality the whole concept of accepting the Presbyterian faith in return for his throne was against the King's strongly held principles.

On 30 January 1647, the Scottish garrison took their leave of Newcastle, handing the keys of that great town and the King to that reliable soldier Philip Skippon, who was appointed governor. If any negotiation was to be made with the King, however, he needed to be brought nearer to London. In many ways Charles was far more dangerous in debate than on the battlefield. What the Earl of Manchester had said about the King still being King if beaten ninety-nine times still held true in 1647. Parliament needed to gain control of not only the King's person, but also his will. The King was carried southward to Holdenby House in the tranquil fields of Northampton-shire. After so many years with rough ill-mannered soldiers, and latterly the dire boredom of the presbyter's tongue, the green fields ·about Holdenby must have seemed like Eden itself. Charles was allowed a surprising freedom at Holdenby, walking freely in the grounds of his open prison. The people of Northamptonshire could watch their King a guest of their Parliament, and wonder at the goodness of his majesty.

If the King had hopes of his restoration, the Presbyterian and Independent parties had further problems with the formation of yet another political voice—the New Model Army. During the winter of 1646–47 an open quarrel with the army looked ever more likely, for the Presbyterian party led by Denzil Holles was set to betray the soldiers. In 1646, Holles had failed to have regiments of the New Model sent to Ireland to crush an Irish Catholic rebellion. It was common knowledge that the Presbyterians desired the almost total disbandment of the New Model to cut the economic budget and remove a certain Independent flow of idealism from the military. The country was in very poor condition: the war had disrupted trade, harvests had failed in a series of cold, wet summers, and even coal was in short supply due to the war stopping a good deal of mining and even its transportation. To put it bluntly, England could not afford to pay its army, and the demob suit awaited.

Since its formation, the New Model Army had changed from a purely military body to become a free-thinking force with its own views on England's freedom and soldier's rights. The soldiers and their Independent officers would not bow to the Presbyterian plan without a say in their own destiny. For an army to disobey the government is mutiny and possibly treason for the officers, but the army of Fairfax and Cromwell thought nought of this, having fought for England and cut their teeth on rebellion. While the likes of Holles had fought a war of words, the men of the New Model had faced pike and shot and through military comradeship had formed a body of free spirit.

In a moment of utter madness, the Presbyterians attempted to withhold the arrears of pay due to each soldier. This folly was a serious act by Parliament, considering the foot were eighteen weeks and the horse some forty-three weeks in arrears. On 30 March, a very moderate petition by certain regiments, supported in London by a political group called by their enemies the 'Levellers', was pronounced to be seditious, and those supporting it were hauled before the Commons. The most noted of the so-called Levellers was 'Freeborn John Lilburne', one-time dragoon commander in the Eastern Association, and a radical pamphleteer even before the war. Lilburne backed those brought before the Commons, and, although already imprisoned for some words he had written about the Earl of Manchester, the underground press of his movement gave vocal support to the common soldier. In a short space of time John Lilburne and Sir Arthur Hesilrige would be bitter enemies, but in the question of justice for the army they were united. Despite calls from the Presbyterian leadership to have the mutinous soldiers imprisoned, those of the Independent party carried the day and all charges were put aside.

The Independents needed the army, for without it they could never hope to stop the Presbyterians upholding any plan they may have regarding the settlement of the nation. The army was a power in the land, and any government needed to either destroy it or have its support.

Ireland was again the stumbling block between the army and the Presbyterians. English soldiers would not accept Irish service unless by choice, and certainly not until their arrears were paid. The Holles-led Presbyterians now attempted to force the issue. Regiments were by late May ordered to divide from the army and disband. In anger, and totally against the orders of Parliament, the army called a general rendezvous near Newmarket, where their answer to the Parliament would be made.

But what of the King? It could be said that whoever held his royal person held the field. This had been the whole issue since 1642, and the Presbyterians held the King at Holdenby. The King was the key to all negotiation, whose use could unlock the door for any party, military or civil. In an unprecedented step, a plain, buff-coated cornet called George Joyce wrote his name into English history. Under orders, Joyce rode to Oxford to secure from the Presbyterians the 'Trayne of Artillerie', and then had orders to secure the King at Holdenby. What was meant by 'secure' was the problem facing Joyce on 4 June. Having received an audience with Charles, it was plain to Joyce that he could not leave the King at Holdenby. The men guarding the King at Holdenby had gone over to the views of the army, greeting Joyce's '500 troopers' as brothers, their Presbyterian Colonel Graves fleeing rather than be taken prisoner by his own men. In panic George Joyce removed the King from his Northamptonshire prison and began the ride to Newmarket, where the army would protect him. Not knowing what next to do, Cornet Joyce wrote to the Independents in London, as Holles relates:

> Joyce after seizing and carrying away the king, immediately sends up a letter to certify what he had done, with directions that it should be delivered to Cromwell and if he is absent, to Sir Arthur Haslerig or to Col. Fleetwood.[1]

The letter was in fact delivered to Charles Fleetwood, but not before its contents were leaked to Denzil Holles, putting the Independents and particularly Hesilrige, who was not of the army, in a very embarrassing and awkward situation. An entry in the diary of Lawrence Whitacre for 8 June sheds more light upon this dark and secret deed:

> The house was informed by Mr. Holles of a letter was come into his hands written from Holmby by Cornet Joyce with directions that it should be delivered to Lieut.-Gen. Cromwell, or in his absence to Sir Arthur Hesilrige or Col. Fleetwood; whereby Mr Holles would have infered that those three gentlemen held correspondance with that Cornet, and so had intelligence of that party's carrying away of the king and the Commissioners from Holmby; but such Sir Arthur Hesilrige denied any knowledge he had thereof, and the names of none of those gentlemen did appear upon the superscription of that letter, so that there was no further proceeding upon it at that time.[2]

Hesilrige's denial was obviously nothing more than a severe bout of political amnesia, there being no way Sir Arthur could admit to prior knowledge of the King's kidnapping without being impeached or worse. In the eyes of the Presbyterians, Cromwell was undoubtedly behind George Joyce's action. News spread that he had held secret talks with the cornet and the leveller William Walwyn, and with this Oliver felt it safer to join the army at Newmarket.

In the meantime the army had at the general rendezvous undertaken to remain together, swearing by 'The Solemn Engagement of the army' to resist any endeavours to disband or divide them. A new and historic step was also undertaken by the establishment of a General Council of the Army, made up both of officers and men, the men choosing two or three 'Agitators'—the word meaning representative—per regiment to give the soldier's views. Parliament now had a body to negotiate with and consequently sent commissioners to Triploe Heath. Despite all efforts to bring the army back under their control, the Presbyterians were losing at every turn. Presbyterian officers were chased from their regiments, and new, trusted Independents were given command. These Independents, led principally by Cromwell's creature, Henry Ireton, quickly gained control of the Army Council, and with their political wing led by Hesilrige, St John and to an extent Harry Vane, they began to introduce political demands into the army crisis.

At a late night meeting of the Army Council, probably on 16 July,

a far reaching decision was made that the army would take their
rights if all else failed. Regiments were sent from the main body to
secure areas of strategic importance, York, Newcastle, Wales and the
west. The army could claim these areas were in danger from royalist
insurrections, and were vital if an army coup was to come.[3]

The Presbyterians in London now turned as much in panic as common sense to the old army officers removed from the army, and the
trained bands were to support these 'Reformados'. However, when
called upon to act against the New Model, the Independents and
Levellers of the trained bands would not muster, leaving only a mob
of disorderly ex-soldiers and a few of the 'City Prentices' to form the
parliamentary guard. This rough, undisciplined militia was a danger
not only to the Independents but to civil order in London itself.
If the Presbyterians now sheltered under some false sense of security,
the Independents daily grew fearful of their lives, and Hesilrige feared
greatly for his own safety at the hands of this rag-tag mob. Edmund
Ludlow tells of the action of Sir Arthur following an attack on the
Independents by an howling mob of these pro-Presbyterian mercenaries and apprentices:

> (27 July) The next morning I advised with Sir Arthur Haslerig and others,
> what was fittest to be done in this conjucture; and it was concluded, that
> wee could not sit in parliament without apparent hazard of our lives, till
> we had a guard for our defence, it being manifestly the design of the other
> party either to drive us away, or to destroy us. Therefore we resolved to
> betake ourselves to the army for protection, Sir Arthur Haslerig under-
> taking to perswade the Speaker to go thither, to which he consented with
> some difficulty.[4]

The Speaker, William Lenthall, was a timid man of no great courage,
but he loved above all things the honour of his chair. Being 'the
servant of this House', Lenthall should not of course choose sides. Yet
of all men in the Commons he respected Sir Arthur, he being a
supporter of this Parliament's freedom that had given Lenthall the
Speaker's chair.

In a strange, almost identical resemblance to 1642, Sir Arthur
Hesilrige again fled the Commons in danger of his life and liberty.
But this time it was not from the divine right of kings, but from the
self-styled divinity of the Presbyterian Covenant. Hesilrige rode
quickly to Sir Thomas Fairfax and the army near Reading to inform
the General Council of the Army of the flight of the Independent

members, carrying with him a letter from Speaker Lenthall dated
29 July:

> May it please your Excellence,
>   Sir Arthur Haslerig can inform you of my condition. I found the many
> inconveniences I was like to have falne into, not in respect of my selfe, but
> in regard of ye Kingdome Co…of your Army. I am assured it will be
> strange to your Excellencie to heare of my being at Windsor where I
> intend to stay until I find the parliament in a better condition, if in case it
> may be my fortune to sitt any more. I pray God blesse your Excellence
> and all the reste there, that you may be, under God, the Saviour of the
> Parliament and people's libertie, which I wish may be perfected by your
> selfe, which hath always been so wished by.
>   Your Excellencies humble servant
>   Wm. Lenthall[5]

The army had been Parliament's saviour in 1642 and the clock
would now turn full circle for it to be so again. Unfortunately it is
forever the military's bane that it is far more likely to impose a junta
than a free Parliament. With every week that passed, England became
more and more likely to be ruled by the sword. With the Speaker of
the Commons at Windsor and Earl Manchester having fled the
Lords, London was in chaos. Looting by the mob began to spread,
and the vultures of the sword picked their victims' bones clean of
wealth and respectability. The army made its move. Fairfax, pressed
by his officers and the hotter-headed agitators, could wait no longer.
Advancing to Hounslow Heath, the New Model army marched into
London on 6 August, and the cold war between the army and the
Presbyterians was over.

The power now being in the Independents' hands, 'Eleven' of the
leading Presbyterians were impeached, including Sir William Waller.[6]
Waller had long been the darling of the more radical Independents in
the old Committee of Both Kingdoms, but with the forming of the
New Model Army had slowly adhered himself with the moderates like
Holles. It was perhaps not so much the likes of Waller who had
changed, but that England and the Independents had grown harder.
Sadly, the Earl of Essex had died the previous year, but how 'Old
Robin' would have laughed to see Waller and Hesilrige on opposite
sides.

The entry of the army into London caused the 'Eleven' to flee on
12 August. It was unsafe in England for Holles, Waller, Walter Long,
Sir Philip Stapleton, Sir William Lewis and Sir John Clotsworthy, all

great names from 1642. After a terrible sea journey, these exiles finally reached Calais, but Stapleton died of the plague soon after.

With the Independents restored to authority by the army, many of the important civil appointments in places of high security were reappointed. At the Tower, Sir Arthur's brother Thomas was granted a vital post. The Commons giving order:

> That Mr. Thomas Hesilrige be appointed to take charge, and execute the Place of Clerke of the Deliveries in the Office of Ordnance in the Tower: And that William Billers, that now executes the said Place, be forwith removed, and is hereby removed, from the Charge and Execution of the said Place.[7]

In effect the Independents were replacing Presbyterians in strategic posts. Thomas Hesilrige had married Rebecca Sheafe at St Luke's Chelsea on 6 September 1632. Her father was old Dr Thomas Sheafe, Prebendary of Windsor, and Rector of Walford near Newbury. At his death, Thomas Sheafe had reached the grand old age of 80, leaving his flock in 1639 just before the purge of the clergy.[8] Being now very much in the power of the army, the Lords confirmed Thomas Hesilrige's appointment, and he replaced the unfortunate Billers.[9]

From the moment the army marched into London, parliamentary democracy ceased to exist. However, following years of civil disorder the military did restore a sense of stability lacking in the civil government. Although Sir Thomas Fairfax was commander of the New Model, he tried to keep aloof from the political side of his army, this being the domain of Cromwell and Henry Ireton. The Independents and officers were forming a strong civil and military junta to restore some form of authority and preserve their own status quo. In this situation, the so-called Levellers were a disruptive influence, for they spoke of freedom for the poorer classes, votes for most if not all men, equality in law—in fact what twentieth-century man would class as a natural right.[10] But in the 1640s this was revolutionary. If these things were allowed the whole class system could break down, leaving even worse chaos than that made by the Civil War. The Levellers were hostile to authority being solely in those called 'Grandees', the 'Silken Independents', the affluent ruling class system. Hesilrige himself owned large estates that were estimated to be £1,000 a year in rents and commercial value even in 1647. Fairfax was one of the most powerful men in the north, and even Cromwell, who would claim a modest heritage, was climbing high on the social ladder. If these were the great fleas, however, smaller fleas quite often lived off their backs, it being common practice for their servants to indulge themselves in petty corruption. It was common gossip, for example, that Sir Arthur's secretaries would charge anyone wishing an audience with their master the sum of ten shillings, a foul practice frowned upon today, but in 1647 it was common enough and indeed expected.

Cromwell and Ireton entered into discussion with the King during the late summer of 1647, but the King was in no way for sale. In the light of this, and also Cromwell's talks with the Levellers—because Oliver was trying to be all things to all men—it is well to look at an aspect not normally associated with high political debate, the nub of the question being Cromwell's nose. This great copper-coloured feature appeared to fascinate Sir Arthur, or so the pamphleteers would have their readers think. Following a meeting between the Independents and the Army Council, in which the settlement of the nation had been the main topic, Sir Arthur Hesilrige was reported to turn to Oliver Cromwell and, looking him firmly between the eyes, uttered, 'If you prove untrue in this matter, I shall never trust a man with a great nose for your sake...'[11]

Did this mean the future of England rested dangerously upon the large bridge of the General's nose? In many ways yes. Cromwell was of the army and also the Commons, and if he gave too much to the former, the restraint upon the latter would be too great for Parliament to bear without malice or jealousy. Sir Arthur was nevertheless a friend of Cromwell, and close to him. It is extremely easy to find some humour in the quote, Sir Arthur poking a jest at that great bulbous nose that dominated Oliver's broad, ruddy-complexioned face. It is a mistake to imagine either man to be the dour, black-coated puritan with matching joyless religion. Cromwell had an almost childlike humour at times, mixed with the earthy ribaldness of the farmer. Hesilrige, although said to be morose, could laugh heartily with his comrades, and with a sexual undertone hardly befitting the standard picture of the puritan. It is clear that laughter was not the privilege of the cavaliers alone, and they did not have the sole right to such pleasure.

In late October 1647, a General Council of the Army sat in Putney Church—the so-named Putney Debates—during which the Levellers and representatives of the army presented a petition of constitutional reform under two documents. From the army came 'The Case of the

Armie Truly Stated'. From the Levellers, yet signed by the army, came 'An Agreement of the People'.[12] The agreement demanded basic human rights with equal laws for rich and poor alike, it being nothing less than a call for democracy for the common man. The 'Case' was for the army agitators, demanding basic army rights. The soldiers had been producing such pamphlets since March, one of August saying:

> ...we were not merely mercenary soldiers brought together by the hopes of pay and the fortunes of wars; the peace of our country, our freedom from tyranny, the preservation of due liberty, the administration of judgement and justice, the free course of the laws of the land, the preservation of the King, the privilege of Parliament, and the liberty of the subject, were which brought us together...[13]

By October the men of the army were calling for that age-old demand of the soldier, 'Homes fit for heroes', and they had received nothing. The agitators, greatly influenced by the London Levellers with their more professional politics, had even turned from the King, but if they no longer wished to preserve Charles, he had plans to preserve himself. On the night of 11 November, the same day that the Army Council broke up in turmoil, the King escaped from his semi-prison of Hampton Court. After much trouble, Charles found himself free. A boat would take him to France—or would it? Some said it was Cromwell's intention that the King should escape from Hampton Court, he being too near his throne during a particularly uncertain stage in the army debates. The great theologist and monarchist, Thomas Hobbes, held the opinion that Cromwell was behind the movement of Charles. Had not Cromwell been implicated in Joyce's removal of the King from Holdenby. It was vital that the Independents of the army and Parliament had control over the King, because at Hampton Court a swift move by the agitators could again change the tide of the debate. Charles only reached the Isle of Wight and further imprisonment at Carisbrooke Castle, under the safe care of Cromwell's friend, Colonel Hammond.

Sir Arthur says nothing of the King's escape, lightly saying, 'Next we shall find him in the Isle of Wight, where the last propositions were tendered to him. He would not consent, though his sword was broken, and he was in the lowest condition.'[14] Sir Arthur could hardly speak of a plot to move the King without the permission of Parliament or Army Council. Yet it seems inconceivable that an event as important as the escape of the King from custody could be so lightly glossed over without some knowledge by the inner circle of Independents.

Safely on the Isle of Wight, the King was again offered terms but rejected them all. Seeing Charles would never change his mind in dealing with them, Parliament, pressed by the army, passed a 'Vote of No Address'. No longer would they deal with a King so unbending.[15] Parliament no longer trusted this King—this 'man of blood'—the assembly now being far more hard line since the moderate Presbyterians had fled. Rumours of a Second Civil War were strong, Charles had long been in contact with the Presbyterian Scots, and still thought his best strategy was to divide his enemy.

With the storm clouds of war hanging dangerously over the heads of the army and Parliament, Hesilrige was again on the move in support of the war party. At Newcastle-upon-Tyne, the Presbyterian Philip Skippon held the gateway to any Scottish invasion. He was loyal to both the army and Parliament, but after five years very hard service he was tired and had requested retirement early in 1647. Skippon had in effect already been replaced in July by an Army Council decision to send Colonel Robert Lilburne north as stand-in governor. However, Fairfax, knowing full well that Robert Lilburne would soon be needed in the field, made his choice for successor on 29 December 1647: 'A letter from Windsore, on 29th December 1647, from the General signifying. That he had granted a Commission to Sir Arthur Hesilrige to be Governor of the Town of Newcastle, was this Day read. Resolve & c.'[16]

Sir Arthur was an excellent choice for Newcastle, the area needed an experienced administrator, plus someone trusted by the army. Between 1642–44 Hesilrige had faithfully controlled Waller's forces, and was therefore highly experienced in that field. Whoever held or lost the far north held the future of the parliamentary cause in their hands. It needed a man of Hesilrige's abilities to hold this key position. Sir Arthur grasped that key, and locked the gates behind him.

NOTES

1.   *Holles's Memoirs*, p. 96.
2.   *The Clarke Papers* (4 vols.; London, 1891–1901), I, p. xxx.
3.   Henry Ireton's speech on the second day at Putney; see G.E. Aylmer, *Levellers in the English Revolution* (London, 1975), p. 124; B. Denton, *Crisis in the Army, 1647* (Leigh-on-Sea, 1987).

4. *Ludlow's Memoirs*, I.

5. *Clarke Papers*, I, pp. 218-19.

6. B. Whitelocke, *Memorials of English Affairs* (4 vols.; 1853), p. 82; also, 'The Arraignment of Major-General Massie, Sir William Waller, Colonel Poyntz and other citizens of the Presbyterian faction...', TTE 404 (6).

7. CJ, V, p. 267.

8. Money, *First and Second Newbury*, p. 195.

9. CJ, V, p. 267.

10. I am indebted to the work of Dr Christopher Hill, whose work on seventeenth-century political groups has blown away so many of the old cobwebs from previous generations. See C. Hill, *The World Turned Upside Down: Radical Ideas during the English Revolution* (Harmondsworth, 1975).

11. *A Word to General Cromwell* (London, 1647)—I am indebted to Lady Antonia Fraser for bringing this tract to my attention.

12. 'An Agreement of the People', TTE 412 (21); for Lilburne see M. Gibb, *Lilburne the Leveller*, or DNB (John Lilburne).

13. 'Vox Militaris', TTE 401 (24); Denton, *Crisis in the Army*.

14. *Burton's Diary*, III, p. 96.

15. Gardiner, *The Great Civil War*, p. 356.

16. CJ, V, p. 410.

❧ 12 ❧

The Defence of the Nation

And thou shalt stone him with stones, that he die; because he hath
sought to thrust thee away from the LORD thy God, which brought
thee out of the land of Egypt, from the house of bondage.

(Deut. 13.10)

The old town of Newcastle-upon Tyne had suffered greatly under
the turmoil of civil war, but in Sir Arthur Hesilrige would have
an administrator capable of raising it again to its rightful position of
importance. If war with the Presbyterian Scots was in the air,
Newcastle and the other northern defences at Berwick and Carlisle
held the gateway to invasion, and undoubtedly a man of Hesilrige's
unquestionable abilities was required to lock this gateway or suffer his
nation to the return of the monarchy. In the so-called Bishops' Wars,
the Scots had no difficulty invading England, and added to this was
the fresh synopsis of a joint Anglo-Scottish pact between the Scottish
Covenant and English royalist forces. Charles, from his distant position at Carisbrooke Castle, where he had more direct liberty than
Hesilrige at Newcastle to plot and play with his friends and enemies,
was without doubt in a better situation than at any period since
Naseby in 1645. If the Scottish Presbyterians backed their faith against
the King's cause, how many would cross the border in support of the
Covenant? The old leadership of Presbyterian-inspired Covenant
armies—David Leslie included—were to some extent against breaking
the solemn league they had made with the English Parliament, but
others, principally led by the Duke Hamilton, were not so inclined to
English Independency and openly negotated with the royalist agents.
The edge of the balance hung on a point of Kirk law, and if the
Scottish Kirk turned in support of a 'Holy War', the influence
therein would provide an army of many thousands—the north and

the whole English nation must have care in its appointments.

In the period between Skippon's departure and Hesilrige's arrival at Newcastle, the area was governed by Colonel Robert Lilburne. The Lilburne family held a position of some high degree in the Northumberland area, they being of long standing throughout the Tyne and Bishopricke of Durham. Robert Lilburne was not of a Leveller nature like the more famous John, but was a very able soldier well trusted by Oliver Cromwell, and was in fact an extremely good influence in the area during the short time he was in control.

On 15 February 1648, Governor Sir Arthur Hesilrige wrote to the Newcastle major, Thomas Ledgand:

> I have heard so much of your abilities, integrity, and true piety that I presume to put upon you a great trouble. The Parliament is very sensible of your town's sufferings, and are very desirous to take off free quarters. It is, and shall be, my exceeding care to procure money to ease that burden which you have so long groaned under. My resolution is not to receive into my own hands any public moneys. The House (of Commons) doth approve of your being treasurer, and I most earnestly entreat you, as you desire the good of your towne, to accept of that office I do not press you to a burden and loss without some consideration for your pains and charges, therefore you shall receive 3d in the I.l for the moneys you receive and pay out upon my orders (as Governor of Newcastle).[1]

As the situation slowly transformed into the dawn of a second civil war, the army under Sir Thomas Fairfax found itself stretched to restrain the regional outbreaks. A force under Sir Arthur's old friend and falconer, Colonel Thomas Horton, had already been sent to South Wales to police the likely insurrections from royalists and English Presbyterians, and Fairfax himself was watching the situation carefully in the south. It was in this light that Hesilrige rode north, probably in late March. With Sir Arthur went Colonel Paul Hobson, who was to act as deputy governor of Newcastle and command various militia and Hesilrige regiments during his office. Paul Hobson, was said to be by trade a tailor, although other sources call him a surgeon in 1645.[2] It is possible that Hobson was a surgeon, although that profession is not noted for its military skills. He was however a strict Baptist. In 1644, Hobson had been arrested at Newport Pagnell for lay-preaching, and his religious life certainly helped to strengthen the Newcastle group of Baptists in the years to come.

On 14 March, the Committee of Both Houses—as it was now called following the break with the Covenant—wrote from its office at

Derby House to the counties of Lancaster, Westmorland, Cumberland and Northumberland:

> We are informed that Captain Wogan has lately marched with a troop of horse through Lancashire towards the north, pretending an order from Sir Thomas Fairfax for so doing, whereas the General has given no such order, and other troops are reported to march that way. We desire you to take care that no such forces may march into or through your country without the order of this Committee, of the General, Col. Lambert, or the Governor of Newcastle, under their hands and seals. If any attempt to do otherwise you are desired to resist them and hinder their passage, securing the persons of the officers that they may answer for their offence, and the horse and arms of the troopers for the use of the state.[3]

The danger of movement by unauthorized soldiers is evident in all military action, but even more so in a civil war or revolution. Captain Wogan was a known royalist agent, and left to wander the north he could soon raise a troop or two from the known 'delinquents' in those parts ready for the Scottish invasion.

On 22 March, Parliament found in Hesilrige's favour a judgment against the Earl Rivers for a debt of £1,000, this sum being paid forthwith. It was good news for Hesilrige and with it he left for the north.

The 31 March saw Sir Arthur and his old friend, George Fenwick, added to the Commission for Sequestration in the far north.[4] The acts of sequestration were to bring Hesilrige into considerable disrepute, with claims for his enemies of corruption and feathering his own nest with taking advantage of his high office. Whether by fair or foul means, Sir Arthur certainly bought a vast northern estate. George Fenwick was again at his side, and with the great work now upon Hesilrige, Fenwick would be worth a regiment of foot to the difficult northern defences.

With the outbreak of hostilities, John Lambert, a very capable parliamentarian officer was required to watch the north ready for the Scottish advance. Lambert's force consisted of three regiments of horse and one of foot, hardly sufficient to hold a Scottish attack, very mobile in design, but very very weak if the Scots advanced quickly and in strength.

On 16 April, Colonel Lambert, on receiving intelligence from Fairfax, wrote from York to Hesilrige, who was now at Newcastle and taking military control of the borders:

Sir,

I formerly recived a letter from his Excellency appointing mee to wait on you to advise of some way for the securing of Berwick and Carlile from surprisall (to which purpose I also percived by yours this post you received directions from him); in answer to which I gave his Excellency this accompt, that I did not think it possible to secure them except by quartering souldiers therein, and did conceive that the advancing of foote neare thereunto (the proper means to the end) would give too apparent cause of jealousie to the Scotts and indeed rather invite a mischief than prevent it, we having no plausible coulor for quartering of foote thereabout. I likewise desire that if his Excellency thought fitt wee should proceed in this business, he would give mee further directions in it by the next post and in the meantime I would have in readiness a competent number of horse in order to that service, and if I heard nothing would not proceed, since which (though my letters came safely to his hands) I have heard nothing, and therefore think fitt to wave it, unless you (being nearer to the places and upon better intelligence of the condition thereof) shall advise something of the possibility to effect it, which if you shall please to doe, I shall willingly upon three daies notice, meete you at Darlington or North Allerton, my occasions heere not well admitting me to come to Newcastle which otherwise I should willingly doe. I had formerly given you this accompt (SIR) but that I had not assurance of your being at Newcastle. I have this week recived a letter from some fewe well affected persons in Cumberland who informe mee that Sir Wilfrid Lawson hath secured a considerable number of ordnance, arms amunition and other provisions of warre in an iland in that county and that he assessed the country for the payment of the forces of the iland being about forty or fifty foote and also that himself and a captaine that he commands his men whose name is William Buller are both suspected of affect the King's partee but certainly are enemies of the late proceedings of Parliament (though Sir Wilfrid was formerly of the committee of warre at York) so that I conceived it very unfitt and (if I be not mistaken) contrary to the intentions of parliament, that either such garrisons should be kept or levyes made, in regard of your nearenes to the place I desire you will please to inform yourself fully of the particulars, and if occasion and opportunity will give you leave to remove the ordnance and to Newcastle or some other secure place, or at least that you will provide some faithful man of your garrison who may take charge of the iland with a competent nomber of soulders for the security thereof, and I am confident you upon his Excellencys order it will be delivered up to him.

I have nothing more but desiring you to excuse this trouble, and to returne mee an answere to theis particulars, as soone as your occasions will permitt and remayne.

Your very faithfull and humble servant
John Lambert[5]

York 16 April 1648

Lambert's fears were well founded, for, although the opening shots of the insurrection of 1648 were fired in Wales, the echoes of that blast were heard throughout the nation. Sir Arthur Hesilrige now began to relive his actions of the 1643–44 period, riding to and from Newcastle to meet the various parliamentarian officers—John Lambert, Robert Lilburne, John Bright, the two majors serving under Lilburne, Smithson and John Sanderson—these men, aided by Hesilrige's administrative power, were to hold the key to the northern campaign. In 1648, Sir Arthur was to these men what he had been to Sir William Waller—Parliament had chosen its northern grandee commander with extreme care.

On 28 April, only twelve days after Lambert began his correspondence with Hesilrige, the garrisons of Berwick and Carlisle were surprised and taken through neglect by the eminent royalists, Sir Marmaduke Langdale and Sir Philip Musgrave. The towns of Berwick and Carlisle were the hinges to the northern gate, the great lock of Newcastle-upon-Tyne was now all that held the gate in place. By taking these towns, the English royalists held open the advance for the Scots. On 5 May the Derby House committee wrote urgently to Hesilrige and Lambert:

> We are informed there are some ordnance which were lately at Carlisle, were with the arms and ammunition belonging to Cumberland appointed by the Commons Order of 17th June (1647) to be secured. St. Herberts isle, supplemented by an order of the Committee of that county of 13th July to that purpose. Notwithstanding these orders the ordnance are not yet brought thinther, but lie by the way between Carlisle and St. Herbert's Isle, liable to be seized on by the malignants and used against the parliament. We therefore desire you to consult with Mr. Barwis and the Committee of Cumberland, and cause order to be taken for carrying the said ordnance forthwith to that island according to former orders, also that a guard be appointed for that service and care taken for their payment.[6]

This is a classic example of lines of communication being too long. Lambert had already written to Hesilrige three weeks before informing him of the same thing. If the Scots were to be held, this example of the central war committee being too late with orders proves that it would be the heroics of those in the field who would win the fight. If these guns had fallen into Langdale's hands, it would have obviously strengthened the royalists and put further pressure on Lambert. A letter dated Penrith 11 June from Lambert to Hesilrige explains the

situation as it stood at that time, as does another from John Bright
and Major Smithson:

Sir,

You had from Brough a relation of our proceedings against the enimie,
and since that, finding they gave ground and retreated before us, we
resolved to trye all meanes possable to ingage them, before they could
gett to Carlile or any other saife quarter. And there upon marched yester-
day morneing early with our whole bodie to Appleby and from thence
(having there left a party to block up that castle because of keeping that
path open) marched forward with the rest towards Penrith, between
which and Appleby, most of the enimies horse lay, and keept a passe or 2
neare Kir(k) by thure, from which our forlorne beate them, their bodie of
foote being quartered in this town marched off before we came neare, and
most of their horse allso that onely their reareguard stayed to face us, but
did not stand to chardge a very small partie of our forlorne, but gave
ground, and onely 5 of ours being well mounted pursuing killd 2 of them,
and put th'others to run for it, till they came to those bridges att this
towne end where haveing a reserve, and Sir Marmaduke Langdaile with
them, endeavored to maintaine there passes, and barricaded them, but
more of ours comeing to reinforce the rest, presently became maisters of
the passe, and pursued that part of the enimie through this towne, and 3
mile further towards Carlile, whereto their foote and strength of horse is
marched, and would not by meanes ingage or hazard the least party
against us. But a party of theirs being sent to garrison Brome Castle about
a mile from hence, upon a bare sumons, yeilded it upon quarter given
them, and we are in some hopes that Appleby and especially Grastock
will also render upon easie tearmes. The enimies foote scatters and runns
away much, they endeadvour to keepe them together by telling them,
they retreate not from us for feare, but are goeing to joyne with 20,000
Scots and to meete the Prince att Barwick where they shall all recive com-
pleate armes. This day we rest us haveing had sore marches and terrable
weather, and withall seeinge nowe advantage by our further advance, the
enimie having Carlile open to them, and a safe quarter beyond that to live
in, where we cannot come at them, without more forcies, to Damnify or
prejudice them, but more to injure ourselves. I perceive them committy
of Derby House hath sent to his Excellencie and Lieutenant General
(Cromwell) hath sent me word they would presently send me 1500 foote
and 500 horse, which once come up, I hope apresent period would be put
to these newe broyles, and the Scots prevented in their designs, whom I
heare, are prepareing against us what they can and am told by a Scots
man that saith he laitely brought a letter from the Lord Balmerince to
you, and there being 4 more with him you gave them 20s Amonst them,
and tells us that 4 regiments of horse was then (when he came out of

Scottland a weeke agoe) ordered by Duke Hambleton forthwith to advance into England and was upon theire march neare Carlile. I hope to see those 2 companies of foote (you sent) to morrow, or that they wilbe come to Abbleby (Appleby) where I have ordered them to stay. I have sent this messinger of purpose to convey that ammunicon I desired you to send to me by the way of Raby) the nearest way hither, and on horseback for more speed, and lesse trouble, I desire you allsoe to send me 4 or 5 sutes of armour, in regard many officers wante their owne. Haveing nother more att present, but desireing a speedie dispatch to this messinger I rest.

Your very humble servant

John Lambert

Penrith 11 June 1648

Sir,

The horse is returned back from Chillingham; and the officers sent thether for viewing thereof conceives itt nott fitt to place any men therein; for Bambrough itt is atother ruined; and decayed; the low rooms filld with sand; the gates burnt upp; and not one peice of timber in all the castle. By their going thether they have gained this intelligence that two broken troopes of Scots commanded by Major Alexander Hume and Captaine Craw as volunteers tendering their service under conduct of Langdale, be now quartered for recruiting att Cornehill, and Norham: but not by authority from the State of Scotland. They enymie ave declared that eyme att Yorkshire, and have been invited againe and againe by letters from those parts assuring them that the whole county will rise with them. Notwithstanding wee are advised to have a speciall care of our selves, for before Wednesday night they intend us a blow—which we shall (by God's assistance) prevent; disiring a supplie of ammunicion may be sent for that purpose. They confidently affirme they will advance to New Castle; and are sure the towne shall be delivered to them upon the first appearance before itt; and itt is said the designe is managed by one Anderson who is now dwelling in New Castle, itt is whispered that Sir Francis Anderson is the man. Wee earnestly peticion a supply of fourteen dayes pay, whereby the horse, and foote here may be enabled to discharge their quarters which if but taken one weeke, would sett all the countrey in combustion, in this nick of tyme, and breed great distractions amongst the soldiers who express discontents already. Wee doubt not but your interest in the garrison sixteen hundred poundes, may bee procured and sent along for the supply of our necessities, which wee promise shall bee repaid out of the moneyes wee dailuy expect forth of Yorkshire.

Sir wee humbly desire may not bee mistaken in these our addresses, and what it may not bee conceived wee ayme att any particular advantage butt merely the promotion of the publick affaires in these parts; and further desire expresse orders for disposing of our forces to the best advantage of

the publick in relation to this, or any other intelligence. Wee shall further
desire that wee may bee assisted with some faithfull men to bee employed
as intelligencers.

> Wee remaine Your Humble Servantes
> John Bright
> John Smithson[7]

Alnewick 15 May 1648

If the parliamentarians feared the entry of the Scots, they could rely
upon at least some assistance in the north from those loyal to the
rebellion of 1642. Lambert, now very active in the field, wrote to
Hesilrige:

> Sir,
>   I am assured by some well affected men in Westmooreland that they
> will be verie active in raiseing some foote in that country, & desire much
> to be put into good posture, & to have armes att their owne chardges. I
> desire you to send 40 musketts & bandaleirs to Captain Robert Atkinson
> who will pay you for one halfe presently att the raite of 10s a muskett &
> bandileire & th'other halfe with all expedecion. I desire 2 words from you
> concerning those particulars of the forementioned Scots man. Because I
> keeps upon suspition.[8]

Hesilrige mentions these loyal gentlemen and his own fears of the
Scottish advance in a letter dated 15 June:

> My Lord,
>   Some of Westmorland gents are resinge forces for the Parlment; and
> wantinge musketts and bandeliers, they sent to me to buy; but I supplyed
> there wants without money. Langdale was forced upon Satturday last to
> retreat into Carlisle; for he would not be peswaded to fight upon any
> tearmes. He expects the Scotts to assist, I verily beleive they will come
> in.[9]

The letters from John Lambert to Sir Arthur at Newcastle were fre-
quent as the situation grew far more dangerous. Lambert was forced
by events to keep the correspondence up-to-date, for Hesilrige would
be the principal hope of their cause should Lambert be swept aside by
a rushed Scottish advance. He wrote to Hesilrige on 10 June:

> Sir,
>   Since my last unto you from Revensworth we have used all possible
> endeavours to have engated the enemy but cannot, they still gieveing us
> way as we come within a dayes martch of them, upon Thursday last we
> lay neere the Spitted on Stainmore and sent up a party of 300 foote and
> 200 horse to a (have) possed a passage of advantage upon Stainmore called

Maidens Castle (which the enemy might probably have much troubled us if not stopt our passage) which was done and kept without any great difficulty or blowes except in a skirmish betwixt eight of oures and 14 of theirs which indeed was (being) very handsomely performed and one of theirs slaine and another taken prisoner, being both Northumberland gentlemen and reformadoes, one was a De la Veile and the other a Blaxton this without the least hurt to us; next day being very bad and rainy all day from mourning to night we martched to Brough and the enemy being retreted past Kirby thuar (there) we quartered all in 5 townes being the first time we housed since oure meeteing, and this day are upon a martch againe towardes then, towardes Pereth, we are in some want of amunicion and doe earnestly desir you to be assisting to us, that twenty barrells of powder and bullett and match proportionable may be sent to Raby with all speed. I have write to the Bishoprick troops to meete it at Durham and convey it thyther, from whence we shall fetch it as we have occasion, I earnestly desire that if possible it may be there by tuesday at night next. Wee have dayly terrible alarames of the Scots advance into England and some times soe hot as it troubles us in our councells. I desire you will let us heare from you that if you heare any thinge considerable from them, haveing nothinge more at present, but to remaine

Your faithfull and humble servant
John Lambert[10]

Brough 10th June 1648

Two further letters followed in quick succession on 19 and 22 June:

Sir,

I recived yours of the 12th instant and together with it the ammunition mentioned therein, for which I returne you many thanks it beeinge a very seasonable supply, since my last to you beeinge very desirous to acte somethinge upon the enemy we drew forth aboute one attacke at night, and marched with our whole force towards Carlyle and about five in the morninge, came within a mile of the town, from whence wee percived the enemy drawne under the walls with about five hundred horse and as many foote, and marching in from the farre side of the watter severall partyes of horse and foote, soe that wee did beleeve they would have fought us, but it seemes there intencions was otherwayes, for drawinge all there forces close to the walls wee faced them foure hours or above and afterwards drew back, the enemy pursued us with about five hundred horse at a good distance and about one hundred more close upon us which indeed trouble us very much. Wee often drew forth an equall party to them and sometymes a lesse but they would by noe means stand a charge, but beeinge very gallantly mounted would keepe very neare to our last partyes, and upon there weeleing about would careare in upon them fire there pistols and soe backe againe, they dangerously shott two of ours one of which is since dead of his wounds and took one prisoner, wee killed off thers that we know of three and tooke five prisoners. This day Apleby Castle was surrendered unto us upon condicions all to goe home ingageinge themselves never to beare armes against the parliment except one whose name is Carleton who is to goe to Carlyle. Wee are almost at a stand what to doe, wee not beeinge able with these few to ingage any against the walles of Carlyle, yeat we are in hopes that Lancashire Gentlemen will advance with 1000 foote to us, and then with Gods assistance wee shall not doubt to drive away Langdale and his horse from Carlyle, and if wee gett them into the plaine feild we doubt not but in a short tyme to break them. I here you have made good progresse in raiseinge of horse both in Northumberland and the Bishoppricke of Durham, if you bee in that condicion that you can possibly spare both or one of my troops with you, you would still adde to the promotion of this service. And if you send them I desire you lett them bringe alonge with them the backs brests and pottes I write to you for. I pray you lett mee here from you how affaires goe in Scotland and what else you thinke fitt to cominicate to Sir.

Your Humble Servant
John Lambert

Penrith 19th June 1648

Postscript: Wee founde Appleby Castle 300 musketts 6 Barrells of powder and all kindes of provisions necessarie proprtionable.

On the 22nd:

Sir,

Before the gentleman sent by you came to mee I had full in my eye the releife of Northumberland, and before this time had done somethinge effectually for the releife thereof had not our expectation from Lancashire forces stayed us for our conjunction with them in order to the more effectuall carryinge on the service aboute Carlyle, they are not yeate joyned with us but did assure mee by letters they would march towards us this day, but have since desired they may bee excused for one dayes longer tyme and tomorrow they will not faile, I am sorry our depending upon them hath retarded your releife but desire you now to bee confident, that it shall bee speeded to you, as sudainly as our advance to Carlyle will secure the way by Hexam, I have purposely sent this messenger back to you with all speede to desire you in order to the releife of Northumberland, to endeavor what you can to horse one hundred or two of your foote as dragoones, for that expedition which would bee of mighty advantage to our horse, who otherwayes may bee much trouble for want thereof in regard I understand the enemy have above one hundred already, Sir this is all for the present from

Your very humble servant
John Lambert[11]

Penrith June 22nd 1648

Of course Lambert could not engage upon a full battle even if the Lancashire Militia commanded by Colonel Ashton joined with him. It was as vital for Lambert to keep in the field as long as possible, by so doing holding ground and advances otherwise open to a rapid Scottish advance through England. When, on 8 July, the Covenant army under Duke Hamilton finally crossed the border, they were hardly a grand army capable of restoring any throne to the King, because opposition from the Kirks had resulted in a much reduced force crossing the border after the muster was called. The Scottish foot was rare in its will and experience, consisting of low-class Highlanders but principally working city tradesmen raised proportionately throughout the Lowland craft and business sectors. The management of such a rag-tag army would be difficult for the Duke, but even despite the roughness of the force it was more than John Lambert could hope to fight alone.

In Newcastle, Sir Arthur Hesilrige had problems building into a state of emergency, as a warrant dated the very day Hamilton crossed the border shows:

> Whereas the Committee of the Army formerly sent you warrants for the payment of the two regiments of foote which are in this garrison; but of late there is no money come to your hands which causes the wants of the soldiers to grow very great, and will necessitate them to quarter upon the townspeople, which cannot but prove very dangerous, especially at this time when the whole nation is so full of risings and mutinies and this town (Newcastle) so exceedingly disaffected. I therefore intreat you to pay Major Paul Hobson upon account for payment of my regiment of foote, 14 day's pay viz 516.1
>
> Sir Arthur Hesilrige to the Mayor of Newcastle[12]

It would appear from this that the soldiers of 1648 were no better treated with pay than the badly supplied troops under Sir William Waller in the Western Association in 1643–45, or the New Model under the Presbyterian-controlled Parliament in 1646–47. Hesilrige had seen the deterioration of badly paid armies before; he knew he could soon fall a victim of mutiny or ill-discipline if pay grew too many weeks in arrears. The townspeople too would soon groan under the order of free-quarter, for soldiers give blood and expect full bellies in return.

With the arrival of the Scots at Carlisle, Sir Philip Musgrave handed the town over to them. John Lambert meanwhile kept a careful eye on the whole situation aided by his scouts or intelligencers. After six days, the Duke's army marched from Carlisle, and the very capable but totally outnumbered Lambert fell back to Penrith. The Scots did not realize it but they had been led forward not by Duke Hamilton but by Sir Arthur Hesilrige and John Lambert aided by the military war cabinet in London headed by Henry Ireton. On 16 May 1648, Ireton had written to Hesilrige:

Sir,

The General is resolved of a speedy advance into the North, with what forces can possibly bee had from these partes. There is one regiment of horse, which laye about Newarde (Newarke—viz. Colonel Twistleton's) ordered 4 or 5 dayes agoe to march forthwith into the Bishopricke and receive orders from Collonell Lamberte untill the Generall come. Hee intends to follow with 3 regiments of horse more and some foote, but for foote wee must depend most upon the rayseing of a good bodye in the north. For present his advance stayes partley upon the refurnishinge of a small trayne, but cheiflye upon an engagement of two regiments of the horse and one of foote about Bury in Suffolke where there is a considerable strength sette together for the kinge and have begunne to guaryson that place; but I hope through the goodnesse of God that engagement will bee soone well over, and then these forces are soe farre on theyre waye northwards. Sir, that which promts now mee to write to you is cheifly this, because I understande you have advanced a regiment of horse and a regiment of foote into Northumberland as farre as Alnwicke. And in the meane while (Colonel Lamberte with the other regiment of horse lyeing in Yorkshire to keep that country quiett and rayse forces in it) the enemye by the waye of Carlisle hath an open waye and free range, through Cumberland, Westmorlande and Lancashire into the very bowells of Englande or into Wales. Sir I beseach do not weigh Northumberlande in ballance with the wholle kingdome; rather give the enemy for the present all that parte beyond Tyne and the moneys and strength they can rayse in it, then leave them unstopt on Carlisle-side. You had better lett them range from Barwicke to Newcastle walls, for you have all cleare behinde you on this side Tine then th'other waye to annoye the wholle kingdome or to come and plante them selves with a strength on the backe of you betwixt yuu and us. From Barwicke and Northumberland, Newcastle and the River Tyne is a barre to theyre further progresse, but on Carlisle-side, there is no stop to them but by a force in the feild. If wee could regayne Carlisle or keep them in on that side, wee should easyly mayntayne the line betwixt Newcastle and Carlisle and have all cleare behind till wee could rayse a force sufficient or come up with that which is raysed (by Gods blessing) soone to beate them out of Northumberlande and Scottlande, I should not much feare what they could doe. I beseech you therefore (and I have write to Collonell Lamberte to same purpose) lett all the strength you can make out, bee applyed against theyre inciursions from Carlisle, (untill a force can bee gotte up to beseige them there) though for the time you leave Northumberland wholly to them. That God would direct and bee with you in these greate straites is the hearty prayer of

Your affectionate and humble servant
Henry Ireton[13]

Windsor May 16th 1648

The action by Lambert around Carlisle advance had done what Ireton wanted, which was to stop the enemy from advancing south, and, despite what Ireton said, Hesilrige still held Northumberland semi-open with only a handful of troops. But, although Lambert had sealed up the advance of the Langdale party, to hold the Scots was an impossible task and he found himself steadily retreating. The Scottish army crossing the border had grown by as many as 6,000 more raw foot before marching from Carlisle, which meant that the Duke Hamilton was now leading near 3,000 horse and at least 14,000 foot. The directive from Ireton made it perfectly clear that the attack should be made as far north as possible, for Lambert must now buy the Parliament time. He attempted the impossible, which was to hold the Stainmoore Pass and Barnard Castle. Hesilrige now received a further letter from Lambert:

Sir,

By my last I acquainted you with the skirmish wee had with the enemy at Appleby on Monday last, and of our intentions to drawe off to Kirby Stephen, which accordingly after this dispute ended, we did without any disturbance of our enemy in the rere; at Kirby Stephen wee refreasht for an houre or two, and conceiving the enemy might march to Brough, and so prevent us the passe into Yorkshire, wee thought fitt to march to Bowes that night and this night are come to Barnard Castle for a little freash quarter (our men and horses being very much tired and worne) and in order to a conjunction with some other forces; some more horses wee doe expect very shortly to come to us, but our great want is for foote which I perceive wee are like to have but very little supply of, I am therefore forced to renewe my desire that you will spare mee five or six hundred foote out of your garrison, if possibly you can, and to appoint them to march to us with speed, which wilbe a great and seasonable assistance to us at this time for the good of theis parts and the whole kingdome which againe I leave to your consideration and remayne, Sir

Your very humble servant
John Lambert

Barnard Castle 19th July 1648

> Postscript: This inclosed is a coppy of the last intelligence from the enmy
> for which imployment I have imployed Captain Kitson.
>
> Wee are likewise in great want of amunition as I intimated to you in
> my last. My desire is also renewed that you will speed the proposition
> mentioned in my former (which is the same you accomodated us withal
> before) to us to Raby Castle for our supply.[14]

Fully realizing the seriousness of the northern situation, Oliver
Cromwell sent all the forces he could spare from Wales in a swift
march north. Fairfax was heavily committed in a siege at Colchester
by this time, where Lord Capel, Sir Charles Lucas and Sir George
Lisle had declared for the king only to be driven into Colchester.
Cromwell had joined a victorious Thomas Horton, who had defeated
a mixed royalist and mutinous Presbyterian force at St Fagans in early
May. Cromwell had been in Wales since that time, but on 11 July—
in the eleventh hour—the forces under Cromwell were released to
march north when Pembroke Castle surrendered.

A very hurried letter was written to Hesilrige by Lambert on the
morning 3 August. The strain Lambert was suffering is shown in the
fact that the letter is incorrectly dated July:

> Sir,
>
> This enclosed came by an expresse from my Lord General which I
> thought fitt to speed unto you; I have likewise sent you a coppy of the
> Secretaryes to mee which will give you a perfect account of the affaires
> before Colchester, and London; upon Tuesday the enemy marched from
> Appleby to Kendall, and probably intend for Lancashire, or rather for
> Pontefract by the way of Craven, whereupon yesterday I march't from
> Barnard Castle to Richmond, and this day intend for Rippon. What our
> further resolution wilbee I cannot now determine but shall upon all
> occasions give you a further account, which is all from Sir,
>
>   Your very humble servant
>   John Lambert
>
> Richmond 3rd July (August) 1648
> nine a clock in the morning.[15]

Cromwell and Lambert finally joined forces at Wetherby on 12
August, and then from there marched to battle with the enemy at
Preston. With this Sir Arthur's immediate interest with Lambert was
relieved. This was just as well for another problem had reared its head.

On 9 August, Colonel Henry Lilburne, another member of that
famous northern family, the governor of Tinmouth Castle, declared
for the King. The castle lay at the mouth of Tyne Harbour and as

such held the key to Newcastle. It was not long before Hesilrige heard of Henry Lilburne's treachery and he acted positively. Two days after Lilburne declared for the King, Sir Arthur sent a large body of foot and 100 dragoons, and they stormed the walls, surprising the garrison. Finding their ladders too short, they entered the castle at the very mouths of the Tinmouth guns, through port-holes and embrasures. During the fight, Henry Lilburne was put to the sword.[16] The Derby House Committee wrote to Hesilrige on 15 August:

> By yours of the 10th instant we are informed of the traitorous revolt of Lieut-Col (Henry) Lilburne, and of his just punishment. We have great cause to bless God for his goodness to us in so happy a recovery of a place (Tynemouth) of so very great consequence, which if it had continued tin their hands, would have given a very great turn to the Parliament's affairs in those parts. But it pleased God only so far to permit it to proceed that it might be a discovery of an unsuspected traitor, and a demonstration of the watchfulness of His Providence.[17]

After this threat to Tinmouth, Sir Arthur was forced to tighten his grip on the Newcastle royalist sympathizers, but, despite this, his strong government was popular with the larger number of people now sympathetic to Parliament.

On 17–19 August the work carried out by Hesilrige and Lambert reached its ultimate end, when a greatly outnumbered army under Oliver Cromwell and John Lambert destroyed the Scots in and around Preston. The royalist hopes had been quelled by the bravery of the parliamentary soldiers and the vast superiority of the administration and intelligence system. Hesilrige's part in this victory was enormous. He had supplied John Lambert with all he desired, held the north from the royalist threat by securing Newcastle from any surprise, and on 1 Jul, aided by Major John Sanderson of Robert Lilburne's regiment, Sir Arthur had taken a notable royalist force under Colonel Grey and the Northumberland gentry. By retaking Tinmouth Castle, Hesilrige had more than proved his ability, and also proved Parliament totally correct in the appointment.

It is believed Hesilrige visited Cromwell in Edinburgh during October, where they were entertained by old Leven and Argyll.[18]

With the Scots defeated, the Second Civil War was ended, the King's cause lost for all time and the dawn of the English Revolution breaking fast.[19]

NOTES

1. CSP Dom, 1648–49, pp. 17-18.

2. T. Edwards, *The Second Part of Gangraina* (1646), p. 161; *idem, The Third Part of Gangraina*, p. 45; 'The Rev. Colonel Paul Hobson, fellow of Eton', *Baptist Quarterly*, NS 9, pp. 307-10.

3. CSP Dom, 1648–49, pp. 29-30.

4. LJ, X, p. 167.

5. *The Cromwell Letters*, LRO.

6. CSP Dom, 1648–49, p. 59.

7. *The Cromwell Letters*, LRO.

8. *The Cromwell Letters*, LRO.

9. Carte MSS 91 EEEE (Bodleian Library). This version is from Nichols, *Leicestershire*, II, pt ii, p. 745.

10. *The Cromwell Letters*, LRO.

11. *The Cromwell Letters*, LRO.

12. CSP Dom, 1648–49, p. 174.

13. *The Cromwell Letters*, LRO.

14. *The Cromwell Letters*, LRO.

15. *The Cromwell Letters*, LRO.

16. Whitelock, *Memorials*, II, pp. 379-80; *Ludlow's Memoirs*, I, p. 191; Rushworth, *Historical Collections*, II, pt iv, pp. 1226-27; 'Sir Arthur Hesilrige's Letter to the Committee at Derby House', E 459 (26); 'A Terrible and Bloody Fight at Tinmouth Castle', E 459 (4).

17. CSP Dom, 1648–49, p. 244.

18. Rushworth, *Historical Collections*, VIII, p. 1295.

19. Although reference numbers for British Library Tracts are quoted, the author has used Newcastle City Library Tracts throughout this chapter. A fuller, more detailed account of this period will be found in the author's *1648: The Year of Revolution*, currently under research.

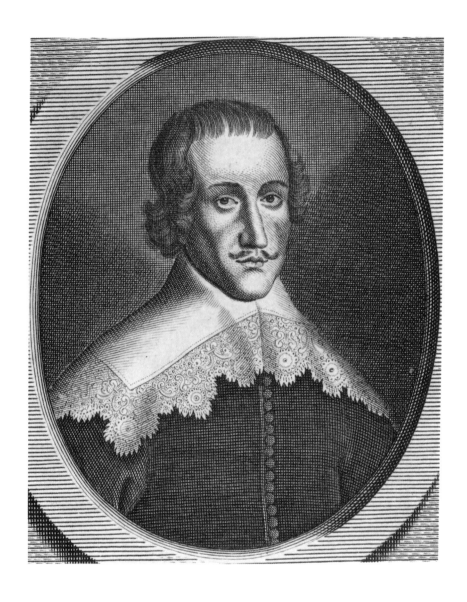

John Lilburne 1614(?)–1657, M. vr. Gucht after an original painting.
By courtesy of the National Portrait Gallery, London.

∽ 13 ∾

Hue and Cry

Thou shalt not suffer a witch to live.
(Exod. 22.18)

When, on Wednesday 6 December 1648, the New Model Army marched on Westminster to the eternal fame of Colonel Thomas Pride and the purge named after him, Sir Arthur Hesilrige was still at Newcastle. The events that led to the purge had nothing to do with Sir Arthur, yet had he been in London he would have undoubtedly sided with the army against the Presbyterians in Parliament. One by one the Presbyterian members who had fled or absented themselves from the Commons in 1647 had returned, and, while Cromwell and Hesilrige had fought the war of 1648, the Presbyterians had re-opened negotiations with the King. All the actions by the Presbyterian majority were against the 'Vote of No Address' and ignored the army completely. The day before the army moved to reduce the Parliament, the Commons had passed a motion to proceed with peace talks with the King, which was too much for the army to bear.[1]

That fateful December morning, Colonel Pride and Sir Hardress Waller arrived at the Commons supported by a guard and arrested one by one the moderate members as they came in.[2] Among those seized were Sir William Waller and John Birch, the man who desired so to fight in 1644 when leading Hesilrige's foot at Cheriton. The Parliament would now consist of those members loyal to a Revolutionary Army—1648 had become the year of revolution. The rest would be 'Secluded', some escaping before Pride, aided by Sir Arthur's Leicestershire neighbour, Lord Grey of Croby, could track them down.

A week after Pride's Purge, Parliament ended all negotiation with the King, and on 15 December a Council of Officers, who now ruled despite the Commons sitting, decided to bring the defeated monarch 'speedily to justice'. Events were gathering pace, and although not involved Sir Arthur relates the story thus:

> Many gentlemen in this House, of great worth, foreseeing our troubles, apprehended their was enough in the king's condescensions for a well-grounded peace. But the officers of the army were otherwise opinioned. Finding the king not sufficiently humbled, they thought the good cause would be betrayed. The officers seized several members. Those that stayed within, asked for them, but could not have them. They seized upon the king, demanded justice, and brought him to judgement. He would not answer, not owning our authority, because he was accountable only to God; whereas, God never made such a creature, to govern men, and not to be accountable to men. Yet he received his judgement, and submitted his head quietly to the block. The edge of justice struck it off. See the wonderful hand of God![3]

In a letter of 21 December 1648, Sir Thomas Fairfax wrote to Hesilrige at Newcastle, but it is interesting to note he said nothing of the King:

> Sir,
>
> Being by credible information soe satisfied concerning Lt. Colonel Halsall now prisoner with you as that I can be content he may be sett at liberty to return home into Scotland upon engagement never to returne in armes into England, I doe nevertheless reserve the manner of his enlargement to yourself to be soe disposed as may be every way most satisfactory and safe. And should any great inconveniency appeare herein I then leave it to you to afford him the most of what other favour you can by permitting him going into Scotland for two or three months upon his paroll, or his continuance there upon caution to render himself within a certaine time after notice given to his suerties or what may else you thinke best respectin this my desire concerning him, soe I remaine,
>
> Your very assured friende
Tho. Fairfax[4]

Sir Arthur had been placed on the list of Commissioners of the High Court of Justice, but at no time did he sit. Why Hesilrige did not take his seat at the trial is a mystery. He claimed years later that he being at Newcastle he did not even know of the fate of the King until after the event. In his later life, Sir Arthur was said to be a republican, but was this an afterthought when monarchy was already gone? It is not impossible that Hesilrige favoured a reduced monarchy up to 1649, in much the same way as Cromwell, but with the axe ending Charles's reign saw an opportunity to build upon a commonwealth system.

However, if Sir Arthur however was absent, his brother Thomas was not. It is said that Thomas Hesilrige was truly the republican, he 'suborning witnesses to valify the king'.[5] Thomas owed everything to the Civil War, because as a younger brother he held little land, and so his duties to Parliament and chiefly the army were vital to him.

With the hand of God striking off the head of the King, a bill was rushed through Parliament to prevent the lawful succession of the Prince of Wales, but young Charles Stuart was proclaimed King Charles II in many parts of the land despite this. Sir Arthur says:

> The king dead, some members of the House, the late General (Cromwell), and Commissary-General Ireton, they would have it determined, (which the wisdom of the House thought to meet) that not only this line, nocent and innocent, but that kingship should be abolished, as dangerous useless and burthensome. Then there was an end of one of the three estates. The Lords, most of them being gone, the remainder, amazed and troubled at this, adjourned their house; but never came again unto it. As they had their beginning from themselves, so they had their end from themselves. The Commons approved the Lord adjornment, and did by them as they had done by the king; and there was an end of that estate. Two of the three estates were thus gone. Then, for the third estate, that knows, had been shattered and broken Force was much upon us, what should we do? We turned ourselves into the Commonwealth. By advice of the soldiers among us, a declaration to that purpose went out from the Army.[6]

These events had moved with the great pace associated with revolutions. The action of the army had transported power to the one estate, aided by the officers of the Army Council. How many of the original Long Parliament in the 1640s could have envisaged the act of regicide in the actions, or the end of monarchy and the Lords? It is difficult to imagine John Pym being a party to killing the King, or the idealistic Brooke destroying the House of Peers. Had he lived it is quite possible that John Hampden would have argued for the King's life. But all these great men had perished, leaving the cold lifeless body of the King as an epitaph to the war. These men had influenced Hesilrige greatly, and only after their untimely deaths had he turned to the more radical politics of the younger Vane and what he saw to be the honesty of Cromwell. However, Sir Arthur was now well into middle age, and it is notable that his actions and speeches were gaining an air of authority, giving the blunt finesse of an experienced leader. Still sharp-tongued, he approached debate with the broad

education of ten years of politics. Sir Arthur had witnessed the testing
of a nation and could not have failed to be influenced by what he
had seen.

To replace the Derby House Committee, a Council of State was
appointed to administer national security, and Sir Arthur was of course
appointed.[7] Having missed the King's trial and execution, Hesilrige
returned to London in the second week of February 1649 and
received the thanks of the Commons for his 'many great and faithful
Services done for the State, at Tynmouth and in the North'.[8] Sir
Arthur had indeed given outstanding service in the defence of the
nation, having held almost total control of an area from North
Yorkshire to the border and kept the vital Tyne secure.

The new Council of State found England in a sorry state, many
areas of national importance being neglected and wasted. On 24
February, the council ordered Hesilrige to see that no horses left
England by way of the north, so many being lost in the war.[9] Horses
were vital in all walks of life: the military needed them, and they were
needed for general transportation and farming. Sir Arthur was a fine
judge of horseflesh, and it was no wonder he took this order seriously.

Three days later Hesilrige was added to the committee appointed
for sending forces to Ireland.[10] Irish service had been the bane of the
Presbyterians in 1647, yet the army under Cromwell now chose to
enter into an expedition against the Roman Catholic Confederacy.
Those who did not wish to serve in Ireland were allowed to retire
from military life without prejudice, many older officers choosing to
do so. Among these was Samuel Gardiner, the old Lobster captain,
who returned to Evesham rather than go to Ireland with Thomas
Horton. The campaign in Ireland was Cromwell's war of religion,
fought bitterly and to his shame. Hesilrige had little direct contact
with this campaign, and to leave Cromwell on route is all a biographer
of Sir Arthur need do.

The next few months were quiet, offering a short period of peace
to the people of England. But for Sir Arthur and Dame Dorothy it
was a time of deep grief after the sudden death of their young son
Arthur. It is certain that the young boy was his father's favourite
child, his joy. The child was buried at Noseley, in the tomb set aside
for his parents. An inscription reads:

This is Arthur Haslerig eldest son of Dame Dorothea.
He was of rare endowments of incomparable learning for
his age both in Hebrew, Greeke, Latin and French of
singular wit and judgement of sweete nature and very
pious.
He died in ye 12th year of his age 1649.

It is unfortunate that the exact date of the boy's death and the cause
is missing. However, the lad was the firstborn son of Sir Arthur and
Dame Dorothy and was favoured over the son and heir, Thomas. Sir
Arthur was a proud father.

By July 1649 the peace between England and Scotland was most
uneasy, and the Council of State once again put Hesilrige on a war
alert at Newcastle, Berwick and Carlisle.[11] If, however, the council
was concerned with the Scots coming in, the people of Newcastle had
invited one Scot to visit them—a witchfinder. During March, while
Sir Arthur was in London, the Newcastle Common Council received
a petition against witches within their area. Acting upon this they sent
two of the town's sergeants, Thomas Shevill and Cuthbert Nicholson,
to hire a Scottish witchpricker, who was to have his travelling expenses
plus 20 shillings for each convicted witch. Unfortunately, these prickers
were notorious for the exposing of witches, especially when paid a
bonus. The witchcraft terror did not begin in Newcastle until later
that year, the first wave of hysteria breaking in December when the
Scot arrived. If he had made slow progress in coming, this vile
professional wasted no time in his work. He sent out a Bell-man to
walk the streets, declaring that all who suspected anyone of witchcraft
should denounce them for testing by the pricker. This was the perfect
opportunity for old family arguments to be raised, jealous neighbours
to point the finger and the game of spite to be played. No one was
safe from accusation.

It was no surprise to find that Newcastle was alive with black magic
in 1649. About 30 poor souls were tested, and at least 15 women and
1 man were hung on the Town Moor. These unfortunates were sub-
jected to the humiliation of being taken in a complete state of terror
to the town hall, stripped naked and intimately searched for the devil's
mark, a blemish or extra nipple with which to feed their familiar or
demonic agent. Then the pricking would begin. The pricking of a
suspect was a devil's art form in itself, the victim being laid naked and
cold on the floor for the ordeal to come. Numb with fear and often
in shock long before the torment began, the victim would be tortured

by the pressing of a long needle into their body. If they screamed and the blood ran freely they were not guilty, just highly abused innocents. However, many prickers were so skilled in their trade that the victim felt nothing, and, because they were cold and often bound, the blood would not flow. For these poor people, the noose was a blessing in its release from pain.

Many innocent victims would have hung had fate not taken a hand. During one examination, the level-headed Baptist, Paul Hobson, attended what was a normal searching and pricking of an accused woman. Hobson stood by as the woman was stripped and searched for marks, and then the needle was inserted into her cold thigh. No blood, no screams of pain, she was guilty. But Hobson was far from convinced. He insisted that the woman was so much in shock it had numbed her mind and that her body was so cold the blood would not flow. In his role of deputy governor he ordered she be moved to allow her circulation to be regained, and then the needle to be used again. The woman screamed and blood flowed from the wound. It could easily be Hobson's experience of war that saved this innocent woman from the noose. He must have seen fear dry the mouths and stifle the cry of pain from men torn by pike and sword, and the cold of night stem the bloodflow of wounds far greater than were inflicted by the prick of a witchfinder.

With Hobson exposing the weakness of this odious Scot, the pricker moved on to Northumberland, where he raised his price to 60 shillings a witch. This greed was his undoing. Again shown to be a fraud, he fled back into Scotland, where he was tried and confessed to the deaths of over 220 victims in England and Scotland.[12]

Why Sir Arthur allowed such a hue and cry after witches is unknown, for it was nothing to his credit. Witch-hunts were common, it is true, and men like the self-styled Witchfinder General Matthew Hopkins had in fact made the art highly profitable, but at a time when men like the astrologer William Lilly called such things 'science', it is amazing that the word 'witch' could be allowed to cause such panic.

While witches swung from Town Moor gibbets in one hue and cry, Sir Arthur himself was a hunted man—the Levellers were out for blood of their own, their sport, the hunting of grandee foxes. Hesilrige's connexion with northern land deals have long been considered dubious, a fact that cannot be denied. He was an excellent businessman and saw the potential of buying ex-royalist land at very cheap prices. Like many old parliamentary army officers, Sir Arthur had not accepted hard cash for his appointment as lieutenant general of horse during 1643–44, but was owed the money on paper. With the war over, many, including Sir Arthur, now accepted in payment the sequestered land of the royalists, and bought still more land with their own money. Hesilrige had amassed a fortune by these methods, and if this is considered immoral, then it was after all how the royalists had obtained the land in the first place, and was therefore just a continuation of history. To the moralist it is without doubt a blot on Sir Arthur's character that he prospered from the war, but few victors in any conflict fail to do so. Where Hesilrige made the mistake was that he inadvertently took away rents from the Lilburnes of all people, when he detained rents for lands in Durham. It was common gossip that Sir Arthur wanted John Lilburne dead, and, with the taking of Lilburne money, the Leveller presses ran hot. In the hands of a master, printing ink is one of the sharpest weapons, and John Lilburne tore into Hesilrige, calling him: '…a Pole Cat, a Wolf [as a subverter and a destroyer of humane society] and may and ought to be knockt on the head thereof'.[13]

Lilburne had borrowed these lines from a 1647 tract by the army mutineer William Thompson, but they summed up John Lilburne's feelings toward Sir Arthur.[14] Hesilrige bought a vast estate in the north and a mansion at Bishop Auckland, but it is a mistake to consider the Lilburne family to have been impoverished, for they were one of the most influential families in and around Durham.

The case of the ownership of Harraton Colliery near Durham brought more charges of corruption against Hesilrige. The mine had been first sequestered in 1644 for the delinquency of the royalist Colonel George Wray. Unfortunately, when a member of the Durham Committee in 1649, Hesilrige had seized the mine believing it belonged to the state under the criteria of the 1644 sequestration order. At this time, a full five years after the initial seizure, three lease owners appeared, one being George Lilburne, the uncle of John. It was now claimed that the lease for three-quarters of the colliery had been granted by Wray to one Josiah Primate in 1629, and further-more George Lilburne and a George Grey had subleased his rights in 1647. Of course, Hesilrige and the committee had assumed that the delinquent George Wray owned all portions of the mine, a situation compounded by five years of silence from Josiah Primate. The whole confusing case was placed before the Committee for Compounding sitting at Haberdashers Hall between 6 November and 12 December 1651, and to George Lilburne's intense fury they found in the favour of Hesilrige. In an autobiographical tract written in 1653, John Lilburne says:

> And so much injustice appeared unto me to have been manifesty done, that I set forth the unworthiness as fully as I was able, and at length the cause being to receive a final determination before that Committee, I with my Client and other his councel appeared daily for many days, proving by undeniable arguments, from point to point, the right to be in Master Primate: but Sir Arthur Haselrige a Member of Parliament and Council of State, and a mighty man in the North and in the Army, so bestirred himself, That when Judgement came to be given by the major Vote against my Client, quite contrary to the opinions of most that heard it, and to my Clients and my understanding, against all equity and conscience.[15]

In reality it is difficult to see how the committee could deliver any other judgement. Wray owned the mine leased to Primate and Wray was adjudged a delinquent, and therefore, in a rather complex case of English law, the fine on Wray was the factor in law, irrespective of any future leaseholder.[16]

Aided by John Lilburne, the primary leaseholder, Josiah Primate, appealed to Parliament in a petition:

> ...where in he supposeth that Sir Arthur had over-awed the Committee to give a corrupt Judgement. And being questioned, avowed the petition to be his own, and cleared me from having any hand therein.[17]

Lilburne denies any part in drafting the petition, or to distributing supernumerary copies before the case was heard, but in reality he is now himself stretching his own credibility. He had no doubt assisted Primate in drafting his petition, and furthermore fails to mention his uncle's investment in the mine. At this John Lilburne sharpened a quill and attacked the committee in print. It would appear that John Lilburne was hell-bent upon his own destruction, for in the tirade of vitriolic rhetoric, he called the members of the committee:

> ...four of the most unjust and unworthiest men that ever the Parliament made judges, fit for nothing but to be spewed out of all humane society by all ingenuous rational men, and deserving to have their skins flayed over their ears, stuffed full of straw and hung up in some public place.[18]

These were very ill-judged words from Lilburne, for Parliament, having grown tired of his eternal criticism, now saw their chance to free themselves from this meddlesome democrat.[19]

The Lilburne family, it is clear, begrudged Hesilrige the governorship of Newcastle, for they had hoped that Colonel Robert Lilburne would hold it, having done so for a short time in 1647. Had this been the case after 1647, Robert Lilburne would have controlled Newcastle and Henry Lilburne the estuary of the Tyne at Tinmouth Castle, which meant that, with George, Richard and John Lilburne owning land and tenancies in and around Durham, the family would have been masters of the far north-east. Perhaps Fairfax had realized this in his decision of 1647, and chose not to put all his administrative eggs in one basket.

Following the attack by John Lilburne upon Haberdashers Hall, and the petition by the long-silent Josiah Primate being presented to Parliament, the former was ordered to attend the House. Parliament had long been concerned by Lilburne's anti-establishment stance, and they wasted no time with this open invitation to martyr him. Lilburne was hauled before the House and accused of publishing without licence. For his crimes, but in reality his politics, Lilburne was fined £7,000, and to rid themselves of him more permanently, he was banished under pain of death if still in the country after 30 days.[20]

One cannot help but feel that, considering George Lilburne had purchased part of the lease of Harraton Colliery (near Chester-le-Street) from Primate during 1647—while the Lilburnes' held control of the area—the morality of the deal was no less murky than that of which they had accused Hesilrige. The origins of the case were almost certainly a classic example of local government corruption. Primate had held his portion of the mine since 1629, and must have known of the sequestration order of 1644, yet had sold on his share to George Lilburne. It seems quite possible that John Lilburne was used by his uncle, and suffered more at the hands of his family than from Hesilrige.

The bitterly exploited argument between Sir Arthur Hesilrige and John Lilburne was still newsworthy in 1653, when the latter published from exile his *Just Defence*. Although now living in the Channel Islands, Lilburne still held lands and leased small farming tenancies around Durham, which were administered in his enforced absence by his father Richard Lilburne. In a belated, and opportune, reply to *A*

Hue and Cry after Sir Arthur Hesilrige, and a timely appearance in regard to *A Just Defence*, the tenants of John Lilburne published their version of the very sad story, here reprinted in full for the first time:

A TRUE
NARRATIVE CONCERNING
OF
SIR ARTHUR HASLERIGS
POSSESSING OF
Lieutenant-Colonel John Lilburnes
ESTATE
in the County of Durham
1653

To the Members of Parliament, and all others that have bowels of pitty towards cruelly oppressed Tenants & c.

You must not expect high language from us who are low borne Tennants: We shall speake plain truthes, And first, we are bold to tell you, That our Fore-Elders were Ancient Tennants to the Dean and Chapter of Durham, who thought they had left unto us that large Birth right which could not legally have been taken from us; but wee find it otherwise, for we are now become (unless God help us) miserable slaves to Lieutenant Colonel John Lilburne: for the Parliament having given unto the said Mr. Lilburne three thousand pounds, and afterwards committed him to the Tower for high Treason; and being acquited him by his Jury at Guild-Hall, he presently assumed, that there was remaining and not paid, fifteen hundred pounds of the said 3000.*l* gift.

The Lord Generall [Cromwell] then coming out of Ireland moved the Parliament to give Mr. Lilburne the said fifteen hundred pounds so owing unto him, out of Deane and Chapters Lands; Which the Parliament immediately granted, and therin began our miseries; for we being poor People farre remote and distant from London, and all, or most of us, within the ignorance of our own business, wanting friends to advise us, or help us, within the small time of presemption the Act allowed us, the said Lieutenant Colonel John Lilburne stept in before us, and made choyce of severall Farmes and Cottages which we held lying in the county of Durham, being the whole livelihood and subsistance of fourteen families. And before the Act passed, the said Mr. Lilburne made large promises of kinde usage to us the Tenants, saying in the presence of severall witnesses, That wee should have our Lands again, paying him the Rates of his purchase (namely the money he paid: but since we have so farre tasted his kindness, as now we have cause to say, The Lord deliver us from such a Landlord.

There are of us fourteen Families and when the Act passed, but two of our Farmes were out of Lease, William Huntington and George Clifton, a poore Prisoner in the gaole, had the other. I the said William Huntington married a Widdow, that was Tennant to the Deane and Chapter, she had a House, Farme, Goodes and Household-stufie, two Cows and four children; I, the said William Huntington after marriage with her was forced to borrow money to Plow and Sow the said Farme, and God gave me a childe by her, that made our numbe five; so soon as our House and Lands were settled by Authority of the Parliament in the said Mr. Lilburne, he immediately came into the County of Durham, and stripped me the said William Huntington, of House, Farme, Cropp, Household-stuffe, Goods, Hay, and Straw, and two Cows; he tooke from me Goods to the value of one hundred and thirty pounds at the least; he thrust us all out of doors, my Wife with her five small children, leave us not one Cow, I may truly say, scarcely one bit of bread; and for my selfe, I could expect no other, but to lye and rot in Prison for the Debt which I borrowed as aforesaid. Next he fell upon me George Clifton, a poor Prisoner in the Gaol of Durham for debt; he likewise cast my poor children out of my House and Farme exposing them to perish in the streets: tooke from me House and Farme, Household stuffe and all that I had; and my children being put by him upon the Parish, he was so farre from allowing them subsistance out of my owne Estate, that he refused to contribute with the Parish towards their maintanance. And thus he dealt with the two Tennants of the two Farmes out of lease. And the said Mr. Lilburne also threatened me Gascoyne Eden, because I would not deliver up my Estate to him, then having seven years in Lease; He write a letter to me wherein he tells me, That he was the Dean and Chapters Successor, and did therein command me to send in a Man and Horse, according to my Lease, in complete Armes, to serve under his Brother Collonell Robert Lilburne in Scotland; and further said in his said Letter, That if I did not give up my Lease to him (having seven years then in being), he would extend all the severall Forfeitures and Breeches of my Lease against me, to make it void: whereby he might weary me out of my Right and Due of years therein. Next after, he fell upon me Robert Christopher another of the poor Tennants, who was always constant and faithfull to the Parliament, and voluntarily set forth Horses and Armes in the Parliament Service farre beyond my Estate; I never offended him in all my life, but in a most humble manner tendering my Rent to him about a week after the day he refused to receive it, and told me, My Lease was forfeited by my failing the just day of payment, and he would take advantage of it accordingly: Yea, after many humble addresses made unto the said Mr. Lilburne by the poor Cottagers and Leasers, divers of them following him to London, and there craving pity and compassion from him upon their poor Wives and Children, offering him his money with an advantage for the said Lands; he (in a great passion) denied, bid them goe home again like as Fools they came, saying, He would out them every man as their Leases expired. Need then made me poor William Huntington to runne from Justice to Justice, complaining of the wrong done unto me by Lieutenant Collonel

John Lilburne; I went to the publique Sessions at Durham where Sir
Arthur Haslerigge was upon the Bench: after the reading of my Petition
there, he told me, it was not in the power of the Sessions to help me, I
then not knowing what else to do, went immediately to London upon
my naken feet to the Parliament, and Printed my sad case and condition,
and delivered it to the Members as they came into the House: at which
Lieutenant Colionel Lilburne was a little moved, and then said the business should be referred to my Lord Generall, Sir Arthur Haslerigge,
Collonel Martin; which made me exceedingly to rejoyce: and in pursuance
thereof, I attended Collonel Martin from place to place according to his
appointment, so long, that weariness and poverty drove me back again
into the Country, having nothing to relieve me, but the Charity of such
as pittied my condition. I then not being able to abide in the Country for
feare of Imprisonment, came again to London on foot, begging my bread
by the way. It being about two hundred Miles, And having no better
success at the Parliament doore after a long attendance, and many being
wearied of me, and my self almost of my life: I returned again to hide my
selfe a while in the Country hoping God might help in the last. Then
when I heard that Lieutenant Collonel John Lilburne was bannished and
that there was a fine to be payed to Sir Arthur Haslerigge, I forthwith
tooke me to my Feet, and again to London, I went and told Sir Arthur,
that it was now in his power to do both my selfe, Wife and Children
good, and that we would pray for him all our dayes, if he would but help
us as God had put it unto his hands. Sir Arthur was pleased to speak to
Collonel Martin, and a time was appointed at Sir Arthur's Chamber at
White-Hall, where Collonel Martin, Mrs. Lilburne, Mr. Richardson,
Mr. Williams, and some others of Mrs. Lilburne's friends met: I had only
my selfe to lay open my miserable case; which when the aforesaid
Gentlemen heard, they lifted up their hands, wondering that Lieutenant
Collonel John Lilburne should deal so cruelly with a poor miserable man,
his Wife, and five small children. Sir Arthur moved, that whereas the
Rent of that Farm had for a long time been but three pounds *per annum*;
And that the Parliament had sold it to Lieutenant Collonel Lilburne, upon
Improvement, at eighteen pounds, that therefore I should give eighteen
pounds *per annum* to Mrs. Lilburne, upon Improvement, which was the
racke Rent valued to her husband, Mrs. Lilburne's friends that came with
her, pittied my case so much that they thought it fit I should have also
the one hundred and thirty pound Goodes restored which Mr. Lilburne
had taken from me. Mrs.Lilburne then replied that she had no money but
I might have one of my Cowes again: Some of her Friends then said it
was fitt I should have satisfaction out of the Rent. And Sir Arthur said
Care must be taken that the poore man have a livelihood from his hard
labour, so he may preserve his Wife and Children from starving; And also
to help Mrs. Lilburne and her children. And further said, That it was
feasible, that John Lilburne ought not to have taken these Goodes from

me, for if any Arrears were due, they belonged to the State, and not to the Purchaser. But said, that now Mrs. Lilburne and her children being in as sad a condition as my selfe and mine: that therefore I should pay unto her, for selfe and children, the full Improvement, which was eighteen pounds a yeare; and that if I did not carefully pay my Rent, Mrs. Lilburne should enter upon the Farme.

This though heavie on my side, to lose all my Goodes, and to be raised up to so high a Rent, as from three pounds to Eighteen Pound *per annum*, the Agreement being signed by Mrs. Lilburne, Collonel Martin, and Sir Arthur Haslerigge, I joyfully tooke it, resolving to labour hard and to pay my Rent honestly; and made haste into the Country and showed the Agreement under the aforesaid hands to Mr. Richard Lilburne, Mr. John Lilburne's father, and desired him to deliver me Possession accordingly: which he absolutely refused. Then some Women, my wives Neighbours desirous to see her in her house again, thrust out the said Mr. Richard Lilburne from amongst them: Which no sooner being done, but the said Mr. Richard Lilburne by his great importunity with the Sherriff of the County, and by colour of an old Warrant, as I understand, procured the said Sherriff to come to my house and thrust us out of possession, and gave it to Mr. Richard Lilburne. Then I forthwith went to London to Sir Arthur Haslerigge, and told him how little Mr. Richard Lilburne valued the Agreement made in his Chamber. He told me he could do no more but get it under Mrs. Lilburne's hand, and Collonel Martin's, and that he knew not what to do or say to Mr. Richard Lilburne. I never durst return into the Country if I had not help from him; and that it was within his power. And really, I had rotted in Prison, and my Wife and her Children had gone a Begging all their days, who was desended of honest Parents, such as had lived in good credit amongst their Neighbours, had I not found pity and compassion in Sir Arthur's brest, necessity inciting me strongly to importune him daily for his assistance; for when he would have put me off I told him I must continue to trouble him. And in truth my condition was so miserable and desperate, having gone upon my bare feet two thousand miles back and again, or thereabouts, in seeking relief, that I thought to hang upon his doors would bring me rest. Sr Arthur then acquainted Collonel Martin what Master. Richard Lilburne had done, and desired him to speak to Mrs. Lilburne, that order might be taken for the performance of the said Agreement, which she and her friends had made and signed; he promised a speedy accompt, and the next day he told Sir Arthur, that she had received Letters from her Husband, wherein he commanded that nothing should be done by her; and thereupon Sir Arthur desired Collonell Martin to tell her from him, That if she would not perform her Agreement, which he apprehended to be juste and reasonable and for her advantage, he thought he was bound in Conscience to preserve the poor man, his Wife and Children, by laying his extend upon the Lands. Collonel Martin immediately replyed, That he would do very well in so doing; and if it was his case he would do the like. Collonel Martin then acquainted Mrs. Lilburne with Sir Arthur's resolution, and returned this answer, that she was John Lilburne's Wife, and that he could not prevail in the least with her, and therefore had Sir Arthur not to expect further. Then we, the rest of the Tennants, hoping there was an opportunity for us and ours, made coyce of one Captain Farrer to be our Solicitor, and sent him to London to Sir Arthur Haslerigge, to entreat, That according to Lieutenant Collonel John Lilburne's promise before he bought our Lands, that we might yet have it as he payd; Thereupon the said Captain Farrer applied himself to Sir Arthur Haslerigge at White-Hall, and acquainting him with the Tennants humble and earnest desires; and as it happened upon some complaints that Mrs. Lilburne had made to Collonel Joyce, against Sir Arthur Haslerigge, there was a meeting appointed at Mr. Peters Chamber in White-Hall, and thither came Mrs. Lilburne, and her own Father; and there were present Mr. Peters and Collonel Joyce; and Sir Arthur Haslerigge took the said Captaine Farrer along with him. Then did Sir Arthur Declare in the presence of all before mentioned That he never had a thought of getting one penny out of John Lilburne's Estate, and that Mrs. Lilburne had compelled him to lay his extent upon the Land, because she would not perform the Agreement under her own hand, whereby Huntington his Wife and Children might live. He then declared the great complaints of the Tennants And this offer was made by Sir Arthur to Mrs. Lilburne. That the Tennants should pay the summe of money, for which the Parliament gave him that Land, being nine hundred and forty pounds, with consideration from the time of passing the Act. She deducting what Rents they had received. Afterwards Sir Arthur told her, the Tennants should give her a thousand pounds at one entire payment; that the present Rent was but three and fifty pounds *per annum*: And then Mr. Peters assured her to help her to a hundred pound *per annum* for ever, and in present possession for that thousand pound. Sir Arthur told her that if she was his own Sister, he would advise her to take it; for if she did, she was then certain to goode maintainance for her self and her Children, and no Act her Husband either had done or should do could take it from them, for she should have it upon this Extent; and for his part he did not expect or desire thanks.

Then Mr. Peters and Collonell Joyce much approved the motion but Mrs. Lilburne would not consent. Then Sir Arthur said, He would do the Tennants what good he could, and never take one penny for his own advantage, from Mrs. Lilburne or her Children. All which the said Captain Farrer is ready to overre and attest, upon his own knowledge: And further, that Sir Arthur Haslerigge hath been at great trouble and charge out of his own Purse; But never received one penny out of Mrs. Lilburne's Estate. Nay, when the Tennants desired the said Captain Farrer to present him with a Breeding Mare, as a small token of our thankfullness, in answer to his great trouble and charge; Sir Arthur replied No, he would not gaine the Hayre of a Horse by Lieutenant Collonel Lilburne's Estate: notwithstanding he bought the said Mare of Mr. Thomas Davison, at the Rate of forty pounds. And all we Tennants do witness That Sir Arthur Haslerigge never received one penny of our Rents; but the same or most part thereof hath been payd to Lieutenant Collonell John Lilburne, or to his Father Mr. Richard Lilburne, for his use since the time of his Grant, until of late, that the said Mr. Richard Lilburne refuses to receive any more Rents off us, saying, That he would not be ordered by Sir Arthur Haslerigge to receive any Rents at his appointment meaning this Order here under written made and signed by Sir Arthur Haslerigge.

I Do hereby appoint the several Tennants that hold and Possess any of the Farmes and Cottages within the Manor of Billingham in the County of Durham, lately extended by virtue of an Act of P. to and in my name; That they forthwith pay unto Mr. Richard Lilburne Gent, for the Wife and Children of Lieutenant Collonel John Lilburne, all the severall and respective Rents, according to the Inquisition returned upon the said Extent, being the same with his purchase, due at Whitsuntide last pas; and payable unto me; taking acquittance under the said Mr. Richard Lilburne's Hand, upon the Payment thereof aforesaid.

Dated the 21 of June 1653.

ARTHUR HASLERIG

Thus we have declared the truth of Sir Arthur Haslerigge desposing of all Lieutenant Collonel John Lilburne's Estate to his own use and the World may see, that Sir Arthur Haslerigge is as much wronged by Lieutenant Collonel John Lilburne publishing the taking away of his Estate, as he was in setting forth a *Hue and Cry* (when he was imprisoned by Parliament for treason as aforesaid) to all persons to assist him for the knocking of Sir Arthur Haslerigge on the head, as they would a Fox or a Poulcat, because he had robbed him of the fifteen hundred pounds, which the Lord Generall procured, as aforesaid; when in truth he never touched or tooke from him one half penny or farthing in all his life, as honest men that are able to make it good, do and will affirme and prove. Now we humbly beseech all Parliament men and others whom it may any way concerne, to preserve us poor Tennants from the cruelty, oppression, and tyranny of Lieutenant Collonel John Lilburne.

AMEN

Gascoyne Eden	Matthew Grey	Robt
Christopher		
William Busby	Jo Maddison	Jo Mason
Wil Huntington	Rob Shepperd	George Clifton
of Billingham	Rob Wilson	John Salter
Will Huntington		
of Coopen		

FINIS[21]

How much Hesilrige influenced the writing of this vindication of his conduct in the Lilburne affair has been debated far and wide, but if the words were intended to whitewash the case they did not altogether succeed, because historians have rightly or wrongly chosen to support the martyrdom of John Lilburne rather than the entrepreneurial but less romantic lifestyle of Hesilrige. Yet it is clear that the beginning of poor William Huntington's case predates the 1651 action of Josiah Primate by some months, for he had travelled to London and back before hearing of Lilburne's banishment.

It is not unlikely that Richard Lilburne did persecute his son's tenants, because of the family John Lilburne was the only one with egalitarian views. If anyone suffered from John Lilburne's political ideals, it was undoubtedly his wife and children.

Meanwhile time had elapsed and enveloped the legal struggle between Hesilrige and Lilburne. Sir Arthur was still the busy governor of Newcastle and the far north. On 28 July 1649 the Council of State instructed Hesilrige to take special care of Berwick, and to make sure his deputy there understood the seriousness of his charge.[22] Hesilrige had no worry concerning Berwick, for he had placed his old friend George Fenwick over this vital garrison. To have such a man as Fenwick in control of Berwick was important. Hesilrige could trust his judgement better than that of the impulsive Hobson, and furthermore the latter was needed in Newcastle during his enforced journeys to London.

Danger was forever on the mind of the Council of State, and on 2 September 1649, a letter was sent to Hesilrige warning of planned insurrections by supporters of Charles Stuart.[23] It was believed that the Levellers were plotting to support the new king in return for political advantage. In Newcastle, however, Sir Arthur held no such fears, and he wrote to Speaker Lenthall on 13 September:

> ...these parts att ye present are in a very quiett condicon both soldrs and people, the soldrs contented being constantly paid, and the wasted impoverished People labouring and taking care of their Subsistance and livelyhood & not being devoured by free quarter.[24]

After years of occupation by the Scots, or oppression from royalist levies, the people of Newcastle were enjoying a period of stable government. Hesilrige had settled many of the economic problems the war had brought the district: the Tyne was open and coal could again be moved from the northern mines, the people were paid to feed the soldiers and work and food was more plentiful. Despite this not all people were happy with Hesilrige's administration, and propaganda was spread throughout London. A northern gentleman by the name of John Musgrave accused Hesilrige of favouring Delinquents: '...he takes for his friends favourites, Councellors, and bosome acquaintances such as were professed enemies to the Commonwealth and preferes none other; he slights, derides, and keeps under all the cordial and well affected.'[25]

The differences between who Musgrave and Hesilrige would call 'enemies to the Commonwealth' were obviously diverse, but important.[26] On 31 January 1650 John Musgrave was ordered to attend the Council of State to present his exceptions to Sir Arthur's choice of Commissioners for the Northern Counties. Musgrave was sent away unsuccessful and had published his anti-Hesilrige tract soon after. The affair dragged on throughout that year and into the next, as we shall see.

NOTES

1.   CJ, V, p. 986.

2.   *The Parliament under the Power of the Sword*, BM 669, f. 13, p. 54; 'A Staffe set at Parliaments owne doore', E 475 (29); 'A True and Full Relation', E 476 (14); see also D. Underdown, *Pride's Purge* (Oxford, 1975) for the best and fullest modern account.

3.   *Burton's Diary*, III, pp. 96-97.

4.   *The Cromwell Letters*, LRO.

5.   Money, *First and Second Newbury*, p. 97.

6.   *Burton's Diary*, III, p. 97.

7.   CJ, VI, p. 141.

8.   CJ, VI, p. 141.

9.   CSP Dom, 1649–50, p. 17.

10. CSP Dom, 1649–50, p. 25.

11. CSP Dom, 1649–50, p. 220.

12. W. Notestein, *A History of Witchcraft in England, 1558–1718* (Washington, 1911): E. Maple, *The Dark World of Witches* (London, 1964); see also J. Fuller, *The History of Berwick upon Tweed* (Edinburgh, 1799).

13. J. Lilburne, 'A Preparative to a Hue and Cry after Sir Arthur Haslerig' (1649), E 573 (16).

14. *An Anatomy of Lieut.-Col. John Lilburne's Spirit* (1649), private copy.

15. *The Just Defence of John Lilburne* (1653), reprinted in A.L. Morton (ed.), *Freedom in Arms* (London, 1975), pp. 338-39.

16. Morton, *Freedom in Arms*, pp. 338-39.

17. To this day a leasholder inherits unpaid debts of previous holders appertaining to the property.

18. J. Lilburne, 'A Just Reproof to Haberdashers Hall' (1651), E 638 (12).

19. Although this chapter is set in 1649–50, the story and consequences of the Harraton Colliery Case is told in this one section.

20. *A Juryman's Judgement upon the case of John Lilburne: Lilburne Tried and Cast* (1653); see also, CJ, VIII, p. 71; Haslerig was awarded £2,000 from Lilburne's fine.

21. From the Hazlerigg Collection.

22. CSP Dom, 1649–50, p. 253.

23. CSP Dom, 1649–50, p. 303.

24. Bodl. Tanner MSS 56, f. 103.

25. J. Musgrave, 'A True and Exact Relation of the Great and Heavy Pressures and Grievances the Well Affected of the Northern Bordering Counties Lye under' (1650), E 619 (10).

26. 'Musgrave Muzl'd or the Mouth of Iniquity Stopped' (1651), E 625 (11).

↭ 14 ↭

An Engagement Verie Difficult

Nevertheless for thy great mercies' sake thou didst not utterly consume
them, not forsake them; for thou art a gracious and merciful God.

(Neh. 9.31)

The Hesilriges were busily buying a vast northern estate to add to
the lands of Noseley and Alderton. On 9 November 1649, Thomas
Hesilrige esq. bought Middleham Manor in Northumberland for
£3,306 6s 6½d.[1] Whether this was Sir Arthur's son or brother one
cannot ascertain from the records of the transaction, but it would
seem unlikely the brother required lands in Northumberland, whereas
his son was nearing his twenty-fifth birthday and probably sought an
estate of his own, and with this purchase would consequently re-
establish the Hesilrige's roots in that county. Sir Arthur himself bought
the borough of Easingwood for £5,833 9s 9d on 5 April 1650, and
on 1 June increased his northern holdings by acquiring Wolsingham
Manor for £6,764 14s 4d.[2] The family was fast becoming extremely
wealthy, and great landowners.

Meanwhile, the Scottish situation was being carefully watched as it
reached a critical stage in its development. Although the royalist James
Graham—the romantic hero better known as Montrose—had fought
a brave war and in many respects a highly successful one, his small
army of Scots and Irish loyalists was finally defeated and he himself
hanged in Edinburgh on 21 May 1650. A month later Charles Stuart
accepted the Covenant, and with it Scottish Presbyterian support. The
same men who had butchered Montrose now owed loyalty to the
monarchy he fought so long for. Having taken the Covenant the
young Charles was allowed to land in Scotland, and an army was raised
under David Leslie, although the usual Scottish lack of pace in its
recruitment gave the English Council of War/State some time to

prepare instead of the common scramble to bolt the stable door. The English had long expected this move by Charles Stuart, and consequently they concluded that if the Scots would again enter England in support of an enemy of the Commonwealth, why should they not steal the march on them and take the war to Scotland.

In January 1650, Lieutenant-Colonel Paul Hobson had been forced to take action against the Northumberland cavaliers.[3] No matter how long the war lasted, the old monarchy men would still answer the call to arms for the royal cause. Considering the good service by Hobson early in 1650, a decision by the Council of State on 28 June seems harsh in the extreme and of no service to Hesilrige at a time when administration was at a premium:

> ...the Council (of state) observes by Lieut. Hobson's readiness to serve the Scotch design in giving a pass to Major Grey, that he is unfit to be employed as Deputy Governor of Newcastle, and Sir Arthur is therefore to think of some other person for that trust.[4]

Hobson was among the most trustworthy of any men Hesilrige could choose for this vital post. If he did wrong in allowing Grey, who he did not know as a royalist agent, free entry into England, it is conjecture to account for the mistakes made by the Council of State during the same period. Weighed against Hobson's obvious error must be his popularity in the town and suburbs of the Tyne. If Paul Hobson was guilty of anything likely to bring the area troubles foreseen by the Council, it was his religion, which was Baptist. Although freedom of religion was part of the Commonwealth, the Baptist faith was considered a fringe religion. The Newcastle Baptists were strong and influential and very much left in peace to practise their faith by Hesilrige during his administration. Hesilrige was criticized for his religious liberalism—a liberalism not extended to the Church of Rome—but it was not enough to remove him from office. Nevertheless, Hobson had not the same old war authority and could be martyred for the sake of ignorance.

Colonel, or Major Grey was taken upon his arrival in London and brought before the Council:

> A messenger calling himself Col. James Grey, a Scot, being brought before Council, and examined from whom he came, and by what warrants and what letters he brought with him, answered that he came from the Parliament of Scotland, with letters to the Parliament of England and the Lord General, and being twice demanded whether he had any other

letters, expressly denied that he had any other; yet upon a third demand, he confessed he brought other letters, but they were of no consequence, and produced a pass from the President of the Parliament of Scotland, intimating his repair to the city of London about the affairs of the public; the letter by him pretended to be to the Parliament of England was directed to the Hon. Wm. Lenthall, Speaker of the House of Commons in England. The Council considering hereof, and of the order of Parliament of the 26th inst, refering it to Council to prevent all correspondance, intelligence, and commerce between England and Scotland, thought fit the said messenger should be continued in the custody of the serjeant.[5]

The Council of State was certainly worried about the Scots, almost to a state of nervous paranoid hysteria. Of course they had good cause for concern, being a revolutionary body born from the blood of the King and not the judgement of the people of England upon the blood he had spilt in his royal progress to the end of monarchy. Leveller middle ground in the army had erupted into mutiny during early 1649, some regiments being reduced to ease the public burden, while others were in Ireland with Cromwell, leaving only 12 regiments of horse, 11 regiments of foot, and 6 companies of dragoons for the defence of England.

One by one the options left to the council in the defence of the nation were being eroded by time, but at the eleventh hour Oliver Cromwell once again made a dramatic arrival. By a miracle his work in Ireland was at a stage where he could leave the army and return where history called. By 1 June 1650, Cromwell was back in England. The council, with Parliament's blessing, voted that Cromwell and Fairfax would command an army for the invasion of Scotland, taking the war away from London and therefore preventing a Scottish design upon re-establishing the monarchy. Fairfax, however, would not command an army which was to enter Scotland in war, claiming quite rightfully that it broke the agreement entered into in the Solemn League and Covenant, but he would command if the Scots invaded English soil. In reality Fairfax had not been happy with much the revolution had brought forth: he was not a republican, nor a dictator, and he did not believe in the establishment of the military junta or the act of regicide itself. For Fairfax this was a happy release from the responsibility the army had thrust upon him at a time when England's future was at turmoil and stability at a low ebb. He took his leave of the army and laid down his commission on 26 June. Who but Oliver Cromwell could take command.

Hesilrige was busy in his own right in his far outpost. The Tyne of course led to the sea, and Newcastle watched all shipping with particular interest. Of interest during this period are the adventures of the sea captain Hall and his patrolling of the actual Tyne Mouth. A most vital letter of 4 July tells of Hall's greatest hour:

> Captain Wyard of the Adventure, a merchant ship hired into your service, and one of the squadron, has strayed a vessel bound for Scotland laden with merchants goods and oats intended for the horses over in the ship which we chased ashore. The master of the vessel is a Dutchman, his men Scotchmen, and the goods belong to Scotch merchants. Captain Wyard and his men have taken out of the ship much goods including a box wherein were two bags, an old and a new one, richly embroidered with silver, gold, and pearl, with the arms of Scotland upon it, which I believe was for the Lord Keeper of Scotland. The bags I have ordered Capt. Wyard to deliver to Sir Arthur Hesilrige for your disposal. I have sent the ship to Newcastle to be secured as also the passengers, amongst whom are Mr. Charles Stuarts cook, and coachman. I order Capt. Wyard to convoy her in there, not having put any of my men aboard, lest what his men have done should be attributed to them. This fact is not only a breach of the orders of Parliament and of the Generals of the Fleet, but will also reflect upon all in your service therefore if you please to call him to question about it he may be found at Newcastle.[6]

The good Captain Wyard obviously had something of the 'Buccaneer' about him, and was not exactly a favourite amongst military types, but he had inadvertently gained a great prize. The two bags were from Holland, the new bag being indeed the Chancellor's purse ready for the Scottish coronation of Charles Stuart. Captain Hall, the rear admiral, had taken seven ships, much to the disaster of Scottish power, and in them found pistols, swords and ammunition, all bound for the Scottish army. Hall's action is a minor piece of naval history compared to the heroics of Drake or Nelson, but any strategic or moral victory was invaluable now war was on the horizon, and therefore the deeds of Hall were a prize indeed.

As July progressed, the Scots too were becoming nervous. The Parliament of Scotland had begun to realize that they would soon have an English army on their own soil, and on 7 July this news broke:

> The Scots go on very fast with their levy. The Parliament of Scotland have this day sent an express to Sir Arthur Hesilrige, wherein they would persuade the Army to delay their march a little longer, but we have been deceived too long.[7]

The reply was negative for the invasion was not far off. The new lord general, Oliver Cromwell, began his march north from London on 28 June—over a week before the Scots wrote to Hesilrige. Upon reaching Newcastle, Cromwell and the principal officers were 'entertained with much magnificence' by Hesilrige, which was followed by a fast and prayers for the Scottish expedition.[8]

Changes in Cromwell's army took place before they marched on. John Bright, one of the heroes of Preston two years earlier, resigned his command—remarkably to become a staunch monarchist before too many moons elapsed. To replace Bright, the lord general chose the ex-royalist prisoner, George Monck. It is ironic that it had been Bright's regiment that had captured Monck at Nantwich and led to him serving a term in the Tower. Nevertheless, Monck was cleared of his delinquency and served the Commonwealth loyally almost to the end. The officers and men of Bright's regiment did not however share Cromwell's views on Monck and refused him. Men were therefore drawn from the 'post New Model' regiments of Hesilrige and Fenwick to serve under him.

Newcastle was to be Cromwell's supply depot, sending arms and reinforcements at regular intervals—in theory at least. The English force gathered itself around Berwick on 19 July, crossing the border three days later under the watchful eye of Scottish scouts, who were reporting every move to David Leslie's army, busily assembling to meet the threat. With English troops advancing through Scottish heather, more of the Scottish Highland clans sent troops to add to the Lowland horse and foot loyal to Leslie—it was already estimated that the Scots' 40,000 outnumbered Cromwell two to one. Cromwell needed a port to link with both London and Newcastle and he turned towards Dunbar, arriving on 29 July.

Meanwhile, Sir Arthur was desperately trying to collect reinforcements and arms, a task quite simple on paper but endlessly difficult in real life. On 29 July the Council of State made order: 'To write to Sir Arthur Hesilrige that Council conceives the article for the Act he mentions is clear that they may raise men preportionable, and has given order to have 2,000 muskets and 1,000 pikes...'[9]

Hesilrige was also given consent to raise a force for the northern defence about Carlisle. It was of great necessity that the weaker Carlisle flank was not left unguarded in attacking the Scots along the

Berwick side. On 3 August the Lancashire Militia was ordered as one regiment to Carlisle.

By 1 September, the English Army had advanced from Dunbar, and for once Cromwell had found himself out-generaled by David Leslie. In fairness, Leslie was a far better soldier than Hamilton had been in 1648, and was superior to many of the Irish commanders Cromwell had met in recent months. The bastard son of old Lord Leven, Leslie had fought with distinction with Cromwell at Marston Moor, and was well respected by Oliver as a soldier and commander. Fate and politicians had conspired to put these men on different sides so late in the day. Falling back to Dunbar, the English now had their backs to the sea, and Cromwell must either fight or perform a seventeenth-century version of Dunkirk and evacuate by sea while Scottish guns and muskets cut at them. He chose to fight. In a now quite famous letter to Hesilrige written on the eve of battle, 2 September, Cromwell described his thankless situation:

> Deere Sir,
>
> Wee are upon an engagement verie difficult, the enimie hath blocked up our way att the passe att Coperspith, through which wee cannot gett without almost a miracle, hee lyeth soe upon the hills that wee knowe not how to come that way without great difficultye, and our lyinge heere dayly consumeth our men, whoe fall sicke beyound imagination. I perceeve your forces are not in a capacitye for present reliefe, wherefore (whatever becomes of us) itt will bee well for you to gett what forces you can together, and the south to helpe what they cann, the businesse nearly concerneth all good people, if your forces had beene in a readinesse to have fallen upon the back of Copperspith itt might have occasioned supplies to have come to us, but the only wise God knowes what is best, all shall worke for good, our spirits are comfortable (praised bee the Lord) though our present condition bee as it is, and indeed wee have such hope in the Lord, of whose mercy we have had large expence. Indeed doe you gett together what forces you cann, against them. Send to friends in the South to help with more, Lett H. Vane know what I write, I would not make it publick. Lett mee heere from you, I rest
>
> > Your servant
> > Oliver Cromwell
>
> September 2nd 1650—hast hast...[10]

This letter was sent very early the next morning, for Leslie's advance had not begun. It clearly shows that Cromwell fully expected the worst and was doing nothing more than preparing Hesilrige for the flood of Scots that would cross the border if he and his forces were destroyed around Dunbar. It is interesting to note that Oliver tells Sir Arthur to inform their friend and colleague Sir Henry Vane, but not to make the situation public. If the destruction of Cromwell's army was near, Hesilrige had little chance of stopping the Scots alone, but Henry Vane in London would need time to re-organize the war policy of the Council of State and hopefully recruit enough militia to add to the New Model's remaining regiments to give battle to the Scots further south. The only alternative was a peace settlement and restoration. If Hesilrige made the situation public, armed insurrection by English royalists would follow within days. If Cromwell fell, so did the Commonwealth.

If ever the English needed the hand of the Lord it was at Copperspith on the morning of 3 September 1650—and the miracle was granted. When the smoke and cries of battle cleared, and the sound of drum, pipe and trumpet had dried out the tears of pain, an estimated 3,000 Scots lay dead with a further 10,000 taken. Oliver Cromwell wrote to Hesilrige the next day, relating the glad tidings:

Sir,

You will see by my inclosed of the 2nd of this month which was the evening before the fight the condicion we were in att that time, which I thought fitt on purpose to send you, that you might see how great & how seasonable our deliverance & mercie is, by such aggravacion having said my thoughts thereupon to the parliament, I shall only give you the narrative of this exceeding mercie, believing the Lord will enlarge your heart to a thankfull consideracion thereupon, the least of this mercie lyes not in the adventageous consequences which I hope it may produce of glory of God, & good to his people, in the preservation of that which remaynes unto which this greate work hath opened so faire a way, we have no cause to doubt but if it shall please the Lord to prosper our endeavours we may find oportunities both upon Edenburgh & leith, Starling bridge or other such places as the Lord shall lead unto, even far above our thoughts as this late & other experiences gives good encouragements wherefore that we may not be wanting I desire you with such good forces as you have immediately to march to mee at Dunbarr, leaving behind you such of your new levies as will prevent lesser incursions for surely their rout and ruine is so totall, that they will not be provided for anythinge that is verie considerable, or rather which I more encline unto, that you would send Thomlinson with the forces you have readie & that with all possible expedicion, & that you will go on with the remainder of the reserve which upon better thoughts, I do not thinke can well be done without you. Sir lett no time nor oportunitie be lost, surely its probable the Kirke has done their doe I beleive their King will sett upp upon his owne score now wherein he will find many friends, taking opportunitie offred, tis our great advantage through God, I need say no more you on this behalfe but rest,

> Your Humble servant
> Oliver Cromwell

Dunbarr September 4th 1650.

Postscript: My service to your good ladie, I thinke very fitt that you bake hard bread agen considering you increase our number, I pray you do so.

Sir I desire you to procure about 3 or 4 score masons and shipp them to us with all speed, for we expect that God will suddeinly put some places into our hands which we shall have occasion to fortifie.[11]

Even in a letter following such a great victory, and full of important military logic, there is a much more important message contained therein and of prime interest to this story, as will later be explained. The following day, Cromwell wrote once again:

Sir,

After much deliberacion, we can find no way hoe to dispose of these prisoners that wilbe consisting with these two ends. (to witt, the not loosing them, & the not starving them neither of which would we willingly incurr) but be sending them into England, where the Council of State may excercise their wisedom & better judgment in so dispersing & disposing of them, as that they may not suddeinly return to your prejudice. We have dispatched away neer 5000 poore wretches of them, verie of which its probable will dye of their wounds or so be rendered unserviceable for time to come by reason thereof. I have written to the Council of State desiring them to direct how they shalbe disposed of, and I make no question but you will hastne the prisoners up southward, and second my desires with your owne to the Councill. I knowe you are a man of business, this not being every dayes worke, will willingly be performed by you, especially considering you have the commands of your supervisers. Sir I judge it exceeding necessary you send us up what horse and foot you can with all possible expedicion, especially considering that indeed our men fall verie sicke & if the lord shall please to enable us effectually to prosecute this business to the which he hath opened so gratious a way, no man knowes but that it may produce a peace to England, & much securitie & comfort to God's people, wherefore I pray you continue to give what furtherance you can to this worke, by speeding such supplies to us as you can possible spare, not having more at present, I rest,

> Your affectionate friend & servant
> Oliver Cromwell

Dunbarr September 5th 1650[12]

The English army was in a very sick condition, much as it had been in Ireland. But if sickness was a problem in the English ranks, the condition of the half-starved and wounded Scots was pitiful when Hesilrige received them. The Council of State gave Hesilrige the following order on 10 September:

> Council have referred the disposing of the prisoners to a committee from which he will speedily receive some order, and that it is left to him to dispose of so many as he conceives he may to work of the coal mines.[13]

Not a happy situation for the prisoners, who, it should be remembered were Parliament's northern brothers not a long time before. How many were actually condemned to the pits is unknown. Indeed, it is debatable that any were fit to dig coal under the terrible conditions of the seventeenth-century pits. Despite the stories of Hesilrige's actual brutality to the prisoners, he saw the sorry and desperate state of these men and allowed them to rest at Durham. The stories of Hesilrige's harsh treatment were mainly disclosed in the slur campaign which followed the Restoration. In reality, out of 5,000 prisoners, many were wounded and filthy, hunger ate at their bellies and disease was spreading through them like fire. It is not so surprising that the death rate was high. A large number of these Scots were transported to Virginia as slaves, but this was at the direct order of the Council of State and was only implemented to ease the public burden.

By 9 September, Cromwell was in Edinburgh, where again he wrote to Sir Arthur upon urgent business:

> Sir,
>
> I cannot but hastne you in sending up what forces possibly you can, this inclosed was intended to you on Saterday, but not come. We are not able to carry on our business as we would, untill we have where with to keepe Edinburgh & Leith, untill we attempt & are acting forward. We have not in these parts above 2 monthes to keep the feild, Therefore expedite, what you can, and I desire you to send us free masons, you know not the importance of Leith. I hope your Northerne guests are come to you by this time, I pray you lett humanitie be exercised towards them, I am perswaded it wilbe comely. Lett the officers be kept at Newcastle some, some sent to Lynn, some to Chester. I have no more but rest,
>
> > Your Affectionat Servant
> > Oliver Cromwell
>
> Postscript: I desire as forces come up, I may heare from time to time what they are, how their marches are laid, & when I may expect them. My service to the deere Ladye.[14]

Hesilrige continued to send fresh troops to Scotland. During late September, Colonel Fitch, who was responsible to Hesilrige as his understudy at Carlisle, led an army into the west of Scotland. In Fitch's absence, Hesilrige was to put a reliable person in his place.[15]

The Council of State now found a way to remove further Scots from Sir Arthur's care:

> To write Sir Arthur Hesilrigge, approving his disposing of some of the Scotch prisoners, and to say that the Highlanders, by reason of their affinity to the Irish, are not proper for the service; but if 500 others may be found, he is to send them to Ireland according to former orders.[16]

By using Scottish Lowland troops of the Presbyterian faith to fight Irish Catholics, English troops in Ireland could be released that service and strengthen the home army. Therefore, the Scots that agreed the Irish service were actually engaged in the defeat of their own cause, albeit indirectly. The use of the Presbyterian Scots in Ireland still bears fruit in the twentieth century, for these Scottish volunteers, with added depth from other Scottish landworkers, were the fuse by which sectarian violence was lit.

In December 1650, a very amusing story begins in Carlisle, which was directly governed by Hesilrige during Fitch's absence. On 19 December, the Council ordered:

> Mr. Robinson to write to fit persons in Yorkshire to examine Denton, a pirate, lately taken, and now prisoner at Carlisle, and return the examinations to Council. Also to write the Governor of Carlisle to keep Denton safe, he being a dangerous person, and to be tried for his life[17]

In February 1651, Denton was moved from Carlisle to greater security at York. There he stayed until 8 July when this letter from the council to Luke Robinson tells the sorry tale:

> You certify the escape of Denton the pirate from York gaol, and think the gaoler should answer for it. Order his prosecution at the assizes, that he may be punished for his offence, whether it be negligence or wilful...[18]

It would appear that Denton the pirate made his escape in true Hollywood tradition, by bribing the gaoler—a feat applauded by every reader no doubt. Piracy had not yet reached its zenith, but many old soldiers from the waste of civil war would turn to the path of crime, with highway robbery and 'mugging' becoming commonplace, the disturbance to civilized society reaping a rich harvest in the years to follow.

Sometime during December 1650, Hesilrige and a political colleague from London, Mr Thomas Scot, visited Edinburgh to see Cromwell and assess the condition of the army.[19] Sir Arthur was no stranger to Edinburgh, having been at least once before, but by so going he was not back in Newcastle until 23 January 1651, where terrible news awaited him. Five days later, on 28 January, his beloved wife, Dorothy Greville-Hesilrige, died. It is this biographer's belief that Sir Arthur loved this lady very much, and with good cause, for she was beautiful, had given him a number of fine children and, being Lord Brooke's sister, was a superb match for the puritan side of his nature. But why a premature death? The reason is unrecorded as so many seventeenth-century deaths are. However, does Oliver Cromwell of all the unlikeliest people provide a cryptic clue in his letter of 4 September following the victory at Dunbar? By ignoring the main part of the letter and taking the postscript by itself as a note from one friend to another, indeed, Oliver tells us more than at first examination: 'My service to your good ladie, I thinke very fitt that you bake hard bread agen considering you increase our number, I pray you do so...'

In these lines we see another side to Cromwell. In the Lord's puritan there was also a man of country humour, and Oliver was indeed making a congratulatory sexual jest. To 'bake hard bread agen' being Cromwell's jest at the further pregnancy of Dorothy—a reference to the proverbial bun in the oven, no less. He further says 'considering you increase our number', a direct reference to a child being added to the puritan family, but then adds 'I pray you do so', signifying the danger therein. Historians in the past have, in this biographer's opinion, misread this postscript to mean Cromwell required troops, when in reality he was merely being human. Dame Dorothy was still of childbearing age, being younger than Sir Arthur, and had already given him eight children—seven still living in 1651—and it is not impossible his beloved second wife died of complications during a ninth pregnancy. Things had been difficult for Hesilrige during 1650, and now came this blow when the tide of the war appeared to turn. Dorothy had been a great comfort to her husband, but now all that was left to do was to lay her to rest, the inscription reading:

> Here lies Dame Dorothea Hesilrige Sister to Robert
> Greville, Lord Brooke and Baron of Beauchamps Court.
> God gave to her True & Great Wisdome and a large &

just heart. She did much good in her generation.
Sir Arthur Hesilrige had by her Three Sons and Five
Daughters.
She left this life ye 28th of January 1650[20]

NOTES

1.   Nichols, *Leicestershire*, II, pt ii, p. 745.
2.   Nichols, *Leicestershire*, II, pt ii, p. 745.
3.   Whitelocke, *Memorials of English Affairs*, III, pp. 140-41.
4.   CSP Dom, 1650, p. 221.
5.   CSP Dom, 1650, p. 221.
6.   CSP Dom, 1650, p. 232.
7.   CSP Dom, 1650, pp. 236-37.
8.   Nichols, *Leicestershire*, II, pt ii, p. 746.
9.   CSP Dom, 1650, p. 256.
10.   *The Cromwell Letters*, LRO. This is reprinted in the Carlisle tract and also the Thomas Carlyle 'Letters and Speeches', although the reprint here is in the original style.
11.   *The Cromwell Letters*, LRO.
12.   *The Cromwell Letters*, LRO.
13.   CSP Dom, 1650, pp. 334-35.
14.   *The Cromwell Letters*, LRO.
15.   CSP Dom, 1650, pp. 330, 400.
16.   CSP Dom, 1650, p. 419.
17.   CSP Dom, 1650, p. 474. It is hoped Sir Arthur would not feel the same about his biographer.
18.   CSP Dom, 1651, p. 282.
19.   CSP Dom 1651, p. 17: CJ, VI, p. 527.
20.   Chapel of St Mary, Noseley Hall, Leicestershire. Death in pregnancy was not uncommon, indeed, one of Sir William Waller's wives almost died during childbirth.

∽ 15 ∽

Adam and Eve

> And the eyes of them both were opened, and they knew that they were
> naked; and they sewed fig leaves together, and made themselves aprons.
>
> (Gen. 3.7)

One can but imagine Sir Arthur's feelings at losing his dear wife. It
had obviously been a good marriage, and lasted over 20 years through
a period of history when wives and families played a supportive role
in national events. Dorothy had certainly supported her husband, and
in respect for this Sir Arthur did not remarry again. Instead, he
devoted his remaining life to his family and that fickle yet passionate
lover—English politics. In many ways Sir Arthur followed the path
of his old friend John Pym, who had devoted himself to a political life
and founded a freedom of politics hitherto unknown.

During this sorrowful time, Hesilrige was again attacked in print
by John Musgrave. The Council of State nevertheless supported Sir
Arthur, and reached out to protect him. Musgrave had questioned Sir
Arthur's administration in the far north, and in particular his choice
of lesser administrators. But in this the council found 'that it does not
at all appear that Sir Arthur Hasilrigge has broken the trust reposed in
him by Council'.[1]

To question Hesilrige's administration of the north was easy, for
many aspects of his style were open to criticism, but throughout his
'reign' he had kept the Commonwealth in safety. The Council of
State fully appreciated the difficulty Sir Arthur worked under. He
would quite obviously make enemies because of his position, which
all powerful men do, but weighed against this Sir Arthur had restored
order in the far north, and at Newcastle had helped business and trade
to flourish. In this respect Sir Arthur had achieved a workable relationship with the numerous groups in and around Newcastle. Coal was

flowing from the Durham and Tyne pits, which was important both locally and nationally, and the mouth of the Tyne was open to shipping to enable transportation of coal and goods. The traders therefore were able to resume their business with little trouble, and just as important the people could once more live their lives with some stability even though they were living in the 'front line' of a war zone. Having achieved all this, it is not surprising that Hesilrige was popular with everyone in Newcastle except Musgrave and the Lilburne circle. If this stability was to continue, the Council of State had to support Sir Arthur, and John Musgrave was 'muzzled' once more.

For the first half of 1651 Oliver Cromwell was a sick man, the Scottish climate and hard wear his body had received during the war, plus perhaps a form of recurrent fever contracted in the bogs of Ireland, having brought his health to ruin. Being almost constantly in the field, with one campaign following another, would wear down a young man, let alone a man in his mid fifties like Oliver. With the majority of his army in Scotland, trouble was brewing in England. When the annual election for the Council of State was held in February, Hesilrige was voted back and two new members added to that great body—Charles Fleetwood and Thomas Harrison. Fleetwood was Cromwell's lieutenant general,while Harrison was a 'praying' officer much admired by Cromwell. Since Oliver had replaced Sir Thomas Fairfax as lord general, his favourites had slowly gained upper positions in the nation's administration.

On 20 March, Hesilrige received confirmation from the Council of State, that Harrison was now Major General for Lancashire and Cheshire. Sir Arthur was to keep a constant correspondence with Harrison, and to assist with forces when appropriate[2] Thomas Harrison was hardly of Hesilrige's character, being of a strange religious sect known as Fifth Monarchists. Such men believed the turmoil now in England heralded the second coming of Christ to begin his thousand-year reign on earth. This was not a doctrine shared by Hesilrige, although he did not openly disagree with the Fifth Monarchists.

On 26 May Sir Arthur reported to Parliament the poor condition of Cromwell's health, which had greatly deteriorated over the cold spring of 1651. Oliver's health was becoming critical. Above all things he needed rest, but such luxury was impossible. An alternative was now suggested, whereby George Monck would take command in

Scotland, thus allowing Cromwell leave in England 'where the air is not so sharp'. Monck had grown in Cromwell's favour during the long Scottish campaign, despite having once been a royalist—there no doubt being more joy in a sinner who repenteth. Hesilrige also had a working relationship with Monck, and trusted him perhaps a little too much. There was nevertheless no need for Sir Arthur to worry unduly about his friend's health, for, considerate as ever, the Scots were organizing a southern holiday for Cromwell. On 1 January, Charles Stuart had been crowned King of Scots at the traditional Scone, and, aided by a 'New Modelled' Scottish army under David Leslie, planned insurrection by royalists all over England. The Earl of Derby and Sir Thomas Tyldesly were by July recruiting royalist forces in Lancashire and Cheshire, and on 7 August the Council of State informed Hesilrige that the 'Scotch are marched southward', leaving Cromwell on the wrong side of the border.[3] Oliver at once sent John Lambert hard in pursuit of David Leslie, hoping for a repeat of his brave rearguard action in 1648. Hesilrige, however, was quicker off the mark than the council, because he had met with Thomas Harrison and Colonel Rich the day before his official notification of the Scottish invasion to organize the northern strategy. It was decided that Harrison's forces should immediately march quickly south in aid of Lambert, Hesilrige holding Newcastle like in 1648.

Sir Arthur could now only wait for attack or news of Lambert and Cromwell. The second week of August saw a light skirmish over the passage to the Mersey, Lambert giving way before superior numbers, which had been his orders. Again the Scots were being shepherded down-country through Lancashire, reaching Hamilton's bane, Warrington, where Earl Derby and the small English royalist force met them. Derby once more went recruiting instead of joining with David Leslie, but was defeated in a policing action by Colonel Robert Lilburne at Wigan. The Earl though wounded escaped, but not so Sir Thomas Tyldesly, who was shot diving through a hedge while trying to escape the narrow lanes around Wigan. Warrington was no home for the Scots, nor Charles. Forever a curse upon the Stuart cause, it seems, this area near Preston saw yet another fateful blunder when Charles decided against a march on London, which was perhaps his one hope of victory. By 22 August, the Banner Royal could be seen flying proudly over the great city of Worcester, but the Scots were trapped and did not know it.

On 24 August, Cromwell met Lambert at Warwick. John Lambert had done his job well, London was safe, and with Cromwell's small army plus the regiments of horse with Lambert a fight could be made. The local militia was also called out to swell the parliamentary forces. Cromwell was very badly outnumbered, but he was well prepared and the Scots morale was very low. At Evesham, Cromwell met Samuel Gardiner, the old 'Lobster' captain, who had retired from military life and now sat on various committees.

Meanwhile, completely out of touch with the realities of life, the Council of State ordered Sir Arthur at Newcastle to send George Monck in Scotland a further 1,200 men. Considering the position in and around Newcastle, such action was impossible. The council also ordered Sir Arthur to fall upon the Scots should they retreat and to 'utterly extirpate and destroy them'.[4] The 1,200 men had not been sent by 2 September, and although quick in orders the Council still failed with pay, and Hesilrige was having trouble with deserters.

On 4 September the Church bells of London rang clear with victory, for Cromwell had crushed the army of David Leslie in the fields around Worcester. The council sent the news to Sir Arthur that same day:

> It has pleased God to give us a great victory against the Scotch Army at Worcester yesterday. The slain are estimated at 4,000 but there are not above 100 of ours. It is possible that such as can scatter homewards will endeavour to do so.[5]

Worcester was a great victory, and the Scots, who had been led like lambs to the slaughter, would not fight for Charles again, and indeed why should they? for the English had not flocked to his banner as they had done for his father. Before the war, a poor man working for a great royalist family would carry out his master's bidding, but by 1651 many of the wealthy royalists had fled abroad and the cannon fodder for a royalist army was no longer subject to such bidding. Charles Stuart had totally misjudged the political climate of post-regicide England. Peace was all the common man craved, and he was no longer willing to spill his blood for the glory of kings.

Many of the Scots escaping the Cromwellian troopers along the lanes and ditches from Worcester were taken or died on the journey home. The danger over, Hesilrige was able to send George Monck his soldiers. A great number of Scots were taken around Northumberland, Sir Arthur filling Durham gaol to overflowing, once again many being sold into slavery in Barbados. Yet when Hesilrige was appointed

President of the Council of State for one month on 26 January 1652, one of his first tasks was the arrangements for the release of all Lowlanders imprisoned at Durham. The Council consented to this in March and at long last a more peaceful settlement began to grow in the country.

So far this biography has dealt little with Sir Arthur's views on religion. It has already been said that to Hesilrige the religious question came second to that of a free Parliament. But Sir Arthur was a puritan and therefore life was, because of, to the glory of, and for the greater understanding of God. God was part of life, as bread was to feed the body, so the scripture fed the soul. Every single triumph or defeat was a blessing or judgement of God. It is certain that Sir Arthur had little in common with the Fifth Monarchist or Quaker sects which were strong in the North, or indeed the Baptists, who were the fastest growing group in Newcastle. Hesilrige was not a strict doctrinaire like the Presbyterians, and was noted for his hatred of the old Episcopacy and the Church of Rome. Sir Arthur Hesilrige, like his friend Cromwell, was a free-Churchman, a Congregationalist, believing in religious freedom. Although of course not totally against the more rigid Presbyterian service, Sir Arthur required of his God far greater freedom than the Presbyter preacher could allow, and therefore he himself did not follow that particular path although he had among his colleagues a number of that faith.

During his years as governor of Newcastle, Sir Arthur did actually influence the religious life of the area. In 1653 the Town's principal preacher, old Dr. Jenison, fell ill, and his successor Mr Sydenham was already sick and died within the year. Hesilrige now appointed Samuel Hammond, a man he could control. Hammond had acted as Sir Arthur's personal chaplain at Newcastle before his new appointment, and as early as April 1651 had been rector of Bishopswearmouth, County Durham.[6] Furthermore, Hammond was although only a butcher's son, a fellow of Sir Arthur's old college of Magdalene.

Hesilrige was also mentioned by the congregation of Cumberland in regard to their minister:

> To the right Honourable Sir Arthur Hesilrige, the worthy Governor of New-Castle and one of the commissioners for settling the ministry in the County of Cumberland.

THE HUMBLE PETITION OF THE PARRISHIONERS
OF AICTON

Humbly Sheweth,

That whereas by your honour & the rest of the commissioners Mr.
Nichols was authorized and appointed to be minister at Aicton wee your
humble peticioners whose names are underwritten doe generall & most
hartily thanke you for him, as being one who by his painfulness plainesse
& power in teaching of us (we doe sensibly find) hath done much good
amongst us, & by his meakness, & loving carrage, hath gotten all our
loves & likeing. Wee therefore with one consent humbly & earnestly
intreate that he may be continued amongst us, and we have at this time &
upon this occasion taken the boidnesse upon us to trouble you because
wee hear that Mr. Lampitt who had formerly thrust him selfe upon us, &
upon his triall & examination att New Castle before the commissioners
was found insiufficient is now endeavouring to return upon us, & to that
purpose as we understand doth make use of some of the hands of this
parrish (which att his first comeing before we knew him he gott from us)
in a peticion of his to the Council of State, and gives it out that he hath
gotten an order, for his being again with us. Wee doe most earnestly
become suitors to your honeyr, that (if you see reason) you will please to
take noe such pains for us of the country who truly honour & love you.
That Mr. Nichols our minister may be continued amonst us whom we
doe all approve of, and thinke wee can not sufficiently thanke God for
him.

And wee shall be ever bound to praye,[7]

Sir Arthur kept this petition among his private papers and letters, it
was justification of his work in the north. Despite all that Lilburne,
Musgrave and countless historians have written about him over three
centuries, Sir Arthur's administration was very popular with the people
of Tyneside and the border counties. Even Cromwell approved of Sir
Arthur's religious policy, indeed, during the time he acted as a com-
missioner for such matters, he weeded out all ministers considered to
be undesirable and planted in their place men of good honest religion,
leaving the fringe groups like the Baptists to find God in their way.

In the meantime, the Rump of the Long Parliament—the group
left following Pride's Purge—were not moving very fast with their
work. Instead they began to once more oppose certain areas of the
military's rule. On 19 May 1652, the Rump abolished the office of
Lord Lieutenant and Lord Deputy of Ireland, much to the displeasure
of John Lambert, who held the latter post. During the same period
Hesilrige began to disagree with much of the policy of Sir Henry
Vane, the two men being of totally different minds on many subjects,
but who would work together against a common foe when an emergency arose. It must be true to say that Vane and Hesilrige had a

mutual respect for each other, knowing the strength and power each had within their own groups. It was the question of the American colonies where the two knights were so deeply divided. When the colonist Roger Williams returned from the New World to obtain a new charter for Rhode Island, Vane supported the plans of the settlers, but Hesilrige supported by George Fenwick was more cautious. Unlike Vane, George Fenwick knew the problems of the colonies, and knew Williams, who he perhaps had little affection for. When the Civil War broke out, a number of the Independent colonies had sent their sons home to fight for Parliament, yet others had chosen to sit the war out before declaring sides. Roger Williams wrote of their differences:

> ...the opposition of our enemies Sir Arthur Hesilrig and Colonel Fenwicke, who hath married his daughter, Mr. Winslow and Mr. Hopkins both in great place; and all the friends they can make in Parliament and Council, and all the priests, both Presbyterian and Independent; so that we stand as two armies, ready to engage, observing the posture and motions of each of the other, and yet shy of each other.[8]

Apart from the political stance of Sir Arthur upon the New World, this statement mentions a quite remarkable marriage. When George Fenwick married Catherine Hesilrige in 1652, he was 49 and the girl a mere 17, having been born in 1635.[9] Catherine must have known Fenwick since her earliest years, and it is not impossible that he bounced her upon his knee as a child of two or three. Catherine had grown up during Fenwick's stay at Saybrooke, and perhaps now alone in England he needed a companion as much as a wife. In the seventeenth century it was not uncommon for a man of advanced years to marry a girl of tender ones like in this case, where Catherine must have thought of him as an uncle. Catherine could have married into the best of families in England, so this marriage says more for Hesilrige's friendship for the man than any other act.

The Rump was getting nowhere with its reformation promised in the wake of the revolution. The Long Parliament had sat since its calling by King Charles I. True it had seen changes, mainly enforced by the sword, but the remaining Rump was fast becoming stateless, without direction or drive. It had entered into a war with Holland, which was a situation the economic climate could well do without, although the people had gained a certain national jingoism that brought them together. The Long Parliament should have been growing in maturity, but it was not. In complete contrast, the officers of the army had grown strong since Pride's Purge. These men had grown tired of the Rump, and the Rump blindly carried on down the same path without any consideration of the army. It was the army's desire that a dissolution of Parliament should be followed by elections. Cromwell in the meantime kept a watchful eye on the whole situation. Sir Henry Vane, who all but led the Rump, was in favour of a bill that would ensure the perpetual sitting of Parliament without dissolution, any gaps to be filled by by-elections, enforcing a state of non-democracy. Sir Arthur was at Noseley when the news arrived of Vane's plan for not dissolving. He immediately rode to London, and the bill was defeated—but too late.

On 20 April 1653, Lord General Oliver Cromwell entered the Commons, where he began to speak. Starting with words of praise for the great work done in the war, he recalled their struggle with the King, but suddenly his mood changed. Cromwell stamped up and down the floor of the chamber, admonishing the House for its present state, and as he reached the climax of his speech 20 or more musketeers entered the assembly. Hesilrige, in his own great speech yet to come, recalled the years up to this action:

> We continued four years, before we were put an end to. In which time, I appeal to all, if the nation, that had been blasted and torn, began not exceedingly to flourish. At the end of the four years, scarce a sight to be seen that we had had a war. Trade flourished, the City of London grew rich: we were the most potent by sea that ever was known in England. Our Navy and Armies were never better.
>
> Yet, after these estates were ended, we found a new trouble, the wars were not then ended, waters broke out. A strong remnant got into Colchester (1648). Our brethren of Scotland were not so firm upon that shaking of Kingship, we sent an army into Scotland, to Colchester, to Wales. This noble Lord (Fairfax) went to the gates of Colchester and conquered and put an end to all the English war (1648). Then a general was sent into Scotland. Our late Protector (Cromwell) that died was then Generall of all our forces. You know the great mercy. There we obtained that memorable victory at Dunbar (1650). What care did the Parliament then take to furnish their army from London with all neccessaries by land and in ships: all provided with the greatest diligence. None but a numerous company of good and honest hearted men could have done the like. The King of Scots came in with a great army. Twenty thousand men came suddenly and freely to Worcester. The people voluntarily rise and assist, in the greatest number that were ever read. The Scotch Army

returned, not three in a company. Man by man they returned in rags. This battle (3 September 1651) put an end to all the miseries of war in England and Scotland. Our wars in Ireland were then not considerable.

This done, it is true here was only remaining a little part of that triple cord, and you know what became of them. I heard being seventy miles off, that it was proposed that we should dissolve our trust, an dissolve it into a few hands. I came up and found it so; that it was resolved into a junta at the Cockpit. I trembled at it, and was after, there and bore my testimony against it. I told them the work they went about was accursed, I told them it was impossible to dissolve this trust. Next day, we were labouring here in the House on an act to put an end to that Parliament and to call another. I desired the passing of it with all my soul. The question was putting for it, when our General stood up, and stopped the question, and called in his Lieutenant, with two files of musqueteers, with their hats on their heads, and their guns loaden with bullet. Our General told us we should sit no longer to cheat the people. The Speaker, a stout man, was not willing to go. He was so noble that he frowned and said he would not out of the chair, till he was plucked out; which was quickly done, without much compliment, by two soldiers, and the mace taken: and there was an end of the third estate also. I rejoiced then, from the soul, that the question was not put. But I would have passed the severest sentence upon those that did this horrid business, that ever was passed upon men, and would have been from my heart the executioner of it. But I forgive them now, both the dead and the living. There was no possibility to dissolve this Parliament, the remaining part of the three estates, but by our own officer. He only had power. Our enemies had none.

Surely all the English blood was not spilled in vain? It was a glorious work of our Saviour to die on the cross for our spirituals. This is as glorious a work for our civils, to put an end to the King and Lords. The right is, originally, without all doubt, in the people. Undeniably and most undoubtedly it reverts to the people: the power being taken away. Like the Gordian Knot, it asked but Hercules' (sic Alexander's) sword to cut the knot. This done, our Generall, in 1653, looked on himself as having all power devolved upon himself; a huge mistake! The power was then in the people. If by conquest he had come in, he might have had something to say. It was undoubtedly in the people. It was a mistake in him; you shall see it. He was pleased to select a number of gentlemen, good, honest men, hither brought. He himself gave them power. They came into this House, and voted themselves a Parliament.

They acted high in some things, and soon cracked. Some of them ran to Whitehall, and returned their power, whence it came, thither it went. Judge whether power could pass thus, either to or from him.

This not serving the turn, then there was contrived an Instrument of Government, with our General at the head of it. This was first delivered to him in Westminster Hall. The Judges met that were in town, and the

> Mayor and Aldermen of the City of London, were summoned, for
> knowing what it was for. There was an oath in this Instrument, which he
> took; and after that took upon him the name of Protector.[10]

Throughout his political career Hesilrige spoke of the people's
power. He quite sincerely believed that the people held power and
Parliament administered that power only by their consent. There is
not a scrap of evidence against Sir Arthur in this respect. Whether by
King or Commons, Hesilrige spoke forever of the people's right to
hold the power unto themselves, this being the foundation stone of
democracy, for whoever takes on power without their blessing takes
it by the sword only.

Cromwell had taken the power and betrayed all Sir Arthur believed
in. In 1647, Hesilrige had remarked on the trust he placed upon
Cromwell's nose, and that trust was now broken. The friendship
between the two men was strong, but not strong enough to bear the
full weight of what Hesilrige saw as Cromwell's dishonesty. To dismiss Parliament without calling for its restoration after free elections
was to Sir Arthur undoubtedly wrong.

The Civil War and Revolution that followed in seventeenth-century England had removed an all-powerful king and replaced him
with a commonwealth ruled by Parliament. This was Sir Arthur's
ideal government, the third estate of the people. But with Cromwell's
action, the first estate of kingship had been grasped by a man and
reshaped into a monarchy called Protectorate. There is no argument or
defence against calling the man Protector, the man King. A Protector
can be a King, as much as a King can be a Protector. It is hardly
surprising to find that age-old biblical riddle being asked in 1653:

> When Adam delved and Eve span,
> Who was then the gentleman?

Who indeed? Hesilrige's bitterness at Cromwell's deed can only be
matched by Cromwell's displeasure of the Rump. Sir Arthur was not
angered by the end of the Rump but by Cromwell choosing himself
to lead the country upon a throne. This action had not only robbed
the Commonwealth of its virginity as the figure of Eve, but proclaimed Oliver to be the boldest ploughman since Adam.

Newcastle-upon-Tyne sent Cromwell a congratulatory message
upon his declaration of his protectorate, showing clearly the town's
great ability to run with both fox and hounds. However, in 1654,
Cromwell held elections which he had promised to do. In these elec-

tions the first since 1640, Newcastle returned as their member Sir Arthur Hesilrige, an anti-Cromwellian. Cromwell of course hoped that his position would be rubber-stamped by a landslide victory for his supporters, but when the returns came in, old names were to be found—Bradshaw, Scot, Vane and of course Hesilrige. Even a small number of known royalists found seats. It would seem that Sir Arthur was chosen for more than one place, as a letter from William Vane to his elder brother Sir Henry explains:

> Sir Arthur has been in these parts a fortnight, and seems to have been chosen both in Leicestershire and Newcastle against his will, and is in great straits whether to act in Parliament or keep out, but will stay hereabouts till Michaelmas.

> Ravensworth Castle
> 3rd August 1654[11]

To be chosen in two places was a problem easily overcome. Sir Arthur had always sat for Leicester and he was not likely to change. But he could not sit in Parliament in peace of conscience while Cromwell sat above it, nor could he deny the people their right to be represented by whom they chose. With his soul under a great weight, Hesilrige finally attended the assembly.

The House was split between the Cromwellians and the Commonwealth men. Sir Arthur was a Commonwealth man, and at once began to stir up a great hornet's nest for the belief in a free Parliament. Between 6 and 11 September, a debate was entered into upon whether the supreme power should be in a single person or Parliament. It was plainly against the Protectorate, although thinly disguised as a debate against monarchy. The republican Edmund Ludlow tells the story:

> In this debate Sir Arthur Haslerig, Mr. Scott and many others, especially the Lord President Bradshaw, were very instrumental in opening the eyes of many young members who had never before heard their interest as clearly stated and asserted; so that the Commonwealth party increased daily and that of the sword lost ground.[12]

To hold the Parliament together, the Commonwealth men, both Independents and Republicans, needed at least some support from the Presbyterian members in the Cromwellian group, but Sir Arthur would not betray the trust given to him and cynically cried, 'Let them establish one good religion and suppress all the sects.' With such disharmony in the Parliament, its fate was clear. Sir Arthur continues his story:

After that, a Parliament was called to confirm this, I was chosen one of those that the people sent up. Something was put in the writ, concerning our owning of this government in that Parliament, but come hither, some gentlemen were pleased to say, being in the dark, I remember one learned gentleman, very well read in Scripture, said openly that 'other foundation that that could no man lay'. Others said that the Parliament and Protector were twins, but the Parliament was the elder brother.

I then said no one Parliament could limit or impose upon me in any other. This doctrine was not well liked by the Protector. We were all turned out. Such a thing as never was done! An oath was made without doors to be taken by us, and was set at the door. Those that would take it came in. Those that would not were kept out by pikes. Knowing the privilege, that no power without doors could make an oath, I went away, and divers more gentlemen.

Those gentlemen that did sit, after five months were raised without giving any confirmation. It needed not, if other foundation could no man lay.

They did nothing.[13]

On the fateful 13 September 1654, the leading members of the Commonwealth party attended a sermon in St Margaret's and included in that number was Sir Arthur. Following the sermon, Hesilrige proudly refused to take Cromwell's Oath, and retired from the House without leave of the Protector, taking with him the bulk of the Commonwealth party.[14]

Between the first Protectorate Parliament and the next called in 1656, Sir Arthur Hesilrige refused to return to Westminster and also to pay his taxes. The second part of this act was perfectly valid. Since Sir Arthur had been arrested for refusing to pay King Charles's taxes, why should he pay King Oliver's? For this act of defiance, Hesilrige's 'Oxen of value' were sold for £20 and £40 each.[15] Yet Cromwell dared not imprison Hesilrige even at his most powerful, which was the logical move. Perhaps Oliver remembered too vividly the war they had shared, his message from Dunbar concerning the 'little lady' and the good days of friendship. If Cromwell impeached Sir Arthur, would not his betrayal be with a kiss?

During 1655, a royalist rising was bloodily put down when John Penruddock and a handful of followers declared for Charles Stuart. Hesilrige was thought to be involved in the plot, but upon examination the charge could not be proved.[16] Sir Arthur had nothing in common with Penruddock, except displeasure with Cromwell.

It is simplistic to call Cromwell a despot and ignore the vast number of opportunist followers who formed the junta under him. Sir Arthur was not simply opposed to dear Oliver, but rather to the ideal of the Cromwellians. To Hesilrige the Parliament was sacred, and the ideals instilled in him by John Pym so many years before must be defended. Therefore, when another Protectorate Parliament was called in 1656 Hesilrige was again chosen for Leicestershire. To the dismay of the Protector his supporters did not form the overall government. Edmund Ludlow tells of Cromwell's reply to the election results:

> The court finding by the lists they had received that not withstanding all their menaces, promises, and other artifices, divers persons were chosen whom they knew to be no favourers of the userpation, resolved to clear their hands of them at once. And to that end, under colour of a clause in the Instrument of Government that none should be admitted to places of power and trust but such as were men of sincerity and integrity, they gave an exclusion to Sir Arthur Haslerig, and Mr. Scott, and with as many more as they thought fit.[17]

Again the Cromwellians had broken the trust of the electorate. Out of a total of 400 members, 100 were kept out, half as many again vacating their seats voluntarily.[18] For anyone to question Sir Arthur's sincerity was an insult not only to him but to men like Pym and Hampden, who had instilled sincerity and loyalty to Parliament in him. Hesilrige says:

> Then came the last Parliament, in 1656. I was again chosen but not for any particular place; but for the whole county. When we came I found pikes again; one set to my breast. I could not pass without a ticket from the council. I found in the hall above fifty of us. We joined in a letter to the Speaker, declaring our willingness to serve, and that we were kept out. After two or three days attendance we were sent to the Council for a ticket. I durst do no such thing. I had lifted up my hands to God for the privilege of Parliament. I could not do it. Two hundred were kept out. Upon this, divers that had been admitted left the House.
>
> Then the government fell dangerously sick, and it died.[19]

But the power of the sword was losing ground, because for the second time in two years Cromwell had been opposed by republicans and royalists in his elections. Although of course the voting system in the seventeenth century was far from being one man one vote, those chosen and elected by the method then in use were entitled under a democracy to sit. The Protectorate had refused this right.

Sir Arthur travelled north, staying for a time at his mansion house at Bishop Auckland. Here, away from the public eye, Hesilrige waited for the day when Cromwell must break. The waiting was not long, for in the summer, 1657 the Cromwellians urged Cromwell to take the crown as King, and Oliver, and in a moment of great personal trial, almost gave in. Yet upon hearing of this Colonel Thomas Pride and the army spoke against such a move, and without the army no monarchy was possible. If they would not have a king, what would they have? They chose a king by deed, a lord protector.

The installation of Lord Protector Oliver Cromwell took place on 26 June 1657. One of the many guests of honour was Sir Arthur Hesilrige, or rather Arthur Lord Hesilrige 'who was as much a lord as Cromwell could make him'.[20] Hesilrige had been chosen a lord in the Uxbridge Proposals over 10 years earlier, but now Cromwell was attempting to buy off his enemies, and perhaps offer the olive branch to his old friend. Sir Arthur, although attending this coronation, would have none of it. The grand ceremony was held at Westminster Hall, where Charles was tried for being king, and the coronation chair was brought from Westminster Abbey. Rich velvets and gold could be seen everywhere. Finally came Cromwell, that man who chose men of 'a plaine russet coat' over the sons of gentlemen, in a robe of purple velvet lined in ermine, 'the habit anciently used at the solemn investiture of princes'.[21] What had become of Sir Arthur's old friend Oliver. From a mere captain of horse and Member of Parliament in 1642, he had risen to the throne of England. In 15 years Hesilrige had witnessed the death of monarchy and the birth of Parliament, and now he saw Cromwell crowned.

In his new role of Lord Protector, Cromwell attempted a reconciliation with his opponents from the early Protectorate. A higher House was brought into being, not named the House of Lords yet a House of Lords nonetheless. To this upper chamber Arthur Lord Hesilrige was called, but how could he take a seat in this reintroduced second estate of power. What rage and turmoil were Hesilrige's on seeing a Commons which was not a Commons, a Lords which was not a Lords and a King who was not a King? Well could anyone wonder at the state of Adam and Eve.

NOTES

1.   CSP Dom, 1651, p. 21.
2.   CSP Dom, 1651, p. 98
3.   CSP Dom, 1651, p. 306.

4. CSP Dom, 1651, p. 385.
5. CSP Dom, 1651, p. 409.
6. DNB (Samuel Hammond).
7. *The Cromwell Letters*, LRO.
8. *Memoirs of Roger Williams* (ed. J.D. Knowles; Boston, 1834), pp. 258-59.
9. DNB (George Fenwick).
10. *Burton's Diary*, III, pp. 97-100.
11. CSP Dom, 1654, p. 286.
12. *Ludlow's Memoirs*, p. 391.
13. *Burton's Diary*, III, p. 100.
14. S.R. Gardiner, *History of the Commonwealth and Protectorate* (4 vols.; London), III, p. 34.
15. *Burton's Diary*, III, p. 57.
16. A. Woolrych, *Penruddock's Rising, 1655* (London, 1955).
17. *Ludlow's Memoirs*, II, pp. 17-18.
18. CJ, VII, pp. 424-45; CSP Dom, 1656-57, p. 87.
19. *Burton's Diary*, III, pp. 100-101.
20. *Prestwick's Republica*, p. 6.
21. *Mercurius Politicus*, 25 June 1657.

❧ 16 ❧

The Commoner of England

And, behold, here cometh a chariot of men, with a couple of horsemen.
And he answered and said, Babylon is fallen, is fallen; and all the graven
images of her gods he hath broken unto the ground.

(Isa. 21.9)

The 'other house', that rebirth of the Lords, marched on, and with
its advance into the political area, the return of the country to the
three ancient estates marked the decline of Cromwellian control.
With the requirement of a monarchy established, it only needed the
entrance of Charles Stuart to return the overall constitution to a
point where the royalists had left the struggle in 1649.

Sir Arthur Hesilrige had been named for the other House, but had
been elected for the Commons. He had received the 'summons' by
messenger, who he dismissed without reply. What a great personal
dilemma Sir Arthur faced: the great commoner, the 'zealous asserter
of the publick liberty' called to a place unchosen by the people—a
grave situation. William Lenthall, however, so long Speaker in the
Long Parliament, had not received one. Hearing this, Cromwell
called him to the assembly, as Ludlow relates:

> This grievous complaint coming to the ears of Cromwell, he sent him a
> writ, which so elevated the poor man, that riding in his coach through the
> Strand, and seeing Mr. Lambert Osbalstone, formerly master of the
> school at Westminster, whom he knew to be a great lover of Sir Arthur
> Haslerig, he asked him what Sir Arthur designed to do in answer to the
> writ which he had received? and Mr. Osbalstone answering that he knew
> not what the intentions of Sir Arthur Haslerig were concerning it: he
> replied, 'I pray write to him and desire him by no means to omit taking
> his place in that House, and assure him from me that all that do so, shall
> themselves and their heirs be forever peers of England'.[1]

Hesilrige did not wish to be a peer of England, and he was the only opponent of Cromwell's administration to be called to the second assembly. Oliver was quite obviously trying to trap Hesilrige by using that age-old political ploy of elevating the troublemaker to where he can do least harm. By removing Hesilrige to a place where political obscurity awaited, Cromwell hoped to secure the third Protectorate Parliament from the dangers of breakage which had accursed the assemblies of 1654 and 1656.

When the two assemblies sat on Monday 25 January 1658, only 42 were sworn into the 'New Lords' from a total of 63. Meanwhile, Mr Thomas Burton was greeted upon arriving at the Commons by a famous and truly historic sight, one to gladden the heart of any democrat:

> When I came into the House, I found Sir Arthur Hazelrigge there asking for some one to give him his oath; but a quorum could not be got till prayers were done, which were performed by Mr. Peters.
>
> Prayers being done, Sir Arthur Hazelrigge from the bar took Mr. Francis Bacon by the hand, and said 'Give me my oath', he answered 'I dare not'. Sir John Thorowgood was asked but he said he might first know the sense of the House in regard Sir Arthur was called to the other House. He would not presume to sit till he had taken the oath; but went out and in his passage, said 'I shall heartily take the oath I will be faithful to my Lord Protectors person. I will murder no man'.
>
> After a little stay in the lobby, there came four commoners to swear him, vis. Colonel Purefoy, Major Templer, Mr. Bond and Mr. Bacon and Mr. Smythe, the clerk; when Sir Arthur, Mr. Sicklemore, Colonel Fitzjames and Colonel Briscoe were sworn together.
>
> Sir Arthur Hazelrigge did speak the words very valiantly and openly, especially the latter part relating to the privileges of the people ('of England', which he added.) That done, he went in and sat close by the chair.[2]

Hesilrige had arrived in London as quietly as possible, but the court of King Oliver soon heard of his coming and sent Colonel Howard to see him the next morning. When Howard arrived at Sir Arthur's lodgings, he had flown, and was at that moment taking the Commons oath. Thomas Scot and many others who were excluded in 1656 came and took their seats, an action that shook the roots of the new court and annoyed Cromwell. The Lord Protector now feared an army coup, for a Parliament had taken its seats behind Cromwell's back and in defiance of the Cromwellian statements concerning suitability to sit. Sir Arthur had a steady following in the army, almost equal to Cromwell's own charismatic support. If Parliament was again dissolved, did Cromwell risk a fresh rebellion from factions of the army who were against him? Could Oliver risk allowing the republicans to sit? In the end the latter action was chosen. Debates began on the power of the Protector and the name of the other House. On 28 January, Hesilrige spoke openly of his fears for the Commons:

> We had it yesterday hinted by one of our prophets that we must live long in a little time, and we know not how long we may sit. It may be questioned whether we shall sit a fortnight. We may be all dead. It is hard that we should not have a month to do all this business that is behind. It is not building this or that House that will do. Unless your foundation be sure, I assure you it will not do your work. Princes are mortal, but the Commonwealth lives forever. It is posterity we must respect: as his Highness tells us, the young children in the womb of their mothers.
>
> I sat with a sad heart in the place in the gallery where I have sat seventeen years before, to hear the minister say nothing of what that victorious Parliament did for the ministers by that large allowance given them, and other great things done by that Parliament. I cannot sit still and hear such a question moved, and bide any debate.[3]

These words so elated Thomas Scot that he joined Hesilrige in leading the Commons against the now declining powers of the Protectorate. Scot praised Hesilrige to his fellow Commoners:

> I move that thanks be given to that honourable person that vouchsafes to sit among the Commons notwithstanding his call to another place; that he thinks it his honour to sit amongst the Commons of England, before any society of men whatsoever.[4]

The debate on the name of the 'other House' was still taking its toll of time in the Commons. Hesilrige and his side knew that no business could proceed from one House to the other while this mundane subject was debated. Hesilrige said:

> If his Highness will make you dukes, earls, he may do what he will. Grant once Lords, then you will find tenderness of course, to maintain the privileges of that House as Lords. The Commons of England will quake to hear that they are returning to Egypt, to the garlick and onions of (he called by a slip) a Kingdom. I crave your pardon for that mistake. We are yet a Commonwealth, and I hope I shall many years humbly ask your pardon for that mistake.[5]

Hesilrige again spoke of his love for the Commons in a speech on 2 February:

> I thought not to have troubled you, but now I am up, I will tell you truly why I will not take the Bishop's seat because I know not how long after I shall keep the Bishop's lands. For no king no Bishop, No Bishop No King. I like your company well, gentlemen; and I do aspire no higher than to be a commoner of England. I had an estate left me, besides my own acquisition, that will maintain me like a gentleman. I desire no more.[6]

The state left him was the family estate at Noseley, the Bishop's lands were part of his northern estate. Sir Arthur's brother, John, still had the estate at Alderton and had purchased a great estate from the sequestered lands of royalists in Northamptonshire, including lands belonging to the Dyvve family at Harlestone and Northampton itself. Other members of the family had purchased land, indeed, the Hesilrige's had done extremely well from the revolution. Nevertheless, good business sense was not then a crime, and if his wealth had increased during the period, it was certainly not at the expense of his own Hesilrigian sense of loyalty to the Commonwealth and the people of England. Sir Arthur could not forget his old friends on another occasion: 'Well it is for Pym, Strode and Hampden, my fellow traitors impeached by the King, they are dead! Yet I am glad I am alive to say this at this day.'[7]

At the age of 57, Hesilrige could demand the respect of his political brethren in the manner of John Pym, could support his party like Strode and had learned the good wisdom of John Hampden. Simply by reminding the Commons of the great work undertaken by himself and these famous political figures, Hesilrige could earn the love of the young bloods who were still wet when Hesilrige fought in the name of liberty. On 3 February the Lords sent two judges to the Commons seeking answers to questions their House desired. The inexperienced members were in favour of calling them in, but Hesilrige, using all the power of his many years of experience of debate, which was absent from many new members, spoke hard and pithily:

> I move against calling them in…This looks like a House of Lords. I tremble to think of wardships and slavery. I am against it; and I could speak till four o'clock. If I had been of the other House, I should not have advised to have sent another message till you had resolved in this. I can suffer to be torn to pieces, and to have ropes tied to me. I should endure that, but to betray the liberties of the people of England, I cannot. Having spoke my conscience, I will say no more.[8]

This was heroic speaking and it could not fail to lift the hearts of those undecided. Would not men take up the sword for such liberty?

Would Cromwell allow it? The answer came the next day when the Lord Protector dismissed the Houses and took the government upon himself. In this action, Cromwell assured the members of the other assembly that their peerage status was intact.[9]

With the power back once more in the first estate, Cromwell decided to purge the army of all disloyal to the Protectorate. Even under King Charles, the Commons had sat for more than a few days. The Commons had truthfully goaded the Protectorate, but Cromwell had cut off the purse from his power by doing away with them, for the lower House still held control of the national wealth, as it had blissfully done for generations. Cromwell needed a Commons to supply the revenue for any economic or military programme, as Charles had before him. Even if chosen by Cromwell, and thus a mocking of the liberty of that assembly, a Commons would have to sit to sign the national cheques.

The free members, those not chosen by Cromwell, now decided to challenge his power in the 'civil court' like Hampden had done for ship money. Mr Henry Nevil, a Commonwealth man, had sat for election in 1656 for the county of Berkshire. Since this time, many dubious methods had prevailed to keep such Commonwealth men from taking their seats. The sheriff of Berkshire had managed to keep Nevil from taking his rightful place and now Nevil sued the sheriff in a test case. At the trial Hesilrige and Scot added their considerable weight behind Nevil. Sir Arthur's time at Grey's Inn held well at such times. Despite Mr Nevil proving that the sheriff was not at liberty under law to prevent the natural laws of England's privilege from being upheld without prejudice and therefore winning the case, Cromwell would not budge.[10]

All that Hesilrige could do would not change the fundamental outlook of the Lord Protector, but a greater judge than any England could produce changed the whole picture with a single wave of his hand. On 3 September, the anniversary of Dunbar and Worcester, Oliver Cromwell, Lord Protector and once saviour of the Commonwealth died. No record of Hesilrige's views upon Cromwell's death are recorded, although Hesilrige, in the great speech used throughout this biography, forgives him in death as he could never forgive him in life. The end of Oliver meant in no uncertain terms a power struggle, but without his strength to resist the Parliament's return the Commons could sit once more. Hesilrige and Cromwell had become firm friends that day long ago when Manchester spoke against fighting at Newbury. They had seen the birth of the New Model Army and breathed life into its embryonic frame until it took the field fully fledged. Cromwell and Hesilrige had saved the country from Scottish invasion on two occasions, and been leaders of political constitutional change to save the Commonwealth and preserve the nation under a free Parliament. It had been a black day for England when these two men had taken different paths. Maybe Hesilrige and Cromwell were too alike to understand the other's viewpoint. Oliver had sought salvation for England through a dictat ordered by the sword, and in so doing turned his back on the ideals set out by Pym and his followers. Sir Arthur, however, had cherished the ideal of a free government. In many respects Cromwell's rule by the sword did not differ from Hesilrige's views early in 1640, but Oliver had chosen to rule by the sword alone and had relied upon the power of a junta to retain supreme power. Oliver Cromwell was no John Pym, Hampden or even Robert Lord Brooke, those great constitutionalists of the puritan leadership during the heady days of the rebellion. The Lord Protector was a man apart, great, but despotic and alien to Hesilrige's vision of democracy. Cromwell had done much good during his rule, but in so doing had robbed England of its freedom under Parliament, which was something Hesilrige could not stomach.

Cromwell's constitution, which was laid down in the Humble Petition and Advice that was passed by his puppet Parliament on 25 May 1657, and in the Humble Additional and Explanatory Petition passed 26 June 1657, allowed for his successor to take the Protectorate upon his death.[11] In the true spirit of monarchy, Oliver Cromwell named his son Richard to be heir to the throne. Richard Cromwell was an unfortunate choice to replace a man of Oliver's stature, and seems to be the final joke from his ribald humour. Richard or Dick Cromwell, aged 33, was the same age as Hesilrige's son Thomas.

On 27 January 1659, the new Lord Protector's Parliament met for the first time, and now Hesilrige was oddly enough recognized leader not only of his group but the whole House. When the members of the Commons House were then summoned to attend the 'other House' in their chamber, 150 led by Hesilrige remained seated in open defiance of recognizing them as Lords, therefore continuing their views from the time of Oliver.

Even before the Parliament met, Richard Cromwell had been busy.

The most interesting point concerning Sir Arthur again involved the problems of Elizabeth Lilburne, the widow of the late John. On 21 January, six days before the sitting of Parliament, Mrs Lilburne petitioned the young Protector:

> Having long suffered heavy afflictions, I hoped that my Husband's death would have been the last of my piercing sorrows. But I find the means for my children's maintenance perplexed by an unexampled Act of Parliament of 30th January 1651–52, fining my husband 7,000.l–3,000.l assigned to the state and 4,000.l to 5 gentlemen—vis 2,000.l to Sir Arthur Heselrigg, 500.l each to Messrs Winslow, Russell, Squibb and Millins—when his debts duly weighed, he was not worth 500.l. The only provocation for such a fine was his delivering a petition for Josiah Primate, for whom he was counsel, about a colliery, which Sir Art. Heselrigg would have had sequested. The Commissioners for Compounding gave the case against Primate, and he petitioned Parliament for relief. My husband did not draw the petition but only delivered it. Primate was fined 7,000.l and sent to the Fleet, but he soon got out, and gained his colliery, and this adds to my vexations.
>
> Your late father professed very great tenderness to me, and persuaded Sir Arthur to return the estate he had taken from me, and this he lately did (though the perverseness of tenants prevent my having much profit drawn from it). His Highness also remitted the parts allotted to the state, and willed the commissioners to remit the parts allotted to them. He also granted me a pension which by your great favour is continued, or I and mine might have perished. Sir Art. Heselrigg has relinquished 2,000.l and Mr. Squibb 500.l their shares of my husband's fine, but the other assignee's will not follow their example. I was advised to address Parliament to repeal the act, but omitted it in your father's life-time. I beg you to discharge the 3,000.l due to the State, and to recommend Parliament to repeal the Act, that after my year's sorrows I may have a little rest and comfort among my fatherless children.[12]

Elizabeth Lilburne had simplified the case somewhat, since her husband of course had been fined for political reasons, and too many of Lilburne's adversaries had been in powerful places for him to be left to roam the political backwaters of the Leveller cause. It had hardly been because of Josiah Primate's petition that Lilburne was fined, but the Leveller pamphlets which attacked the establishment. Sir Arthur had no quarrel with this poor woman. He was a man of great wealth and did not need to acquire more at the cost of a widow's misery. It must be said that Mrs Lilburne would have benefited from her tenants had her father-in-law, Richard Lilburne, left his opinions out of the situation, for he was less a friend to his son's wife than many who were bitter enemies of John.

The real enemy of Hesilrige was the Protectorate itself, not Richard Cromwell, who was a political babe compared to Sir Arthur. The Petition and Advice was worded to perpetuate a whole line of Cromwells. Hesilrige could not let this act rest unquestioned, and on 7 February, during a debate on an act entitled 'An act of Recognition of his Highnesses right and title to be Protector and Magistrate of the Commonwealth of England, Scotland and Ireland...', he spoke for two or three hours, in which time he recalled the history of England and the rebellion.[13] Thomas Burton explains what happened:

> The bill being read, Sir Arthur Haslerigg, moving himself upon his seat was called up, as if he had an intention to speak which he had not, but being so great a work and prefacing something of weakness then upon him, yet hoping that if he had anything to deliver, that God would enable him, he began a very long harangue.

Hesilrige began his speech slowly:

> I wonder not at this silence in a business of this weight I have much weakness upon me.
>
> The business that we are about, is the setting up a power over this nation. It will be necessary, for methods sake, to consider what we have been, what we are and what we shall be. I beg patience to look far back. Time was...[14]

Sir Arthur told of the ancient kings, Magna Carta, bishops and the power of the Norman line, the war of his youth and that Godly Axe that sought justice. As he reached the Protectorate, Hesilrige's tone became bolder, with the true strength of the man building up a picture for all to see. The narrative became more detailed:

> Another foundation was laid: A Petition and Advice; and this must be the law and the foundation of all! And these must be the fruits, all we must enjoy, after the spilling of so much blood and so much treasure. Pardon me, if I thus make bare my mind to you.
>
> This was a forced Parliament, because some of us were forced out: an imperfect Parliament, a lame Parliament, so much dismembered. We are here, the freest, and clearest and most undoubted representatives that ever were since the desolation of the three estates, King, Lords and Commons. I know not one member kept out: If I did, I would on my knees beg his admittance. I hope God direct us how to get out of this great darkness, as the minister told us that we have been in since this great desolation. What

was done in the last Parliament is not a sufficient foundation to bring peace and settlement to this nation. The people of England were never more knowing and sensible of their privileges and liberties, nor better prepared to have a settlement from this free representative. We can do here whatever is for the good of the people. We have power over their purses and persons; can take away whole laws, or part of them, or make new ones. I will tell you what we cannot do. We cannot set up any power equal to the people; either in one person, or another House. We are trusted with no such power. God is the King of this great island, as Mr. Calamy told us. I hope he is King of our hearts. God has done this work. King, Lord and Commons: It was not in our thoughts at first. Let not us set up what God has pulled down; not plant what God has rooted up, lest we be said to build against God.

We see what a confusion we are in. We have not prospered. Our Army at Jamaica prospered not. The trade and glory of the nation are much diminished. The Council have been exceedingly bewildered. The government you see twice set up, presently pulled down. The strange oppression by making Acts of Parliament without a Parliament, raising monies, denying fiabeas corpus, sending learned long robe gentlemen to the Tower, for asserting Magna Carta, such as all the Kings of England never did; all this because we knew not the good mind of God. We were in darkness. It is Gods mercy that we are here to declare ourselves in this place.

I shall now come to speak to the bill, whether to be committed or not. I confess, I do love the person of the Lord Protector. I never saw nor heard either fraud or quite in him. I wish only continuance of wealth, health, and safety to his family. I wish the greatest of honour and wealth of any man in this nation to him and his posterity, but this bill to recognise is a hard word. I never heard of such a bill but in King James case; which was to declare him of the undoubted line to the crown, and so having a right to succeed. We must here take for granted the government, the Petition and Advice, which was not done in a free Parliament. It may be skinned over for a time, but will break out. The people are not pleased. What foundation soever is built, let it rise from us, that are the clear representatives. For the authority itself, it appears by that Petition that the Protectorate was for his life; but it appears not how he appointed his successor, we must not take that upon trust, but be fully satisfied. I would not have this committed at present; but let it lie here. Never begin with the person first, but agree what trust he shall have. I forget not the great cause of our mischiefs the influence of the King over the Judges. To make the King judge of neccessity; that cut all our purses, that brought all our evil upon us. I would have us seriously advise and consider what we may do, as the peoples representatives. The way of wisdom is everlasting peace. There is no danger to the nation, so long as the representatives sit here. They are the supreme power. The way to prevent fire is to do our duties. We shall be preserved from the fire of hell and the fire of men. Let us let this rest, and consider of foundation stones. If a single person be thought best, to be accountable to the people for mal-administration, I shall submit to the majority.[15]

With this, after almost three hours, Hesilrige sat down. If this example was Hesilrige speaking from 'weakness', it was a powerful speech. By reminding the Commons of their most illustrious past and the consequence of a single ruler, he had opened their minds and hearts. Moreover, Sir Arthur's statements on liberty and justice inspired lesser men to continue the debate in questioning the Protectorate. The following day Hesilrige threatened to make another long speech, but Sergeant Maynard begged him to keep it shorter and to oblige the House he did.[16] Sir Arthur Hesilrige was now in complete control of the country's destiny, not fearing Richard (Tumbledown Dick) Cromwell, for this puppet Protector had little support from the military.

Since the Purge in 1648, the Army Council had demanded some respect, and even Oliver Cromwell had not dared to upset this wild beast too much. But, like Hesilrige, the army held no fear of the new Protector. A strong group of army officers, including such influential men as Fleetwood and the 'old Ironside' Disbrowe, had been meeting at the home of Fleetwood, Wallingford House, thus receiving the name of the 'Wallingford House Party'. This group was highly respected by all sides, for by the power of the sword they could, if they so desired, break or bless both Commonwealth or Protectorate. The army was split down the middle, some having gained greatly from the Protectorate, others still holding the 'good old cause' to their hearts. Only Charles Stuart could benefit from the total confusion that spread daily. Hesilrige knew that the army was again in arrears of pay, and so on 14 February—St Valentine's Day—he wooed them by saying the army must be paid although the nation was in debt.

Three days later the Lord Protector wrote to the Commons, this letter bringing yet more words from Hesilrige, expressing that he hoped the 'young Prince may have good and wise council about him'. Sir Arthur feared another war with Holland. Oliver Cromwell's war with the Dutch had been a mixed success, but, like all wars, had cost the country dearly in men and economic growth. Again, only the party of Charles Stuart could benefit by a war.

Meetings between the Commonwealth men and the officers at Wallingford House were mistrusted by Richard Cromwell. Ludlow

was in contact with the officers, and in his memoirs relates how
Fleetwood and his party desired to meet with Hesilrige and Henry
Vane, Ludlow acting as 'go-between':

> I acquainted Sir Henry Vane and Sir Arthur Haslerig with what had
> passed and they approved the way that was proposed, and promised that
> when they saw it seasonable they would be ready to assist them in all
> things tending to the publick service.[17]

Vane and Hesilrige had joined together once more against a
'Common-foe' and would back the Wallingford House Party in a
coup when time was at a minimal fortune for the Protectorate. The
Wallingford Party persuaded Cromwell to call a General Council of
the Army Officers to discuss the maintenance of the military. By the
second week of April, the situation had deteriorated. The Commons
did not trust the Army Council, and Cromwell, not having his father's
strength or foresight, ordered that the council should disband and
Fleetwood to attend Whitehall. The officers would not stand such
treatment and with Fleetwood at their head a grand parade was held
at St James on 21 April. Fleetwood and Disbrowe then demanded a
dissolution of Parliament which Cromwell could do no more than
grant.

The army sword had again put an end to a Parliament, but this time
in order to deliver it. Within a fortnight the Protectorate was over,
the Commons and Commonwealth was now restored, and, despite all
the hopes of a free republic ruled by the Parliament of England,
Charles Stuart would do well to practise the role of King of England.

NOTES

1. *Ludlow's Memoirs*, II, pp. 31–32.
2. *Burton's Diary*, II, pp. 346-47.
3. *Burton's Diary*, II, pp. 375-76.
4. *Burton's Diary*, II, p. 399.
5. *Burton's Diary*, II, p. 403.
6. *Burton's Diary*, II, pp. 423-24,
7. *Burton's Diary*, II, p. 407.
8. *Burton's Diary*, II, p. 437.
9. *Ludlow's Memoirs*, II, pp. 33-34.
10. *Ludlow's Memoirs*, II, p. 35.
11. *Constitutional Documents of the Puritan Revolution*, pp. 447-63.
12. CSP Dom, 1658–59, pp. 260-61.

13. This is the powerful speech cited throughout this volume. Quite obviously Thomas Burton could not take down every word as spoken by Hesilrige, but in the same manner that William Clarke took a synopsis of words spoken at Putney in 1647, Burton gives the fullest transcript of parliamentary speeches for this period.

14. *Burton's Diary*, III, p. 87.

15. *Burton's Diary*, III, pp. 101-105.

16. *Burton's Diary*, III, p. 141.

17. *Ludlow's Memoirs*, II, p. 65.

∽ 17 ∾

For Civil Government

For the LORD knoweth the way of the righteous; but the way of the ungodly shall perish.

(Ps. 1.6)

The Protectorate gone, a well-known situation appeared which gave fresh hope to the cause of Charles Stuart despite the restoration of a Commonwealth. With the factions of the original 1649 Common-wealth badly at odds among themselves, the royalist cause had good reason to formulate new designs upon the vacant throne. During this period after the peaceful fall of Richard Cromwell, Sir Arthur met frequently with Ludlow and Harry Vane in trying to build a working constitution for the rebirth of the Commonwealth. At this time, Hesilrige and Vane were not close and did not trust each other. Vane's actions before the usurpance of Oliver Cromwell had not endeared him to Sir Arthur, and in matters of politics Hesilrige was not quick to forgive anyone he felt had betrayed his trust. On 30 April 1659 news broke that important changes in the civil and military govern-ment were being debated by the army grandees at Wallingford House, saying: 'They have spent much time in considering of a new Govern-ment, and incline to the calling of the Long Parliament, and nomi-nating a council, who are said shall have a check or negative upon them, others say nott.'[1]

By desire of the Wallingford House Council of Officers, the Long Parliament was indeed recalled, but to say the country was in dire straits would be an understatement. In 10 years the government had gone from Monarchy to Commonwealth to Protectorate back to Commonwealth ruled by the ghosts of the Long Parliament and the self-proclaimed Council of Officers. At no time since the beheading of the King had power been in more than a few hands. That is not to say that the Long Parliament had not and could not govern the country well, but that it needed to be free to do so.

In the period between Richard Cromwell's abdication and the new sitting of the Long Parliament, a Committee of Safety made up of 'Sir Henry Vane, Fleetwood, Sir Arthur Haslerigge, Lieut. Gen. Ludlow, Col. Sydenham, Maj. Salway and Col. Jones' sat for the public safety.[2] These moves in England gave much encouragement to Charles Stuart, for one false move and he would be but a stone's throw from coming in. It is possible that Charles's followers understood this better than some of the Commonwealth men, who tried hard not to see the signs of history. On 6 June, a royalist supporter wrote a coded letter to Edward Hyde, in which he gave the political views in England disguised in religious terms:

> Among the Annabaptists are Fleetwood and Vane. Harrison is an enthu-
> siast, Fleetwood is a Presbyterian Annabaptist: Desborough and Bury
> are beasts of prey of no congregation; Lambert if anything, is a Catholic;
> Salloway and Sir Arthur Haslerigg are more Presbyterian than anything:
> H. Nevill is of no religion.[3]

From this it seems the royalists now thought Sir Arthur to be more stable of mind and moderate in comparison to the views of John Lambert. A large number of these cryptic letters were collected by Hyde and shed some light upon the murky darkness of their expectations. A letter from Brodrick to Hyde on 17 June continues the view of Hesilrige's new-found moderation:

> Sir Arthur Haslerig professes he never understood what a Commonwealth
> was till now; he was a violent persecutor of the Caligliers but is changed
> for the better and will preserve all from oppression, and (into this) intro-
> duces equality as far as it consists with moderate government.[4]

Surely this statement is consistent with Sir Arthur's political stance throughout the period. The King's rule prior to the Short Parliament was to Hesilrige's viewpoint oppressive and unequal in the civil government. The events following the army coup in 1647 and again in 1649 had taken the country far beyond the boundaries set by John Pym, and so in saying he would 'preserve all from oppression' he was clearly stating his line on freedom and liberty, whether from King or Protector or any junta.

Following a brief period of control by the Committee of Safety, it was stood aside and a new Council of State was called in which Hesilrige was a member. On 31 May, the Commons passed an order for a regiment of foot that was formerly Colonel Howard's, to be Sir Arthur's. At the same time Charles Fleetwood was appointed commander-in-chief of the forces in England.[5] The Commons had hoped to live in harmony with the military, but Hesilrige knew that Parliament only sat by the consent of the army and watched for a method of bringing the military back under civil control. By 6 June, Sir Arthur had convinced Parliament that control of the army was in them. Ludlow relates the mood of the Commons:

> Another bill was brought in to constitute Lt. General Fleetwood Commander-in-Chief, and was resolved that his commission should continue during the present session, or till the Parliament should take further orders therin; and instead of authorizing the Lieut. General to grant commissions to such officers as should be appointed by Parliament, it was ordered that the said commissions should be subscribed by the Speaker, and received from his hands, by which it was endeavoured to bring the military sword under the power of the civil authority, as it ought to be in a free nation. But observing that these things were greatly disliked by the officers and knowing how much it imported the very being of our cause to maintain a good correspondance between the Parliament and Army, I earnestly pressed the House not to insist upon the restrictions before mentioned. Sir Henry Vane and Major Soloway were of the same opinion, but Sir Arthur Haslerig, Colonel Sidney, Mr. Nevil, and the majority of the House carried it.[6]

Of course, in an ideal society the army should not govern the country through Parliament, but after so long Sir Arthur must have realized that the army would not be easily brought under civil control. In this matter Hesilrige was obviously being not a little bull-headed, trying to rush through measures that may be possible in time but were far from simple in 1659. That same day, the Commons also resolved that Parliament should not continue beyond 7 May 1660, when hopefully elections would be held.[7]

With this stop to their power, the army officers held a meeting at Colonel John Disbrowe's house, where Hesilrige and Ludlow attended them to hear their views. John Lambert claimed the Parliament had been untrue to the army 'contrary to the promises made to them before the restitution of Parliament.[8] Sir Arthur and Ludlow spoke in favour of a free Parliament, as one would expect. Since working closely with Hesilrige in 1648, John Lambert had grown in influence within the army, until at this time he held many keys of power. Sir Arthur knew Lambert very well indeed, and knew he was a strong character and a certain danger to Parliament if the army chose fresh leaders.

With this in mind, Hesilrige began to choose military allies, men to whom Parliament and liberty were the cause and not power. On 8 June, Colonel Hacker with the officers of his regiment went to Parliament after talks with Sir Arthur. Here they received commissions from the Speaker's hand, to signify they were commissioned by the civil and not the military. The next day Ludlow's regiment did likewise, and with these breaches of army solidarity others reconsidered their position. Fleetwood took his commission the same day for a regiment' of horse and foot and as commander-in-chief. On this day it seemed that Sir Arthur had won a great democratic victory, but had he?

An act of indemnity was progressing through Parliament to pardon those who had benefited from the Protectorate, and a clause was inserted to the fear of old Cromwellians.[9] Lambert was particularly upset by the act, for he had done very nicely from Cromwell's rule, and no doubt Hesilrige would also have prospered had he sided with Oliver. On the morning of 13 July, Ludlow met with Lambert, who complained that honest soldiers were now liable for their service in the Protectorate. Ludlow relates what followed:

> Sir Arthur Haslerig joined us, and the conversation continuing on the same subject, Sir Arthur affirmed that the Act was as full and comprehensive as could justly be desired; but the Major-General (Lambert) said that it signified nothing, and that it left them at (our) mercy. 'You are' said Sir Arthur, 'only at the mercy of the parliament, who are your good friends'. 'I know not', said Lambert, 'Why they should not be at our mercy as well as we at theirs', and then Sir Arthur contented himself only to shake his head, because divers officers were there present; yet meeting me the next morning in the Speakers chamber, he told me, that if the two regiments had not already been given to Major General Lambert he should never have them with his consent.[10]

It is clear from Lambert's statement that he did not consider that Parliament should be the master of the military, unless, that is, the military was Parliament. Sir Arthur, on the other hand, viewed Parliament to be the saviour of the nation from an oppressive military. In no way did Hesilrige trust Lambert's ambition, because it was not unlike that he saw in Cromwell six years earlier and was a danger to the Commonwealth.

Another danger to the Commonwealth were the royalists or

monarchy men, whose fresh activity was worrying, for many of these
new supporters of Charles Stuart were the very backbone of the 1642
parliamentary leadership. Such names as Sir William Waller and the
Earl of Stamford were known royalist supporters. The Sealed Knot,
the royalist secret society, were hoping the rifts between Parliament
and the army would widen to where a royalist rising would find
popular support. This was the hope of the Sealed Knot's inner
council, but those who made up this group were men of little action
who were more inclined to enjoy their own voices than to fight a
war. On paper Charles Stuart could expect great deeds and thousands
flocking to his banner, but in reality action did not speak louder than
words. One rising nevertheless was planned in North Wales. The
former parliamentarian, Sir Thomas Middleton, prepared to join the
royalist Sir George Booth. Believing himself to be part of a great rising,
Booth declared for Charles II, but Sir George was a poor judge of
timing and had declared too soon. Parliament, having learned of the
planned insurrection, acted quickly and ordered arrests. It was, however too late for Booth to abort his part of the whole comic affair.
On Sunday 31 July 1659, Sir George with 500 men made muster at
Warrington, marching to Rowton Heath before turning towards
Chester. Sir Thomas Middleton, who was ready to join Booth on
the march, declared in Wrexham.

Who could Parliament and the Council of State send to extinguish
this little spark of royalist fire? The choice was obvious, none other
than John Lambert, a better choice being difficult to imagine. Sir
Henry Vane having managed to patch the tear in the association of
Lambert and Hesilrige for the sake of unity, Sir Arthur did not oppose
such a plan and encouraged Lambert in the preparation of his force.
The royalists, knowing John Lambert's views of the way Parliament
was treating the army, had asked Mrs Lambert to persuade her husband
to join the risings, but the Lamberts were no traitors. John Lambert's
small army marched north on 6 August, and Parliament waited.

During this time Hesilrige began a fourteen-day appointment as
president of the Council of State.[11] One of his first tasks was to
inform General George Monck in Scotland of Booth's action to keep
Scotland secure in case of risings there, and that Parliament was considering an act of union between England and Scotland to rule the
two countries as one.[12]

The following day, 18 August, Sir Arthur wrote to his friends at the committee of Leicestershire, ordering that the Earl of Stamford be sent to the council for examination of his part in the rebellion.[13] Sir Arthur had little personal liking for Stamford, following the Earl's attack on him years earlier.

By 20 August, news reached London that Lambert had defeated Booth near Nantwich, the scene of two earlier battles during the first Civil War. In a letter dated 22 August, Sir Arthur wrote:

> Sir George Booth hearing that Lambert was only fifteen miles off, sent his trumpet, with a letter saying he was surprised to see him at the head of an army against him who had only declared for a free Parliament, offering to confer on an accomodation. The General said his orders were to reduce him and all others to obedience, and the only way to avoid effusion of blood was to lay down his arms. The answer, and the design of the levies to gain time and join Middleton in Wales, made them draw towards Lancashire, under cover of a river, but Lambert seized the bridges, after a feeble resistance, and on 19/20th there was a fight in which the levies were routed, the cavalry having fled, and abandoned the infantry, to the number of 1,700: 50 or 60 were said to be slain, 400 or 500 taken prisoners.[14]

Booth in fact made his escape and, disguised as a lady's maidservant, travelled to a nearby town to rest. Unfortunately for poor Sir George, a sharp-eyed inkeeper became suspicious when his companion asked for shaving knives. Within 10 days of Booth's defeat, Lambert had quelled all insurrection in Cheshire, and Hesilrige recalled him.

While Lambert was away, saving the nation from further civil war, it was suggested by Charles Fleetwood that for a reward Lambert should once more have the rank of major general restored to him. It would seem a reasonable prize for such service, yet Sir Arthur would have none of it, and said openly that there was no need for more generals. Hesilrige still did not trust John Lambert, and the bitter quarrel began again.

Lambert returned to London on 20 September. Before he arrived, however, Sir Arthur received information that the officers under him had met to prepare a petition to Parliament, outlining their grievances at the refusal to make Lambert a major general and saying that Parliament had not kept faith with the army.[15] The humble petition was sent to Fleetwood. Sir Arthur heard this and demanded that the commander should produce it, which he did. The petition was a demand rather than a request, and, upon hearing the hectoring tone of the words, Hesilrige flew into a rage, shouting feverishly for the impeachment of Lambert and that he should be sent to the Tower.

This was a fatal error, for it broke one of the locks keeping Charles Stuart out.

John Lambert tried to disown the petition, asking to resign his two commissions, but this was impossible while the army was so heated. A new petition milder in its manner was drawn up and John Disbrowe presented it to the House on 5 October. It was put open to debate, and the seeds of mistrust in Hesilrige's heart, burst forth in full bloom when he heard his old colleague Harry Vane speak in favour of Lambert. Was he planning to bring John Lambert in as Protector? He raged at Vane with such violence that the House, carried along by his tide of indignation, reduced nine officers and ended Fleetwood's command of the army.

Entering the House on 12 October, John Okey, the one-time major in Hesilrige's Lobsters and a loyal friend of Parliament's cause, told those assembled that the officers had published and circulated their petition.[16] The Parliament now felt in danger and ordered the regiments of Colonel Morley and Colonel Okey 'and so many of Colonel Mosse his Regiment as attended at Pauls, be, and are hereby, required to guard the Parliament, and Places hereabout, this Night'.[17] It was a desperate position for the Commonwealth, for one turn would bring in the army, and another Charles Stuart. Either direction the Parliament was lost. Edmund Ludlow, who was a great supporter of the ideals of the Commonwealth, puts the blame for the present problems firmly on Sir Arthur's shoulders, saying,

> Neither did it a little contribute to this disorder, that Sir Arthur, who took it upon him to be principle manager of affairs in Parliament, was a man of disobliging carriage, sower and morose of tember, liable to be transported with passion and to whom liberality seemed to be a vice. Yet to do him justice, I must acknowledge, that I am under no manner of doubt concerning the rectitude and sincerity of his intentions. For he made it his business to prevent arbitory power whatsoever he knew it to be affected, and to keep the sword subservient to the civil magistrate.[18]

The next morning, 13 October, John Lambert marched upon Westminster at the head of his two regiments. He was met by Colonel Morley at the head of his forces, pistol in hand, barring Lambert's way. The tension grew as the two sides faced each other. Morley raised his pistol and pointed it at Lambert, threatening to shoot him if he continued his march—Lambert turned another way. Moss's regiment now barred him again, but Lambert spoke to them and many went over to him. Then came Parliament's own guard under Major Evelyn, riding up to Scotland Yard Gate, these too joined Lambert. The situation was a step away from a bloodbath and totally desperate for any force sent against Lambert. Suddenly old Speaker Lenthall's coach appeared and was stopped by the unruly mob with Lambert. Lenthall, who had been such a servant to the army and Parliament, was jeered at and insulted, and for his physical safety turned away. At the Council of State, Hesilrige, Scot and Bradshaw opposed Lambert, but the sword was again in control and John Lambert with his faction of the army ended the Parliament, taking the power unto themselves.

If the recipe for the Commonwealth was wrong, perhaps the royalist satirists had a better one, although the number of cooks were apt to spoil it:

A CORDIALL RECIPE, FOR CAUSING ADHERENCE TO PARLIAMENT

Beg of Sir Henry Vane's affection to the ministery.
Of Sir Arthur Haslerigg's honesty...take two drums.
The whole to be boiled the length of a fast sermon
of Dr. Owen's, before the House.
And close stopt with a paste made of Scott's chastity and
the Speaker's religion.[19]

A strong mixture, no doubt highly fattening for the adherents of the monarchy, but of a stomach turning richness for Lambert. The next round of this stale old mixture would undoubtedly bring forth more troubles for a tired nation.

NOTES

1. *Clarke Papers*, III, p. 196.
2. CSP Dom, 1658–59, p. 341.
3. Cal. Clar. SP, IV, p. 232.
4. Cal. Clar. SP, IV, p. 239.
5. CJ, VII, p. 670.
6. *Ludlow's Memoirs*, II, pp. 88-89.
7. CJ, VII, p. 673.
8. *Ludlow's Memoirs*, II, pp. 89-90.
9. CSP Dom, 1659–60, p. 21.
10. *Ludlow's Memoirs*, II, pp. 100-101.
11. CSP Dom, 1659–60, p. 117.

12. CSP Dom, 1659–60, pp. 119-20.

13. CSP Dom, 1659–60, p. 125.

14. CSP Dom, 1659–60, p. 136.

15. The Humble Petition and Proposals of the officers under the command of the Lord Lambert in the late Northern Expedition.

16. Carte, II, p. 225.

17. CJ, VII, p. 796.

18. *Ludlow's Memoirs*, II, pp. 133-34.

19. Cal. Clar. SP, IV, pp. 403-404.

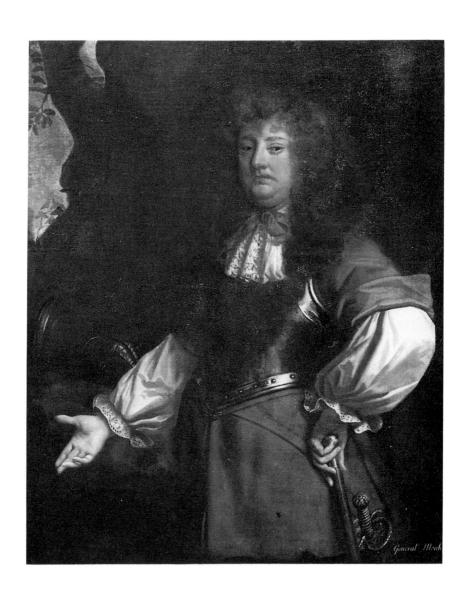

George Monck (Duke of Albermale), Hazlerigg Collection.

❧ 18 ❧

A King for Two Pennies

And Joseph made ready his chariot, and went up to meet Israel his father, to Goshen, and presented himself unto him; and he fell on his neck, and wept on his neck a good while.

(Gen. 46.29)

The Rump yet again dissolved and the sword the power once more, Hesilrige must have feared the outcome. The new supremo, John Lambert, told Edmund Ludlow that he believed Sir Arthur wanted him dead. Ludlow relates:

> I endeavoured to take him off from that opinion, by telling him, that being assured of Sir Arthur's sincere affection to the Commonwealth, I could not think that he would do anything to the prejudice of those that were friends to it. I told him also, that according to my notion of things, the aim and design of Sir Arthur Haslerig was good, even in the matter which had been the first occasion of differences between them concerning new titles and powers, which had proved so fatal to the Parliament in former time, and which he thought very unsafe under an equal and mode-rate Government. I assured him that Sir Arthur had a personal respect for him, which he had manifested on several occasions, particularly I desired him to remember that he had prevailed with the Parliament to grant him the command of two regiments; and also with those members who were for the greatest sum to be given him in acknowledgement of his service in Cheshire. In conclusion, I told him that Sir Arthur was well known not be of an obliging carriage and therefore if ever he had been used too roughly by him, it would become him to pardon it, and to charge it upon his temper.[1]

The old Council of State was no longer recognized by the army, being replaced by an Army Committee of Safety. However, nine of the council chose to continue to sit as a government in exile, namely, Scot, Morley, Wallop, Walton, Ashley-Cooper, Nevill, Barnes, Reynolds and of course Hesilrige. On 24 November 1659, this shadow group declared George Monck to be Commander-in-Chief of all Armies in England and Scotland. Monck had a month earlier stated his favour to be in the Rump and not John Lambert's phoney Protectorate. Those in Monck's army who favoured Lambert were replaced by men he knew to be loyal to him. Monck then had sent letters to England on 20 October in which his terms to the shadow group were outlined. He also wrote to Fleetwood, urging him not to ruin the nation out of personal ambition, and warned Lambert that England would not submit to the sword and that true English soldiers would oppose it.[2] George Monck had made his stand and the Commonwealth men could feel hope in being saved from the sword, but should they fear Monck's old cause of monarchy?

Hesilrige, despite Ludlow's words to Lambert over him, was rigid in his views, continuing with the opinion that Protectors should not bring the sword to Parliament's door. Ludlow was right in believing that Sir Arthur had some respect for Lambert, perhaps dating from the campaign of 1648. But Hesilrige did not trust Lambert, because he had been too involved in army politics too long not to have influence or ideals. Sir Arthur trusted few men by now, so many having proved false to him, Harry Vane included. Ludlow, forever trying to smooth over arguments, asked Sir Arthur to think better of Vane, saying he thought he had taken the wrong course of action. Sir Arthur replied that 'if ever he returned to sit in Parliament and thereupon showed himself revengeful to any man, he would permit me to spit in his face'.[3]

During November, negotiations between Monck and Lambert reached nowhere, and with this Monck decided to march south from Scotland, arriving in the borders on 8 December. Meanwhile, to back Monck in his plan, the old Rumpers sent Hesilrige, Colonel Walton and Colonel Morley to Portsmouth, where Governor Colonel Whetham was friendly and admitted them. Hesilrige, again the military man, declared:

> We came hither on Saturday the third of December instant at four of the clock, myself and my son, Colonel Morley, Colonel Walton with divers other gentlemen some whereof were neighbouring inhabitants to this place.[4]

Hesilrige's son-in-law Herbert Morley was a rigid republican and totally loyal to the Rump, so it is not difficult to see why Lambert held such a low opinion of Sir Arthur.[5] Once inside Portsmouth,

Hesilrige, Morley and Walton quickly declared for Parliament against Lambert and the army. The navy followed their example, removing the possibility of a siege from both land and sea. This move by Hesilrige was a severe blow to Charles Fleetwood, who was by now confused and without guidance from Lambert, who had marched north against Monck. A force was sent against Portsmouth, but on 20 December, five troops of horse and a like number of foot went over to join Hesilrige, with Lambert's other supporters submitting.[6] Writing to a friend, a local gentleman, Mr Nicholas Love, said, 'Sir Arthur Hesilrige and Colonel Morley have behaved themselves very gallantly...the siege is raised and the town at liberty without a drop of blood.'[7] With these new troops at their disposal, the three heroes were ready for the next move. That Sir Arthur could still hold such power after nearly 20 years in Parliament was a vindication of others' esteem for him. No one could ignore him in their plans.

The army was in utter confusion. Lambert needed either to defeat Monck in the field or come to peace with him, and neither was possible. In the meantime Fleetwood was dithering. Bulstrode Whitelock told him he must restore either Parliament or Charles Stuart. Fleetwood chose a king, but, upon meeting with the old Ironsides John Disbrowe and James Berry, he changed his mind and declared for a free Parliament. The officers and George Monck had already declared the same to Hesilrige on 19 December:

OFFICERS AT COLDSTREAM TO
SIR ARTHUR HESILRIGE
& OTHERS

Right Honourable,

Itt is not unknown to you that since the late force upon the Parliament wee have put ourselves uppon our duty as English men and faithfull soldiers for the preservation of the freedome and priviledges of the Parliament, since which tyme there hath bin a treaty between us and the authors of that force to prevent the effusion of Christian bloud, and that not comeing to the desired effect there hath bin a continued overture and endeavoure to bring the matter to a happy composure: but haveing received intelligence that you Honoures are now in Portsmouth, where you have declared for the same cause with us, and that you act as Commissioners by Act of Parliament beareing date the eleventh of October last, wee finde ourselves disinabled to treate any further uppon our owne single accompt. Wee have therefore sent this Gentleman to your Honoures to receive your commands in this business, assuring you that itt is our earnest desire that things might be composed in an amicable way, and that the Common

Enimy might not reape the benefitt of our contentions. And in this wee doubt not but wee shall have your Honoure's complyance, and shalbee speedily furnished from you with such directions and instructions as may sufficiently inable us for that worke.

Wee remaine

Your very humble servants

Charles Fairfax

Tho. Reade

I. Lytcott

John Clobery

R. Knight

Coldstreame 19 December 1659

With the Parliament restored by a hamstrung Charles Fleetwood, Sir Arthur's triumph was complete. On 29 December, Hesilrige, Morley, Walton and the loyal army rode to London. The three leaders entered the Commons amid cheers 'in their riding habits, and Haselrig was very jocund and high'.[8] Sir Arthur no doubt remembered that day he had ridden from Newbury to announce another victory, and there is little wonder that he was again high with the passion of a victor. That same day the House gave thanks for Hesilrige's great work and approved his removal of several officers loyal to Lambert, replacing them with men loyal to Parliament.[9] But even while the Speaker gave thanks, the country was balanced upon a knife edge. The country was simply ungovernable, and if Hesilrige was elated it was short-lived.

To Sir Arthur's horror, members were again purged and turned from the House. Even Harry Vane was removed, despite Hesilrige's pleading that he should stay. Hesilrige knew that men of Vane's experience and political ability, not to mention his knowledge of the navy, were vital in the national security. Sir Arthur had stirred up a great hornet's nest he could not now control.

Upon their return, Hesilrige, Morley and Walton began to reorganize the army in preparation for the advance of Monck. The army was purged of 1,500 officers, a task not seen since the forming of the New Model. On 1 January 1660, Monck ordered his forces to cross the River Tweed at Coldstream, bringing fresh troops into the political arena.[10] By 11 January, Monck had reached York, and arrived in London on 3 February. Before Monck arrived, the troops already garrisoned around London had been moved further afield, including a regiment of horse under Sir Arthur. Hesilrige was losing ground in

Parliament, and with it the cause of Charles Stuart grew daily. Edmund Ludlow visited Sir Arthur at this time and relates the frame of mind he found him in:

> Sir Arthur was unwilling to enter into any discourse concerning what had lately passed, saying it was too late to recall things now and then told us how his enemies thought to ensnare him, by Monck's motion to the Parliament for removing his regiment from London, thinking thereby to create a difference between him and Monck, wherein he had disappointed them by desiring their removal himself, contrary to their expectation; entering into a prolix commendation of Monck and assuring us that he was a person on whose fidelity they might safely rely. And if I may be permitted to deliver my sense touching this discourse of Sir Arthur Haslerig I conjecture it proceeded partly from an apprehension that things were already gone so far, that he doubted whether he come put any stop to them; and partly from some sparks of hope that Monck could not be such a devil to betray a trust so freely reposed in him. For he kept a constant correspondence with Sir Arthur, and in all his letters repeated the engagements of his fidelity to the Parliament, with expressions of the greatest zeal for a Commonwealth government.[11]

Even at this stage, Monck was playing a foul double game with Sir Arthur and Charles Stuart. He had assured him of his trust, and in return Hesilrige had freely given his sincerity—but in his heart Sir Arthur tasted the bitterness of Monck's lies.

As Monck entered London, Edward Massey, the one-time parliamentarian, but now Presbyterian royalist, wrote to Edward Hyde:

> Sir Arthur Haslerig (whose second son two days past married Cromwell's daughter, Lord Rich's widow, and has settled £5,000 per annum on her) and some other Parliament men lay private in the City and borrowed £30,000 to pay the soldiers. Haslerig fears and hates Monk lest he, as a twig of the Plantagenants, should set up for himself.[12]

Massey was correct in calling George Monck a Plantagenet, for he was of that line of kings. But the same could not be said for Massey's knowledge of London marriages. Frances Cromwell, the widow of Lord Rich, had married Sir John Russell of Chippenham. Sir Arthur's second son, Robert, did not marry until 1664, when he settled in Northampton.[13] Hesilrige's first son and heir, Thomas, married Elizabeth Fenwick, the daughter and co-heiress of Sir Arthur's old friend George Fenwick, who had died in 1657. George Fenwick's widow, the young Catherine Hesilrige, married again, this time to Colonel Philip Babington.[14]

Throughout February 1660, Sir Arthur Hesilrige deluded himself of Monck's honesty. The Commonwealth men had asked the general if he would join with them against any attempt by Charles Stuart, to which he had taken Sir Arthur's hands and with false witness replied,

> Sir Arthur, I have often declared to you my resolution so to do—I here protest to you in the presence of all these gentlemen that I will oppose to the utmost the setting up of Charles Stuart, a single person, or an House of Peers.[15]

The Rump of the Long Parliament had been brought back by Fleetwood before Monck's return, but places were still empty. These places were of those 'Secluded members' who were kept out. Monck held meetings with these men, much to the distrust of Hesilrige, for they were pro-monarchy men and certainly now an extreme danger to the Commonwealth. The army also began to mistrust Monck, and, when the danger grew too great, the general sent the officers in London back to their regiments. In connexion with the growing unrest in the army, Sir Arthur was called before the Commons to answer allegations that he had stirred up the officers against the interest of Monck. Instead of his usual fire and courage in his speech, Hesilrige was but a shadow of himself, saying limply that he was always loyal to the civil authority. This was not of course to say he was loyal to Monck. Although a member of Parliament, Sir Arthur's heart had gone from the place and he attended on few occasions. Hesilrige's high states were transformed to bouts of extreme depression. By his actions Monck had robbed him of pure joy in a way Cromwell had never done. The Protectorate had been a challenge to fight, Cromwell doing things openly and with one face, Monck did not.

It is highly probable that Sir Arthur's general health was not good. He appears to have suffered from bronchitis in his later years, due no doubt to the long period he spent in the north, and he had increased in weight from the slimly built knight of Robert Walker's portrait. Like Cromwell before him, Sir Arthur's health was suffering from the hard usage his body had taken during the war, and, with Monck betraying him too, he had not the will to fight on.

On 6 March, John Lambert was committed to the Tower. But just over a month later, on 9 April, he escaped. Monck was now in direct communication with Charles Stuart, and the death throes of the Commonwealth were plain to see. John Lambert was intent on one desperate attempt to save the nation from the Stuarts. A number of the displaced officers rallied to Lambert, including John Okey, who had four months earlier been an opponent of his. This small band of army men assembled their force near Edgehill, the site of the first major battle of the Civil War. The site was ironically fitting, and how many of the ghosts of 1642 joined with Lambert as he rode with his force? and how many that rode now with him would join the army of the dead if battle ensued once more? With John Lambert rode captain Hesilrige, son of Sir Arthur. There is conflicting evidence as to which son this was, for family tradition says that Thomas Hesilrige was a captain in 1660, whereas state papers state it was the 19-year-old Robert.[16] With Lambert in the field, Monck sent Colonel Ingoldsby to Northampton to observe the next move. The morning of 22 April—Easter Sunday—Lambert and Ingoldsby faced each other at Daventry. A few shots crackled from the ranks spread thinly across the field, then, in almost a replay of Sir Faithful Fortescue's act at Edgehill, Captain Hesilrige rode forward and by a prearranged plan surrendered to Ingoldsby. With this John Lambert's force had no fight left in it, and after trying to escape Lambert himself was taken and returned to the Tower.

Totally defeated, Sir Arthur Hesilrige began to consider his safety and the future of his family. The Rump was dissolved on 17 March, and with it Hesilrige's political life. By now Sir Arthur was in a severe state of melancholy. He had asked Monck again if he would be true to the Commonwealth, to which he replied: '…how he could expect anything from him whom he had endeavoured to make less than he was before he marched to London'.[17]

On 30 April, a letter arrived before Monck, and enclosed within the packet were two pennies—

> My Lord,
> I beseech your lordship to lett the Council understand that I have neither directly nor indirectly done anything in opposition to the present authority settled by the Parliament in the Council of State. Neither was I knowing in the least degree of the disturbance made by Lambert. I have always acted with the authority of Parliament, and never against it, and hold it my duty to submit to the authority of the Nation and not to oppose it, and have hazarded my all to bring the military power under the civil authority. I forgott to give you the two pence it is here enclosed, and being assured by your lordshipp's promise, I hope to end the remainder of my days in peace and quiet.
> Arthur Hesilrige[18]

Sir Arthur had told his friends that if Charles Stuart came in 'it was but three wry months and a swing for himself'. Monck had offered Hesilrige help in return for his pledge not to cause trouble. The token of this pledge were two pennies. For these two small coins Charles Stuart would receive a crown, his kingdom being based upon no greater sum than tuppence.

On 26 May 1660, George Monck held out his arms and took unto the nation a King once more. With Charles II landing at Dover, the 'Good Old Cause' was undone, and the tragedy of the Stuarts was returned to England.

Sometime before 7 August, Sir Arthur was arrested and sent to the Tower. Sir Harry Vane was seized and would pay the full price through losing the peace. Other noted old parliamentarians were also taken, Bradshaw, Okey, Scot, the list grew daily. The pretext for arresting Hesilrige and Vane was that they had tried to persuade the old army officers to oppose the Restoration. It was a weak charge, with no more of a disguise than the dagger in the back. The new leaders of the nation sought revenge, and these men who had been their bane for so long were being removed as quickly as possible. Betrayed by Monck, Sir Arthur was left to petition the King:

TO THE KING'S MOST EXCELLENT MAJESTY
THE HUMBLE PETITION OF
SIR ARTHUR HESILRIGE

Shireth,

That your petitioner was never in field service with the Army since the Year 1644. Nor had any thing to do with the Generall Councell of Officers after that time.

That your petitioner was not in least measure guilty of contriveing or so much as knowing of his late Majesties death before it was past, he being long before and then at New Castle.

That he had neither Councell nor Vote in the change of the Government into a Commonwealth.

That the Government being so changed, your petitioner finding the Court of Justice settled Judges acting and a General Obedience to that Government. And conceiving it could not have been altered without great effusion of blood. He acknowledgeth he acted in the support of that Government.

That your petitioner opposed Cromwells Usurping to his Utmost from the begining to the end, & refused to accept from him both honour and profit, publiquely affirming and Declaring. That if the Nation had a King he ought to be the right King as is notoriously known. And for which Cromwell vowed to ruine Your Majesties petitioner and to make him suffer in his Estate.

That your petitioner was against all Usurpers and did therefore labour to bring the chief Officers of the Army under the power of the civil Government by taking their commissions from the then Speaker. The chief officers not being able to bear that, took government upon themselves wch proved a great stop to your Majesties return.

That your petitioner assisted the Lord Generall Monck in keeping the officers in Scotland in their commands according to his desire who otherwise had been turned out of the Army.

That your petitioner hazarded his life and his all, injoyning with the Ld Generall Monck against Lambert and the Army under him, and through the blessing of God was not a little instrumentall in his overthrow and afterwards your petitioner removed all the forces out of this town his regiment of horse being parked and brought the Generall and his army into their Quarters.

That after the Members were brought into the House your petitioner was use full to the Generall in keeping the army quiet and in preventing the spilling of much Blood in your Majesties Kingdome, and to submit to that and not to fight against it. And although your Majesties petitioner was Colonell of a Regiment of Horse and also of a Regiment of Foote and well aquainted with many officers then of the army yet his judgement then was and still is that he had rather yeild up his own life than occasion the death of one man in opposing the authority of the kingdome.

That your petitioner being very tender of blood never had anything to do with any high court of justice.

That his excll the Lord Generall for some of the reasons afore said promised your petitioner that he should be an excempted person and that he would procure him your Majesties grace and wished your petitioner to be advised by him and your petitioner relyed upon him otherwise your petitioner had most humbly supplicated your Royal Majesty with the first upon your return into your Kingdome.

And the God almighty having by wonder full dispenstone restored your Majesty to your Kingdome in peace your petitioner doth rejoyce in the good hand of God in bringing it about without the effusion of blood. And much bewaileth & unfeigned by sorrowfull for his many provocations giving your Majesty and promiseth for the future by exemplary obedience and faithfulness to redeem his former miscarriages.

And if your Majesty will please graciously to pardon your petitioner as it will be an Act of Infinate clemency & to the Glory of your Mercy so it will forever inguage him in a peculiar manner to be serviceable in all faithfulness and pray for your Majesties long and happy reign.

Your petitioner most humbly castes himself at your Royall Majesties foot desiring rather to be a prisoner all the remainder of his few days if your Majesty cannot be confident that he will lose his life before he will be ungratefull disloyall or false to your Majesty.[19]

The wording of Sir Arthur's petition was clever, for all details in it were true, but it was the things left out that condemned him. Sir Arthur says little about pre-1653, the fact that he had sought the deaths of Strafford and Laud, or spoke of the 'Wonder full hand of God' beheading the King. To petition the King was pointless. Sir Arthur could only escape the vengeful axe or worse if Monck betrayed his trust no longer. One by one Hesilrige's friends and family implored Monck to speak with Charles on his behalf, and a slowly building tide of popular opinion grew in his favour. The vital question was, however, had Monck promised too much on the King's behalf when he had not the power to do so. Pressed on all sides, George Monck wrote to the King via Sir Edward Turner:

Most honoured Sr,

After I had admitted the secluded members of the longe Parliament to sitt with the others, in order to the callinge of the last Parliament. I found my selfe involved in many and great difficultyes, because they that satt before them had modelled the Army in England to their owne principles of a Commonwealthe's Government. And although I had divided the quarters of the troops into very distinct stations, yet their correspondence was such that I was very much distracted in my endeavours for the peace and settlement of the nation, and putt to severall and distraict postures in the manginge of them. I was forced to youse the force of power to some, and friendshipp and faire promises of security to others, till att last I had reduced matters to such a consistancy that all were removed from commande and trust in armes that would not inguage to acquiesec in whatsoever the then succeedinge Parliament should act. Att this conjunture of tyme noe man was soe capable to obstruct my designe as Sir Arthur Haselrig, whoe had in his immediate commaund the government of Berwicke, Carlisle, New-Castle and Tyne-Mouth, with a regiment of foote and one of the best regiments of horse in the Army, and had an influence upon all the rest of the regiments in England. Hee havinge had the chief hand in modelling the regiments before my cominge into England. Hee was very jealous of the intended revolution of governmt to his Majies advantage, and came to me to discover his apprehensions, urging that hee perceived all tended to the restitucion of the Kinge, and that there would thereby ensue a ruin to his person, family and fortune; to wch I told him that if hee would engage to mee to goe home to his own house and lyve quietly there, I would undertake to secure his life and

estate; whereupon hee did soe engage; and shortly after upon Collonel
Lambert's defection, when there was soe great a disposicion to mutiny in
the army, and his conjunction wth him might have hazarded the hope of
all, hee decloyned all manner of action and adhered to his engagement
made to mee, and upon my letter to him freely delivered up his garrisons
to my Lord of Carlisle and his regiment of horse to my Lord Faulconbridge.
I confess the commaund I had that tyme of the army and strength of the
kingdome was but a possessory and noe legall power, and what I did must
bee submitted to his Majies gracious clemency and favour to mee. My
unwillingness to hazard his Majies restitution by engageinge in blood
induced me to venture further in my use of itt than perhaps some may
thinke well of. But I knew in matters of soe great importance second
councell would bee too late, and therefore I chose to leave as I could to
the uncertainty of event.

Att the request of Sr Arthur Heselrig's friends I am desired to give you
the diversion of this narrative wch I thinke not most to send to you in
your publique capacity to bee communicated to the house, but as a private person that from hence you may bee informed of what passed
betwixt my selfe and that unfortunate man, which I leave to you to make
use of as you in yor high judgmt shall thinke fitt and am,

Your most affectionate friend & servante
ALBERMARLE (Monck)

Cockpitt 4th July 1660[20]

Monck had therefore kept his promise, although hardly pressing
the matter too far. The main interest in Monck's statement is that he
knew how dangerous Sir Arthur could have been, and the lack of
Hesilrige's spirit to continue with a government that relied upon the
sword. Ludlow states that Hesilrige was sent to the Tower in August.
However, it is clear from Monck and two petitions from his children
during July to visit their imprisoned father that he was taken not long
after the return of the King.

There followed much haggling whether or not Sir Arthur should
be included in an act of indemnity, and eventually, by section 40 of
the act, he was exempted for pains and penalties not extending to life,
to be imposed by a future act.

Their father imprisoned, Sir Arthur's children were divided in their
loyalty to him. Sir Arthur's daughters Catherine and Dorothy were
always devoted to him, and his second son Robert also loved his father.
But with the Restoration, Thomas, the son and heir to the title and
estate, turned from him, denouncing his actions and like Pilate washed
his hands of his family's involvement with the Commonwealth.
Whether this action, was understood by Sir Arthur is unknown, but

perhaps such action was necessary to keep the great estates of his father. If most of Hesilrige's children were proud of their father and followed his puritan fashion, the Restoration brought out the less puritan side of one daughter, who, according to one broadsheet, was seen enjoying the less sexually austere London of Charles II. It reported that the 'young daughter of Sir Arthur Hesilrige was currently enjoying the company of a number of gentlemen and bringing disgrace upon his family' and upon another occasion that she was 'caught with a stableboy'.

This England was no place for Sir Arthur, and the mental agony of his imprisonment in the Tower must have been great. The physical side of his nature also began rapidly to deteriorate. Sir Arthur had not expected to live long, this much he had expressed to Monck before the King returned. He was weary after so much hard work, and fever struck. One can but imagine the anguish of the man, the ghosts of Strafford and Laud mocking his misfortunes, the spectres of Charles and Cromwell pointing knowing fingers at their fallen foe and Lilburne watching fever that greatest of levellers tear at him. Pym, Strode and Hampden all gone, leaving Hesilrige to play a game so difficult that in the end even he had broken, losing all to men like Denzil Holles and George Monck.

With the fever burning hot inside him, the wonderful hand of God so beloved by Sir Arthur extended to the Tower, and with infinite mercy carried him through that heavenly cloud to eternal peace.

NOTES

1. *Ludlow's Memoirs*, II, pp. 143-44.
2. *Old Parliamentary History*, XXII, pp. 4-7.
3. 'A letter from Sir Arthur Haselrig in Portsmouth etc. 1659'; also several letters from Portsmouth by Sir Arthur Hesilrige to the Lord Fleetwood, Newcastle Central Library Tracts.
4. Nichols, *Leicestershire*, II, pt ii, p. 746.
5. *Publick Intelligencer*, 19–26 December 1659.
6. BM 669, fol. 22 (3).
7. *Clarke Papers*, IV, pp. 207-208.
8. Whitelock, *Memorials of English Affairs*, p. 636.
9. CJ, VII, p. 799.
10. Modern calendar.
11. *Ludlow's Memoirs*, II, pp. 212-13.
12. Cal. Clar. SP, IV, p. 543.

13. A house still stands in Marefair, Northampton, called Hazelrigg House where Robert Hesilrige lived after the Restoration. Robert was very instrumental in the rebuilding of Northampton after the town's Great Fire, obtaining wood from the forests of Charles II for the rebuilding of All Saints Church when the fire burned its great roof. Robert in due course became the fifth baronet of Noseley and Northampton.

14. The marriage settlement between Thomas Hesilrige and Elizabeth Fenwick forms part of the Hazlerigg Collection, LRO.

15. *Ludlow's Memoirs*, II, p. 237.

16. C.H. Firth and G. Davies, *Regimental History of Cromwell's Army* (Oxford, 1940).

17. *Ludlow's Memoirs*, II, p. 251.

18. Egerton MSS 2618, fol. 71.

19. Hesilrige Petitions, LRO.

20. *Clarke Papers*, IV, p. 302. I am indebted to Newcastle City Library for tracts relating to the letters from Monck to Hesilrige which were used throughout this chapter.

☙ Select Bibliography ☙

The reader will find the following secondary source list of use in understanding aspects relating to the English Civil Wars. They are also referred to in the notes which contain the primary sources to the period covered.

Aylmer, G.E., *The Levellers in the English Revolution* (London: Thames & Hudson, 1975).
—*Rebellion or Revolution? England from Civil War to Restoration, 1640–1660* (Oxford: Oxford University Press, 1986).
Ashley, M., *The English Civil War* (London: Alan Sutton, 1990).
Carlton, C., *Going to the Wars* (London: Routledge, 1992).
Coward, B., *Oliver Cromwell* (London: Longman, 1991).
Denton, B., *Naseby Fight, 1645* (Leigh-on-Sea: Partizan Press, 1991).
Firth, C.H., *Cromwell's Army: History of the English Soldier during the Civil Wars, the Commonwealth and the Protectorate* (repr.; London: Greenhill Books, 1992 [1902]).
Fraser, A., *Cromwell: Our Chief of Men* (London: Mandarin, 1973).
Gardiner, S.R., *Oliver Cromwell* (London: Longmans, Green, 1909).
—*The History of the Great Civil War, 1642–1649* (4 vols.; repr.; London: Windrush Press, 1987 [1893]).
Gaunt, P., *The Cromwellian Gazetteer* (London: Alan Sutton, 1987).
Gentles, I.J., *The New Model Army in England, Ireland and Scotland, 1645–53* (Oxford: Basil Blackwell, 1991).
Hill, C., *God's Englishman* (Harmondsworth: Penguin, 1970).
—*The English Bible and the 17th Century Revolution* (London: Allen Lane, 1993).
— *The World Turned Upside Down: Radical Ideas during the English Revolution* (Harmondsworth: Penguin, 1972).
Hirst, D., *Authority and Conflict, England 1603–58* (London: Arnold, 1986).
Morrill, J. (ed.), *Reactions to the English Civil War* (London: Macmillan, 1982).
—*The Impact of the English Civil War* (London: Collins & Brown, 1991).
Newman, P.R., *Companion to the English Civil War* (Oxford: Oxford University Press, 1991).
Ollard, R., *This War without an Enemy: A History of the English Civil Wars* (London: Hodder, 1976).
Roots, I., *The Great Rebellion* (London: Batsford, 1966).
Roberts, K., *Soldiers of the English Civil War. I. Infantry* (London: Osprey, 1989).
Russell, C., *The Causes of the English Civil War* (Oxford: Oxford University Press, 1990).
—*The Fall of the British Monarchy 1637–42* (Oxford: Oxford University Press, 1991).
Sharpe, J.A., *Early Modern England: A Social History, 1550–1760* (London: Arnold, 1987).
Tincey, J., *Soldiers of the English Civil War. II. Cavalry* (London: Osprey, 1990).

Wedgwood, C.V., *The King's Peace, 1637–41* (London: Collins, 1955).

—*The King's War, 1641–47* (London: Collins, 1958).

Woolrych, A.H., *Battles of the English Civil War* (London: Pimlico, 1991).

—*Soldiers and Statesmen* (Oxford: Oxford University Press, 1987).

Young, P., and R. Holmes, *The English Civil War: A Military History of the Three Civil Wars, 1642–51* (London: Methuen, 1974).

☙ Index of Names and Places ☙